S0-EJV-445

CORYNEBACTERIUM PARVUM

**Applications in
Experimental and Clinical Oncology**

International Conference on the Effects
of Corynebacterium parvum in
Experimental and Clinical Oncology,
1st, Paris, 1974,

CORYNEBACTERIUM PARVUM

Applications in
Experimental and Clinical Oncology

Edited by

Bernard Halpern

Collège de France

RC 261
A1
I 57
1975

PLENUM PRESS · NEW YORK AND LONDON

312506

Library of Congress Cataloging in Publication Data

International Conference on the Effects of *Corynebacterium parvum*
in Experimental and Clinical Oncology, 1st, Paris, 1974.
Corynebacterium parvum.

Includes bibliographical references and index.
1. Oncology — Congresses. 2. Oncology, Experimental — Con-
gresses. 3. *Corynebacterium parvum* — Congresses. I. Halpern,
Bernard N., 1904-   II. Title.
RC261.A1I57   1974   616.9′92′0145   75-16310
ISBN 0-306-30837-1

Proceedings of the First International Conference on the
Effects of *Corynebacterium parvum* in Experimental and Clinical Oncology,
held in Paris, May 9-10, 1974

© 1975 Plenum Press, New York
A Division of Plenum Publishing Corporation
227 West 17th Street, New York, N.Y. 10011

United Kingdom edition published by Plenum Press, London
A Division of Plenum Publishing Company, Ltd.
Davis House (4th Floor), 8 Scrubs Lane, Harlesden, London NW10 6SE, England

All rights reserved

No part of this book may be reproduced, stored in a retrieval system, or transmitted,
in any form or by any means, electronic, mechanical, photocopying, microfilming,
recording, or otherwise, without written permission from the Publisher

Printed in the United States of America

Preface

In his introduction to the Ciba Foundation Symposium on "Immunopotentiation," Sir Peter Medawar stated that, "for the past twenty years the control of the immune response has been virtually equated to immunosuppression because the great goal of applied immunology has been the transplantation of tissues," and that, "with the discovery of tumor immunity—the focal point of immunological control has changed from immunosuppression to immunpotentiation and correspondingly the great prize of applied immunology has become the prevention and control of malignant growth." *Corynebacterium parvum* is now universally recognized as being the most potent presently known immunopotentiator.

C. parvum is at the center of almost all papers presented at this conference and it has been analyzed from various viewpoints: taxonomy, pharmacology, immunopotentiation, stimulation of host resistance to tumor invasion in experimental models and in human therapeutics. Almost all data reported in this volume are original and recently obtained. The discussions were spontaneous, stimulating, and highly enriching, and the results already established and reported here are in many respects unique. Discussions at the conference revealed many other aspects which require further exploration.

Nonspecific immunopotentiation has strongly penetrated into immunology, immunopathology, and, recently, oncology. Undoubtedly, this area of research will witness important developments in the near future.

This book offers the first synthesis of presently available knowledge and emphasizes future prospects.

These proceedings should interest immunologists working in basic and applied immunology, as well as those concerned with the mechanism of tumor immunity and cancer immunotherapy.

Paris, June 1975
Bernard Halpern

Contents

Part VII: Concluding Remarks

Opening Address

It is a great pleasure for me to welcome you to the College de France, one of the oldest and most universal schools of thought and science throughout the world. May I remind you that the College de France was founded in 1531 by King François I, at a moment when the western world was emerging from the Middle Ages and when the breath of the Renaissance was illuminating civilization. The ambitious motto of the College de France is *Docet omnia,* and the institution has not failed to live up to this device so far.

This meeting, devoted to the study of the effects of *Corynebacterium parvum* in experimental and clinical oncology, comes at the right time. It so happens that this year is the tenth anniversary of the first paper published Halpern *et al.,* 1964 on the strong stimulatory effects of *C. parvum* on the reticuloendothelial system. Since then, much information has been reported from different laboratories concerning the immunopotentiating properties of this bacterium, such as potentiation of antibody synthesis, stimulation of cell-mediated immunity, and antibacterial and antiviral activities.

There is also now accumulating evidence that *C. parvum* affects neoplastic growths and inhibits metastatic dissemination. Although this evidence originates mainly from experimental data, the flow of clinical data corroborates the experimental findings to a great extent. However, *C. parvum* is of a highly complex nature, and the mechanisms which are instrumental in its antitumor activity are only hypothetical at the present time. It will be the aim of this meeting to analyze this essential problem in the light of available data, and to suggest new experimental models that are likely to illuminate this field.

This meeting brings together bacteriologists, biochemists, pharmacologists, biologists, oncologists, and clinicians. It may be hoped that the data presented will be of mutual interest and that the discussions which will follow will suggest new avenues of investigation.

BERNARD HALPERN, Professor of Experimental Medicine, College de France, Paris (France).

Recent advances in immunology have stressed the complexity of immuno-competent-cell interactions. The results which will be reported here must find their explanation in the light of these fundamental facts. While *C. parvum* is known to activate macrophages, and probably also B lymphocytes, the effect on T lymphocytes is less evident.

Another important aspect which should be discussed is the real importance of the so-called enhancing antibodies in the antitumor effects of *C. parvum*. Finally, this conference should lay down some principles for clinical applications and criteria on which the appreciation of clinical results should be based.

Nonspecific immunopotentiation is a new breakthrough in fundamental and applied immunology, particularly in oncology. The ground rules of this approach have still to be established. It will be the goal of this conference to accomplish this.

Acknowledgments

I wish to express my very great thanks to Professor Etienne Wolff, President of the College de France, who kindly put at my disposal for the purpose of this conference the lecture room, the personnel, the cafeteria, and many other facilities which made this conference successful.

I am also addressing, in your name as well as my own, sentiments of gratitude to Dr. Charles Mérieux, Director of the Institut Mérieux, and to his deputy director, Dr. R. Triau, whose generous financial support made this conference possible. Dr. Mérieux is a true Maecenas in the biomedical sciences, and countless are the conferences and research programs which he has subsidized so generously. His sentiments of personal friendship and kindness toward me are deeply appreciated.

I would like to express my best thanks to my secretaries, Mrs. Elisabeth Launay, Mrs. Betty Sossler, and Miss Ghislaine d'Hérouville, for their devoted and untiring help in the organization of this conference and their assistance in my editorial endeavors. I must also congratulate Palantype, London, for the splendid job they did in transcribing the recorded tapes.

Part I
Bacteriology
and Taxonomy

1

Bacteriological Aspect
of Anaerobic Corynebacteria
in Relation to
RES Stimulation

A. R. PRÉVOT

Background

Anaerobic corynebacteria have been known since 1897, when Roux first described *Corynebacterium pyogenes*. Roux, a veterinary doctor practicing in the Ile-de-France, observed an enzootic disease of purulent abscesses affecting cattle (hence its incorrect name of *C. pyogenes bovis*). Roux isolated the germ which caused the disease and studied it at the Pasteur Institute. In 1908 and 1909, in Metchnikoff's laboratory at the Pasteur Institute, Jungano was studying fecal microflora and discovered three species of corynebacteria: *Corynebacterium liquefaciens, Corynebacterium diphtheroides,* and *Corynebacterium granulosum.*

The first notion of their pathogenicity was revealed in 1913 by Massini, who isolated several strains of *Corynebacterium anaerobium* from cases of septicemia, mastoiditis, and purulent adenitis. *C. anaerobium* later proved to be the most frequent and most pathogenic of the anaerobic corynebacteria. As the type of this subspecies, we chose *C. anaerobium* for our experiments.

It was Torrey who, in 1916, first stressed the reciprocal affinity between

A. R. PRÉVOT, Institut Pasteur, 25 rue du Dr. Roux, 75015 Paris, France.

anaerobic corynebacteria and the RES when he described the *Corynebacterium lymphophilum* species.

In 1926, Mayer described *Corynebacterium parvum*. In the work carried out in my laboratory, *C. parvum* was the first species to reveal the secret of its pathogenic mechanism and, therefore, its capacity to stimulate the RES. Later on, other, less important species were described: *Corynebacterium hepatodystrophicans* (Kuczinski, 1929), *Corynebacterium renale cuniculi* (Manteufel and Herzberg, 1930), and *Corynebacterium avidum* (Eggert, 1935).

Personal Research

It was in 1938 that I undertook my research on this interesting group of bacteria. I began by publishing a first attempt at classification of the species already described, taking as the basis for their taxonomy the morphological and physiological characteristics briefly outlined by the various authors (Prévot 1938; 1946). That classification attempt showed that the various species of corynebacteria clearly differ in their enzyme patterns. Since at that time, the still existent axiom, "1 enzyme = 1 gene," had already been recognized, it may be hoped that they are genotypical rather than phenotypical species. The classification enabled me gradually to account for all of the species, to complete their description, and to study their pathogenicity, which was so unexpected, and, consequently, their capacity to stimulate the RES (Prévot *et al.*, 1949; Prévot, 1960). One of the observations which impressed me most and was to lead me to study in depth the relationship among these anaerobes and certain malignant RES diseases dates back to 1949. With Courdurier (Prévot *et al.*, 1949), I isolated by anaerobic hemoculture a strain of *C. avidum* in an elderly woman suffering from episodes of recurrent septicemia, lasting seven days, from whom it had been impossible to isolate any of the anaerobic organisms normally looked for in such cases. For several months, this recurrent septicemia resisted all treatments, leading to the death of the patient. The postmortem revealed a malignant lymphogranulomatosis, the characteristic symptoms of which had never appeared. At a later stage, this coincidence enabled us to find a relationship between the anaerobic corynebacterial septicemia and certain malignant RES diseases, which (in our statistics) accounted for as many as 11% of the cases.

We observed a second case of septicemia caused by *C. avidum* (Prévot and Huet, 1951) and published a study (Prévot and Tardieux, 1953) on the pathogenicity of anaerobic corynebacteria. In 1960, I was able to present a comprehensive study of these infections (Prévot, 1960), in which endocarditis played an important part (Prévot *et al.*, 1954a; Prévot, 1956; Prévot *et al.*, 1956a). Our coworker, Mme. Mandin (1956), reported approximately thirty cases (observed in the clinic of Prof. Janbon at Montpellier) in which recurrent septicemia led to a malignant RES disease.

The study of the culture characteristics of our 600 strains of anaerobic corynebacteria showed some peculiarities of this group and, above all, their great variability. We will stress here only two such characteristics: first, they can be isolated only under strict anaerobiosis. Second, the very first colonies isolated are exempt from catalase; however, in the second subculture, a catalase appears, and the strict anaerobiosis is no longer necessary.* In deep gelose, the levels of the colonies rise progressively, first appearing at a depth of more than 1 cm below the surface and rising to within a few millimeters from the surface. Some strains may even give facultative anaerobic mutants but, on the whole, they remain preferential anaerobes (Prévot and Thouvenot, 1952). Another aspect of their variability is that most strains, even when isolated in a pure state from serious microbial septicemia, lose all experimental pathogenicity as early as the first culture. This led several authors who had studied only a few strains—which were precisely such apathogenic mutants—wrongly to deny the pathogenicity of anaerobic corynebacteria. Other strains which retain this pathogenicity during the first cultures gradually lose it with successive subcultures. It is probably because of this variability that the understanding of their unexpected pathogenicity was delayed for so long.

Study of Pathogenicity

This study could be carried out only when we were able to use strains which were pathogenic to animals and remained so. The study was undertaken with Dezest and, in particular, with Levaditi and his team (Levaditi *et al.*, 1965; Prévot *et al.*, 1954b; 1955; 1958), and also with other authors. When a guinea pig is injected intramuscularly or intravenously with 1 ml of a 24-h culture of a highly pathogenic strain, the animal dies either rapidly within 24–48 h, exhibiting local infectious reactions and purulent metastasis (purulent adenitis, pleurisy, peritonitis, etc.), or within 10–12 days. In the latter case, there are no massive reactions, and only the histopathological examination of the lungs, liver, spleen, and kidneys reveals an acute histioreticulosis with large multinuclear macrophages showing intense hyperergia. In the former case, anaerobic corynebacteria are easily isolated from the lesions, but this is very difficult and sometimes impossible in the latter case where the reactions are, in fact, due to self-sterilizing experimental infections. In both cases, we then observed—and this is pathognomonic—a hypercytosis in the four clones of the RES: reticulated Aschoff cells,† lymphocytes, reticulocytes, histiocytes, and macrophages. Thus, the injection of living anaerobic corynebacteria induces a lethal stimulation of the RES. However,

---

*Some authors thought they could assert the existence of a catalase in the first culture after isolation. It seems that the technique they used was not sufficiently discriminating to detect the absence of initial catalase.

†At that time these cells were called reticulocytes. This word now has another meaning in hematology: reticulated red cells.

when we tried with Linzenmeyer (1954), to obtain sera to agglutinate these corynebacteria by intravenously injecting cells killed by heat or formaldehyde, we found that the high doses required for the 9th, 10th, and 11th injections killed the rabbits and that the histological examination revealed the same epithelial hyperergia, the same lethal stimulation of the RES, and the same hypercytosis of the four clones of RES.

Therefore, it is not the virulence of the anaerobic corynebacteria that is at the basis of their pathogenicity, but the action of one of the components of their cells, whether living or killed. We tried to determine with Tam (Prévot *et al.*, 1968) which substance was responsible for the pathogenicity. We identified it as being one of the constituents of the bacterial cell wall. This was later confirmed while working with another team (Prévot *et al.*, 1972), and we initially suggested calling the pathogenic component reticulostimulin (Prévot, 1965a) to express its potential to stimulate the RES.

When we successfully titrated this substance (Prévot *et al.*, 1963; Prévot, 1964) by using the Halpern and Biozzi method, our research changed from qualitative and became quantitative. We were then able to define the pathogenic substance as being "a parietal constituent of pathogenic anaerobic corynebacteria which, at high doses, is capable of causing a lethal hyperergical histioreticulosis and, at the therapeutical doses, brings about a beneficial stimulation of the RES, involving a remarkable increase of the natural defenses of the system."

Before describing the research which followed this turning point in our investigations, it should be noted that one of the most serious anaerobic corynebacterioses is Whipple's disease, which we showed to be an infection of the lamina propria by *C. anaerobium* (Caroli *et al.*, 1963; Prévot and Morel, 1964). This disease always reveals itself to be a fatal mesenteric histioreticulosis; when treated with specific antibiotics, in particular chloramphenicol, this infection can now be cured (Prévot, 1965b). It has two characteristics: It is self-sterilizing and, at that stage, not only is it impossible to isolate the organism, but a large number of intestinal bacterial species are expelled. This is the reason why many authors dispute the corynebacterial origin of infection, having only studied the disease after self-sterilization (Prévot, 1965b) and after associated reinfection.

With regard to recurrent septicemia ending—sometimes after a very long delay—in a malignant RES disease, we formulated the assumption that these recurrences finally blocked the RES after repeated stimulations, causing the system to become the prey of unknown agents of malignancy (oncogenic viruses in particular) (Prévot, 1972).

Research on Reticulostimulin

The titration of reticulostimulin (RS) by the colloidal carbon method enabled us to carry out the following research:

1. Selection of productive strains: As the 936B strain of *C. parvum* had undergone a noticeable decrease in its potential of RS synthesis, we tried to replace it with more active strains. Originally we used strains of *C. anaerobium*. This species has been isolated from Whipple's disease for several years for the preparation of RS ampoules intended for human therapeutic trials (Kouznetsova *et al.*, 1972). We later found a strain of *C. granulosum* isolated from nonstreptococcic endocarditis which was more active, and we still use it for our preparation.

In the meantime, we showed (Prévot and Tran Van Phi, 1964) that all the pathogenic strains of anaerobic corynebacteria were producing RS to various degrees, whereas aerobic corynebacteria never produced any RS.

2. Having demonstrated with Mandin, Giuntini, and Thouvenot (Prévot *et al.*, 1956b) that the lysis areas around the colonies of strain 1452 were due to a typical bacteriophage, we studied this phage (Prévot and Thouvenot, 1959). It is a 65-μm bacteriophage, with a tail approximately 140 μm long. It is capable of lysing other strains.

Having succeeded in isolating six other anti-*Corynebacterium* phages from filtrates of spontaneous lysogenic strains, we undertook phage-typing tests on 212 strains. We found 11 phage types.

Later, after isolating two new lysogenic bacteriophages, we reacted our collection of nine bacteriophages with 50 new strains of corynebacteria which we were in the process of studying for their reticulostimulating potential. We observed that all the phage type III strains were stimulants, whereas none of the strains resistant to all the phages had the slightest stimulating potential (Thouvenot, 1967). During this work we found, with Thouvenot, that contrary to the Freeman phenomenon, the lysogenicity of anaerobic corynebacteria prevents all synthesis of RS.

3. Mechanism of the stimulation of the RES by RS: With Levaditi and his team, we found that the increase of the four antixenic clones of the RES was considerable, rapid, and durable. This is in line with the cellular theory of immunity. We wondered if a parallel humoral mechanism also existed. We showed (Prévot and Thouvenot, 1972) that in mice there is, in fact, a marked increase in the serum proteins, corresponding to the increase in the number of cells.

Conclusions

1. Although clearly different (Prévot, 1969), all the pathogenic strains of anaerobic corynebacteria are reticulostimulants to varying degrees.

2. Reticulostimulin is a parietal component of nonlysogenic anaerobic corynebacteria. Lysogenesis prevents its synthesis.

3. *C. parvum* was the first strain to be studied with respect to its RS synthesis potential. Although it is a classical example, it is not the most active reticulostimulant.

4. Strains of *C. anaerobium* isolated from Whipple's disease and *C. granulosum* isolated from nonstreptococcic endocarditis are much more active.

5. The stimulation of the RES antixenic clones runs parallel to the stimulation of certain serum proteins, indicating that in the natural defenses of the system, the aspecific immunity is due both to cellular and humoral mechanisms.

References

Caroli, J., Prévot, A. R., Eteve, and Sebald, M. (1963). Contribution à l'étiologie et au traitement de la maladie de Whipple (Contribution to the etiology and treatment of Whipple's disease). *Sem. Hop.* **39**:1457.

Kouznetsova, B., Bizzini, B., Cherman, J. C., Degrand, F., and Raynaud, M. (1972). Immunostimulating activity of whole germ cells, cell walls, and fractions of anaerobic Corynebacteria. *Proceedings of C.N.R.S. Symposium.*

Levaditi, J., Prévot, A. R., Caroli, J., and Nazimoff, O. (1965). Particularités histologiques de la maladie expérimentale provoquée chez le lapin par inoculation de souches de *C. anaerobium* isolées de la maladie de Whipple (Histological peculiarities of the experimental disease induced in rabbits by inoculation of *C. anaerobium* strains isolated from Whipple's disease). *Ann. Inst. Pasteur, Paris* **109**:144.

Linzenmeyer, G. (1954). Etude sérologique des Corynébactéries anaérobies par l'agglutination (Serological study of anaerobic corynebacteria by agglutination). *Ann. Inst. Pasteur, Paris* **87**:572.

Mandin, J. (1956). Les Corynébactéries anaérobies en pathologie humaine. Thèse de Médecine, Montpellier (Anaerobic corynebacteria in human pathology). Thesis, School of Medicine, Montpellier).

Prévot, A. R. (1938). Etudes de systématique bactérienne. III (Studies of bacterial systems III). *Ann. Inst. Pasteur, Paris* **60**:285.

Prévot, A. R. (1946). Etudes de systématique bactérienne. VII (Studies of bacterial systems VII). *Ann. Inst. Pasteur, Paris* **72**:2.

Prévot, A. R. (1956). Corynébactéries anaérobies et affections diverses du SRE (Anaerobic corynebacteria and various RES diseases). *Rev. Fr. Etud. Clin. Biol.* **1**:201.

Prévot, A. R. (1960). Les corynébactérioses anaérobies (Anaerobic corynebacterioses). *Ergeb. Mikrobiol. Immunitaetsforsch. Exp. Ther.* **33**:1.

Prévot, A. R. (1964). Système réticulo-endothélial et corynébactérioses anaérobies (The reticuloendothelial and anaerobic corynebacterioses). *J. Reticuloendothel. Soc.* **1**:115–135.

Prévot, A. R. (1965a). Etat actuel des recherches sur la réticulostimuline. (Present position in the research on reticulostimulin). *Pathol. Biol.* **13**:321.

Prévot, A. R. (1965b). Etiologie et traitement de la maladie de Whipple (Etiology and treatment of Whipple's disease). *Monde Méd.* **75**:961.

Prévot, A. R. (1966). La maladie de Whipple est une corynébactériose anaérobie (Whipple's disease is an anaerobic corynebacteriosis). *Volume jubilaire du Pr. Nicolau.* Bucharest.

Prévot, A. R. (1969). A propos de la classification des Corynébactéries anaérobies (About the classification of anaerobic corynebacteria). *Int. J. Syst. Bacteriol.* **19**:119.

Prévot, A. R. (1972). La réticulostimuline. Son utilisation en thérapeutique anticancéreuse (Reticulostimulin. Its use in cancer therapy). *Med. Biol. Environ.* **1**:21.

Prévot, A. R. and Huet, M. (1951). Second cas français de septicémie à *C. avidum* (Second French case of *C. avidum* septicemia). *Ann. Inst. Pasteur, Paris* **80**:94.

Prévot, A. R. and Morel, C. (1964). Nouveau cas de maladie de Whipple à *C. anaerobium* guéri par l'antibiothérapie (New case of *C. anaerobium* Whipple's disease cured by antibiotic therapy). *Bull. Acad. Nat. Med., Paris* **148**:540.

Prévot, A. R. and Tardieux, P. (1953). Recherches sur le pouvoir pathogène des espèces anaérobies du genre *Corynebacterium* (Research on the pathogenicity of anaerobic species of the *Corynebacterium* genus). *Ann. Inst. Pasteur, Paris* **84**:879.

Prévot, A. R. and Thouvenot, H. (1952). Signification de la présence paradoxale d'une catalase chez les anaérobies strictes (Significance of the paradoxical presence of a catalase in obligatory anaerobes). *Ann. Inst. Pasteur, Paris* **83**:443.

Prévot, A. R. and Thouvenot, H. (1959). Nouvelles recherches sur le bactériophage 1452 actif sur les Corynébactéries anaérobies (New research on bacteriophage 1452 acting on anaerobic corynebacteria). *Ann. Inst. Pasteur, Paris* **97**:234.

Prévot, A. R. and Thouvenot, H. (1961). Essai de lysotypie des Corynébactéries anaérobies (Tentative phage-typing of anaerobic corynebacteria). *Ann. Inst. Pasteur, Paris* **101**:966.

Prévot, A. R. and Thouvenot, H. (1964). Inibition de la réticulostimuline chez les souches lysogènes de Corynébactéries anaérobies (Inhibition of reticulostimulin in lysinogenic strains of anaerobic corynebacteria). *C. R. Acad. Sci.* **259**:1447.

Prévot, A. R. and Thouvenot, H. (1972). Influence des injections de la réticulostimuline à la souris Swiss sur les protéides sériques (Influence of injections of reticulostimulin to Swiss mice on serum proteids). *Bull. Acad. Nat. Med., Paris* **156**:68.

Prévot, A. R. and Tran Van Phi, J. (1964). Etude comparative de la stimulation du SRE par différentes souches de Corynébactéries anaérobies et d'espèces voisines (Comparative study of the stimulation of the RES by various strains of anaerobic corynebacteria and similar species). *C. R. Acad. Sci.* **258**:4619.

Prévot, A. R., Courdurier, J., and Aladame, N. (1949). Recherches sur quatre espèces anaérobies de *Corynebacterium: C. liquefaciens, C. diphtheroides, C. avidum, C. parvum* (Research on four anaerobic species of *Corynebacterium*). *Ann. Inst. Pasteur, Paris* **76**:232.

Prévot, A. R., Siguier, F., Zara, M., and Funck-Brentano, J. L. (1954a). Maladie d'Osler à *C. liquefaciens* (*C. liquefaciens* Osler's disease). *Bull. Soc. Med. Hop., Paris* **70**:344.

Prévot, A. R., Dezest, G., and Levaditi, J. (1954b). Reticulose experimentale mortelle du lapin à *Corynebacterium* anaerobie (Fatal experimentally-induced anaerobic *Corynebacterium* reticulosis in rabbits). *C. R. Acad. Sci.* **238**:1937.

Prévot, A. R., Levaditi, J., Tardieux, P., and Nazimoff, O. (1955). Caractères histopathologiques de la réticulose expérimentale mortelle du lapin provoquée par les Corynébactéries anaérobies. I (Histopathological characteristics of the fatal experimental reticulosis induced by anaerobic corynebacteria in rabbits. I). *Ann. Inst. Pasteur, Paris* **88**:537.

Prévot, A. R., Gonzales, C., Pierson, R., Robin, A., and Levaditi, J. (1956a). Nouvelles recherches sur le pouvoir pathogene de *C. liquefaciens* (New research on the pathogenicity of *C. liquefaciens*). *Sem. Hop.* **32**:755.

Prévot, A. R., Mandin, J., Giuntini, J., and Thouvenot, H. (1956b). Etude d'un phage actif sur les Corynébactéries anaérobies (Study on a bacteriophage acting on anaerobic corynebacteria). *Ann. Inst. Pasteur, Paris* **91**:766.

Prévot, A. R., Levaditi, J., Tardieux, P., and Nazimoff, O. (1958). Caractères histopathologiques de la réticulose expérimentale mortelle du lapin provoquée par les Corynébactéries anaérobies. II (Histopathological characteristics of the fatal experimental reticulosis induced by anaerobic corynebacteria in rabbits. II). *Ann. Inst. Pasteur, Paris* **94**:405.

Prévot, A. R., Rouillard, J. M., Masius, N., and Wilhelm, J. (1960). Deux nouveaux cas de corynébactéries anaérobies suivies de tumeurs malignes (Two new cases of anaerobic corynebacteriosis followed by malignant tumors). *Pathol. Biol.* **8**:721.

Prévot, A. R., Halpern, B., Biozzi, G., Stiffel, C., Mouton, B., Morard, J. C., Bouthillier, Y., and Decreusefond, C. (1963). Stimulation du SRE par les corps micorbiens tués de *C.*

parvum (RES stimulation by killed *C. parvum* microbial organisms). *C. R. Acad. Sci.*
257:13. (Also in 1964 *J. Reticuloendothel. Soc.* **1**:77–96.

Prévot, A. R., Tam Nguyen-Dang, and Thouvenot, H. (1968). Influences des parois cellulaires de *C. parvum* 936B sur le SRE de la souris (Influence of the cell wall of *C. parvum*
strain 936B on mice RES). *C. R. Acad. Sci.* **267**:1061.

Prévot, A. R., Raynaud, M., Bizzini, B., Cherman, J. C., Kouznetsova, B., and Sinoussi, F.
(1972). Activité réticulostimulante des parois de Corynébactéries anaérobies (Reticulostimulating activity of the walls of anaerobic corynebacteria). *C. R. Acad. Sci.* **274**:
2256.

Thouvenot, H. (1967). Nouvelles recherches sur les lysotypes des Corynébactéries
anaérobies et leur rapport avec la production de réticulostimuline (New research on
phage types of anaerobic corynebacteria and their relation to the production of
reticulostimulin). *C. R. Acad. Sci.* **265**:86.

2

Acute and Chronic Toxicities in Mammal and Subhuman Primates with Inactivated *Corynebacterium* Suspension

M. ROUMIANTZEFF, M. C. MYNARD,
B. COQUET, C. GOLDMAN, and G. AYME

Introduction

Before studying the potential activity of immunostimulant preparations, it is necessary to examine their actual toxic effects carefully. Although this approach is a very general obligation for any kind of pharmaceutical preparation, it is especially important to enforce this rule for immunostimulants since the potentiation of the host defense system leads to radical transformations of the host itself. Therefore, subtoxic effects and stimulant activities must be clearly separated. The immunostimulant activity of *Corynebacterium parvum* suspensions was first discovered by Halpern *et al.* (1963), after the studies done by Prévot and Tardieux (1953) on the pathogen activity of anaerobic corynebacteria.

M. ROUMIANTZEFF, M. C. MYNARD, G. AYME, Institut Français d'Immunologie, Marcy l'Etoile, 69260 Charbonnières-les-Bains, France. B. COQUET, IFFA-CREDO, Saint Germain sur L'Arbresle, 69210 l'Arbresle, France. C. GOLDMAN, Institut Mérieux, Marcy l'Etoile, 69260 Charbonnières-les-Bains, France.

Table I. Different Lots of *C. parvum*, All Issued from Strain IM 1585

Immunostimulant : *Corynebacterium parvum* IM

Strain	Classification
Prévot 3607	*Corynebacterium parvum* (Prévot, 1954)
IM 1585	*Propionibacterium avidum* (Cummins and Johnson, 1974)

Bacterial suspension, 2 mg/ml (dry weight), $65°C$ for 1 h inactivation and formaldehyde

Experimental lots : 1 − 2 − 5 − 6 − 7 − 8 bd − 11 a.g − 14 a.g − 16 b − 17 − 18 b − 19 − 21 − 22

Pilot lots : 4 − 7 − 8 − 10 − 12 − 15 − 16 − 18 − 20 − 22

Experimental lots for clinical use (SO) : SO195 − 225 − 260 − 274 − 282 − 301

Materials

The material used in this study is always a *C. parvum* suspension. Table I illustrates the different preparations: experimental, pilot, and clinical-use lots. All were prepared from strain Prévot 3607, which we have designated as *C. parvum* (Prévot and Coudurier, 1948) until a new taxonomic denomination is universally adopted. This strain biochemically belongs to anaerobic corynebacteria group IV, also designated as *Propionibacterium avidum* (Johnson and Cummins, 1972; Cummins and Johnson, 1974). These preparations were always totally inactivated by heating and, generally, by formaldehyde.

Methods and Results

In this report, we present results concerning different aspects of acute, subacute, and chronic toxicities of inactivated *C. parvum* suspensions in different laboratory rodents and monkeys.

Acute Toxicity

Acute toxicity was studied in mice. The standardized, final concentration of *C. parvum* used for experimental and clinical trials, 2 mg (dry weight)/ml, never killed male or female (OF_1) Swiss mice, even by intravenous or intraperitoneal routes. Using inactivated, but concentrated, raw material, it was possible to demonstrate acute toxicity. Table II summarizes the results observed. By the intraperitoneal (i.p.) route, no mortality was observed in OF_1 mice up to a dose of 150 mg/kg, which is equivalent to about 2100 human doses. By the intravenous (i.v.) route, mortality was observed, thus allowing the establishment of the lethal dose for 50% of the mice (LD_{50}). Even if no mortality had been observed, acute-toxicity assays revealed pathological effects at high doses administered by i.v. and i.p. routes. Figure 1 shows the transitory sublethal effect by i.v., i.p., and intramuscular (i.m.) routes for three different doses in OF_1 female mice. Toxic sublethal activity was observed with i.p., and especially the i.v., route between 8—72 h after the administration of a 145 mg/kg dose. There was no observable effect with the i.m. route at the same dose.

Despite these results, the observations made in other laboratories working on tumor activity have indicated that acute toxicity can be more severe for some inbred strains of mice. For this reason, we ran the same acute toxicity assays previously described (Fig. 1) on different inbred mice. We used mice of the same weight, 18—20 g, of both sexes from strains Balb/c, AKR, and $C_{57}Bl$. We used the intravenous injection route, which is the most severe for acute toxicity (Table II and Fig. 1). For both sexes, $C_{57}Bl$ and Balb/c mice were definitely more sensitive to the toxic effects of concentrated *C. parvum* preparation. AKR mice showed a sensitivity intermediate between $C_{57}Bl$ or Balb/c mice of OF_1 or Swiss mice. Figure 2 illustrates and compares the acute toxicity with mortality and toxic sublethal effects of a single intravenous injection of three

Table II. Acute Toxicity on 18—20 g ♀ OF_1 Mice[a]

Normal *C. parvum* inactivated suspensions 2 mg (dry weight)/ml

i.p. route	} 0.5 ml {	1 mg/mouse	No mortality
			$LD_0 > 50$ mg/kg
i.v. route		50 mg/kg	$LD_0 >$ about 700 human doses

Inactivated concentrated raw material

i.p. route:	Up to 3 mg/mouse	No mortality
	150 mg/kg	$LD_0 > 150$ mg/kg
		$LD_0 >$ about 2100 human doses

| i.v. route: | Mortality observed: | $3.1 < LD_{50} < 4.7$ mg/mouse |
| | | $2200 < LD_{50} < 3300$ human doses |

[a]Toxic effect observed during 7 days after single 0.5 ml intraperitoneal or intravenous injection at time 0 with: (a) normal *C. parvum* inactivated suspensions and (b) concentrated *C. parvum* inactivated raw materials. 50% lethal dose (LD_{50}) established when possible.

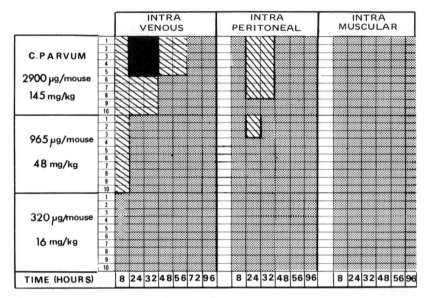

Fig. 1. Acute toxicity in 18–20 g ♀ OF₁ mice. Acute toxicity without mortality was observed 96 h after a single 0.5 ml intravenous, intraperitoneal, or intramuscular injection at time 0. Effects (very sick ■ ; sick ▨ ; and perfectly healthy ▦ mice) observed for the 3 routes with 3 threefold dilutions of the same concentrated raw material (*C. parvum*, lot 20).

twofold dilutions of a heavily concentrated raw material in 20-g male mice of strains C_{57} B1 and AKR.

Subacute Toxicity

Subacute toxicity in mice was studied by measuring the growth variation on young, 12–14 g, female OF₁ mice. For accurate comparison, a quantitative test was used with one or several concentrations of *C. parvum* and a control group inoculated with saline dilutant. The weight of each mouse was registered on days 0, 1, 2, 3, and 4. For each dose, the growth curve defines a surface when compared to the control curve. Figure 3 illustrates this subacute mouse weight-gain test; its quantitative expression being determined by surface growth variation and its significant value by the Student's *t*. This assay is a very accurate tool, giving a precise comparison of different batches. The limit dose, leading to no significant variation, was 20–100 µg in a 14-g mouse, which is equivalent to 1.4–7 mg/kg or 20–100 doses in humans.

Pyrogen Activity

As a bacterial suspension, concentrated preparations of *C. parvum* generally show a pyrogen activity. Table III gives the results observed with four pilot lots:

pyrogen activity was clearly evident with dose-effect response. However, a *C. parvum* suspension demonstrates a remarkably weak pyrogen activity for a crude bacterial material, and doses up to 100 μg/kg are within the nontoxic limits of the *French Pharmacopeia* rabbit assay.

Sensitization Studies

It seems to us that sensitization studies are crucial before using an immuno-stimulant such as *C. parvum,* and injecting it weekly over a long period of time. Unfortunately, the classical animal models can only provide a rough criterion of sensitization, and only experimental and clinical long-term protocols would conclusively determine whether a substance is a sensitizing agent. However, two tests are available which can give a first indication and which can be used as control assays for routine production. Figure 4 illustrates these tests. Intentionally, the doses are not too high, the equivalent of 2–6 human doses. Examples of reactions observed in the general immediate-sensitization test on rabbits and the general delayed-specific sensitization test on guinea pigs are also shown. Both assays, based on two different mechanisms, did not reveal any kind of local or general sensitization reactions to *C. parvum* preparations.

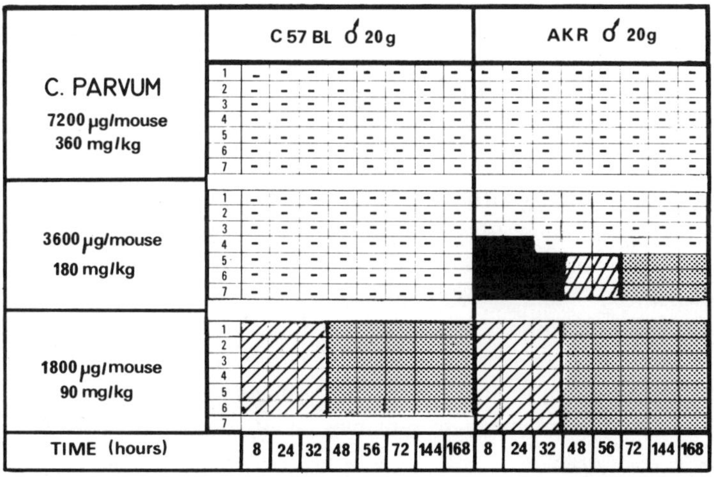

Fig. 2. **Acute toxicity in 20-g mice of 2 different strains.** Acute toxicity and mortality was observed 7 days after a single 0.5 ml intravenous injection at time 0. Mortality ‾ ‾ or toxic effects (very sick ■■■; sick ▨▨▨ ; and perfectly healthy ▦▦▦ mice) observed for 3 twofold dilutions of concentrated raw material (*C. parvum,* lot 5). ♂ C₅₇ Bl (IFFA-CREDO); ♂ AKR (IFFA-CREDO).

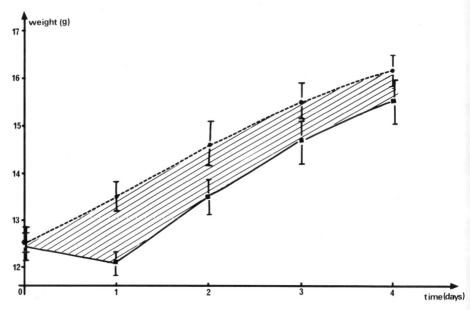

Fig. 3. Subacute toxicity. Quantitative estimation of 4 days growth-variation effect on 12–14 g ♀ OF$_1$ mice after a single 0.5 ml intraperitoneal injection of 1000 μg/mouse of *C. parvum* SO 301 ——. Comparison with control injected with saline – – –. Mean values for 5 mice per group with I ± 2 standard errors. The total variation during the 4 days test can be expressed by ΔS, which represents the variation of growth observed (−3.7). The significance was tested by Student's t (−4.0, sign.) or in percentage (−6.4%), giving the percentage of weight loss during the test as compared to control.

Inflammation Test by Intradermal Injection

The inflammation test is conducted on New Zealand depilated rabbits: a 0.2 ml intradermal injection of four fivefold dilutions is administered at two randomized points per dilution. Observation and measure of local inflammation, erythema, and induration at peak reaction times are recorded. Table IV illustrates one such assay. Maximal reaction to a *C. parvum* suspension was observed between 24 and 48 h after injection. A neat inflammatory reaction was regularly obtained with a 0.2 ml injection containing about 70 μg (equivalent to 1 human dose) of *C. parvum* suspension per point. Many assays to reduce this inflammatory effect did not succeed in abolishing this undesirable side effect.

Chronic Toxicity

To support the clinical investigation dossier, it is necessary to run chronic toxicity experiments carefully. Clinical preparations of *C. parvum* were studied in rats and monkeys. We will report here only some of the more important

Table III. *C. parvum*: Rabbit Pyrogen-Activity Test[a]

C. parvum	i.v. route dose/kg rabbit, µg/kg	Equivalent human doses	Maximal temperature variation $\Delta\theta°$, °C	Variance (expressed by σ) compared to limit in *French Pharmacopeia*
Lot #2	210	3	+0.9	+2
	100	1.5	+0.4	<1
Lot #4	1150	15	+1.3	+2
	230	3	+1.2	+1
	50	0.7	+0.3	<1
Lot #7	820	12	+1.7	+4
	165	2.5	+0.9	+1
	35	0.5	+0.2	<1
Lot #8	1100	~15	+1.2	+3
	200	~3	+0.2	<1

[a]Dose-response effect; doses up to 100 µg/kg are in the limits of *French Pharmacopeia* assay.

M. Roumiantzeff *et al.*

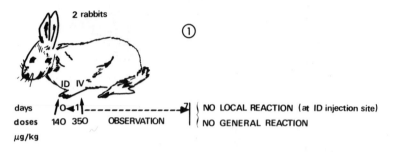

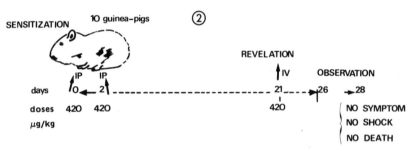

Fig. 4. Schematic representations of two tests for sensitization studies: ① Rabbit test for general immediate sensitization; ② Guinea pig test for general delayed specific sensitization.

Table IV. Inflammation Test by Intradermal Injection in Rabbit[a]

Protocol:	Intradermal injection—0.2 ml per point			
	Serial dilution—2 randomized points per dilution			
	Reactions recorded at maxima (24 or 48 h)			
Results: (max 24 h)	400 μg/point 0.2 ml	80 μg/point 0.2 ml	16 μg/point 0.2 ml	Saline control 0.2 ml
	Reaction diameter (mm): erythema and slight induration			
Rabbit 1: (2 points/rabbit)	8–8	6–6	0–0	0–0
Rabbit 2: (2 points/rabbit)	8–7	7–5	0–0	0–0

[a]Protocols of test and results observed with *C. parvum* lot SO 260 at 3 fivefold dilutions. Each rabbit received 8 intradermal injections on the flanks, 0.2 ml at each point. Reactions were recorded at 2, 6, 21, 24, and 48 h. Clear reactions are expressed by diameters (mm).

Table V. Rat Protocol for Chronic Toxicity Study and Main Results Observed During the Assays[a]

Clinical examination: Local reactions, each day
Weight, twice a week
Hematological examination, weeks 0, 2, 4, 8, 13
Blood biochemical examination, week 13
Autopsies: organs' weight/anatomopathology, week 13

Dose	Clinical state	Local reaction	Leuko.	Hb	Liver	Nodes	Spleen	Injection site
Control	N	0	N	N	N	N	N	N
200 µg/kg	N	0	+ (4th week)	±	+ [♀]	+	+	N
600 µg/kg	N	0	+ (4th week)	±	+ [♀]	+	+	N
2000 µg/kg	N	0	+++ (2nd week)	+	+++ [♀]	++	++	Inflammatory degeneration

[a] Assays on Sprague–Dawley ♂ and ♀ rats. *C. parvum* SO 260, 3 doses: 200–600 and 2000 µg/kg. Two intramuscular injections per week for 13 weeks = 27 injections. Hb = hemoglobin; N = normal; 0 = no reaction; ±, +, ++, +++ show different intensities in reaction; [♀] means more reaction in females.

points revealed by these assays. Table V summarizes the rat protocol with injections at 3 doses: 200, 600, and 2000 μg/kg (equivalent to about 2, 6, and 20 human doses). These injections were repeated twice a week for 13 weeks, so there were 27 injections by the i.m. route. The clinical state was normal; no pain or functional abnormalities were observed after injection; no biochemical variation on serum was detected after 27 injections. However, very significant hematological changes were found: increases in the number of leukocytes and polynuclears occurred as early as 2 weeks after the first injection for females and 4 weeks for males, even at a dose level of 200 μg/kg. A slight decrease of hemoglobin appeared after 8 or 13 weeks. At autopsy, macroscopic lesions were detected at the injection site, especially in animals receiving 2000 μg/kg doses. Reticuloendothelial system organs showed transformation at the end of the experiment: liver, nodes, and especially spleen had increased in weight. Histological examinations revealed images of stimulation for these organs. Some nodes had various degrees of reticular hyperplasia with epithelioid cells in a follicular pattern. Figure 5 shows a typical example: a lymphatic node from a male rat which had been repeatedly injected with 2000 μg/kg doses of *C. parvum* serum. The spleen demonstrates a neat reticular reaction appearing as hystiocytic nodules. The liver shows periportal lymphoid infiltrates and reticular reactions leading to very specific lymphohistiocytic nodules (Fig. 6). The inflammatory effect of *C. parvum* was not revealed on histological screening of the injection site of rats receiving 200 and 600 μg/kg doses, but clearly evident in each animal receiving 2000 μg/kg doses (equivalent to 20 human doses). Inflammation, muscular degeneration, and even microabscesses were observed. Globally, the

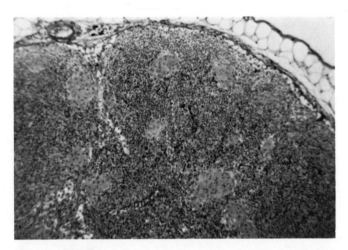

Fig. 5. Lymphatic node from a ♂ rat (dose 2000 μg/kg) after 13 weeks. Staining was performed with Hemalun Phloxin-Safran. (35 ×.)

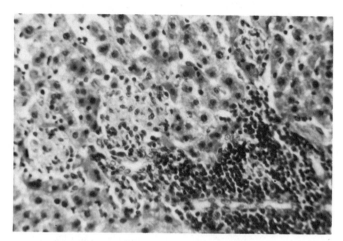

Fig. 6. Liver from a ♀ rat (dose 2000 µg/kg) after 13 weeks.
Staining was performed with Hemalun Phloxin-Safran. (85 X.)

growth curves for the different male and female groups (Fig. 7) did not demonstrate a significant effect on growth, even after 27 injections of the highest dose. The same protocol was used for monkeys but only two groups of four *Macacus rhesus* were used and only 2 doses were administered: 200 and 800 µg/kg (equivalent to about 2 and 8 human doses). These injections were repeated twice a week for 13 weeks; so 27 injections were administered by the i.m. route. Clinical state was normal. No pain or observable reaction was detected at the injection sites. No lesion or organ variation was observed at autopsy. Histological examination did not reveal any pathological transformations. No biochemical variation on serum was detected after 27 injections. The growth curves of the eight monkeys showed no significant variation at both dose levels. Figure 8 illustrates this fact for the highest dose level (800 µg/kg). Two control animals are not represented, but they showed very similar weight curves. Contrary to the results of the rat experiment, even at 800-µg/kg doses, no significant hematological variation or reticuloendothelial organ changes, such as organ weight increase or histological transformation, were observed after repeated injections of *C. parvum*.

Discussion

As with any other immunostimulant, it is very important to control potential toxic effects of *Corynebacterium* preparations. Because of its pathogenic stimulant activity, it is crucial to separate subtoxic effects from stimulant effects clearly. Our work had two very simple and practical aims: to check the different

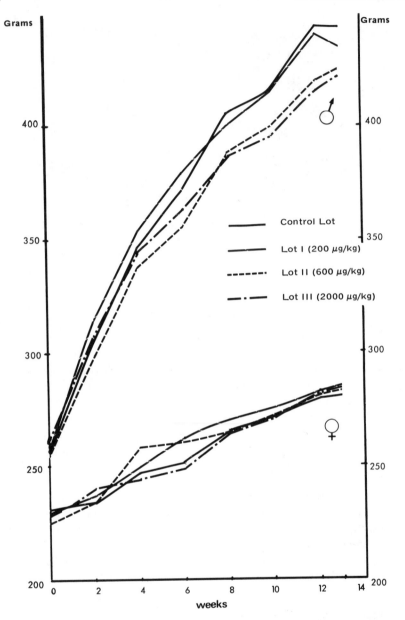

Fig. 7. **Growth-rate curves of rats during 13 weeks of toxicity assays.** Each rat received 27 intramuscular 0.5-ml injections. Eight groups were used: 4 groups of male rats (3 dose levels and control) and 4 groups of female rats (3 dose levels and control). No significant variations were observed.

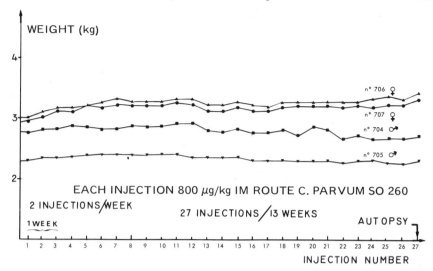

Fig. 8. Weight charts of 4 monkeys (*Macacus rhesus*) during 13 weeks of toxicity assays. Each monkey received 27 intramuscular 1-ml injections. Each injection contained 800 μg/kg of *C. parvum*. Two control animals are not represented in the figure, but show similar weight charts.

aspects of potential toxic activities of totally inactivated *C. parvum* preparations and to obtain reliable, standardized, and quantitative tests to allow a strict control of different batches. Of course, because of the use of *C. parvum* in immunotherapy experiments on tumors in different animal systems, toxicity must be studied with these different models. The potential use of *C. parvum* preparations in human immunotherapy, where repeated injections for long periods of time would be required, makes it necessary to know its effect in long-term treatment.

Our studies clearly demonstrate that it is possible to measure the immediate toxicity accurately. Hopefully, because even concentrated preparations do not kill mice and other laboratory animals, it seems that a quantitative subacute toxicity test, such as the mouse weight-gain test, allows for the comparison of different preparations and the determination of minimum requirements for acute toxicity. Pyrogen activity of *C. parvum* suspensions appears to be very limited for an inactivated bacterial suspension.

Although no experimental and clinical evidence of sensitization effects has been reported, sensitization studies must be performed. Fisher *et al.* (1970) adopted the subcutaneous route for their studies on *C. parvum* sera because they felt possible allergic reaction resulted after i.v. or i.p. administrations. With the abundant results of repeated injections of *C. parvum* without any allergic reaction, it seems likely that what these authors observed was a special sensitivity of their $C_{57}Bl/J$ strain to 500 μg doses of inactivated *C. parvum.*

The inflammatory reaction at the injection site is a side effect which seems difficult to reduce with a plain, inactivated *C. parvum* suspension. For this reason, the suspension must be well-known and carefully measured, as described in our rabbit intradermal-injection assay which provides a very accurate tool for comparing different batches of *C. parvum.*

The problem of special sensitivity of some animal models has to be clearly defined in order to design useful systems for experimental studies, especially in tumor immunotherapy. It seems that no special problem occurs with different laboratory animals, such as the common mouse, rats and hamsters, with the doses normally administered. Our chronic toxicity assays confirm this fact for rat and monkey.

The problem of special sensitivity is real for some mice strains generally used in experimental immunotherapy. Because of the small weight of mice, it is possible to obtain very high doses per kilogram of body weight. Some inbred lines exhibit a very sharp sensitivity. This fact was observed by different researchers and led, in an empirical way, to the doses used for different strains (Halpern *et al.,* 1966; Halpern *et al.,* 1973b; Woodruff and Dunbar, 1973), for AKR (Lamensans *et al.,* 1968), for $C_{57}Bl$ (Fisher *et al.,* 1970), or Balb/c (Halpern *et al.,* 1973a) and those which are avoided by some routes, especially i.v. or i.p. routes (Currie and Bagshawe, 1970; Fisher *et al.,* 1970). This toxicity can also be reinforced if *C. parvum* is associated with some chemotherapy (Currie and Bagshawe, 1970). Our work confirms these previous results, and it seems that quantitative acute or subacute toxicity tests can easily define the workable doses.

Few results about long-term use of *C. parvum* are available in the literature. Only the fundamental work of Halpern *et al.* (1963) gives results after 8 injections of 255 μg per mouse during a 24-day period, followed by another 24 days of observation: apart from a very potent stimulation of the reticuloendothelial organs, no adverse effects were observed.

Our results on rats and monkeys demonstrate that it is possible to repeat intramuscular injections twice a week for a long period, even at high doses, without observing any local or general adverse reactions. This confirms the clinical observation of Israel and Halpern (1972) in patients given 4-mg doses weekly. The dose of the *C. parvum* suspension is clearly limited by the inflammatory reaction. It seems that the usual human dose, calculated on a 1-mg/kg basis, could be repeatedly injected (6–8 times) without involving macroscopic or microscopic lesions. The inflammation test on rabbits which we described earlier, allows a quantitative estimation of the local reaction. However, another factor, which is difficult to estimate with animal models, limits the dose injected into patients: pain at the injection site. This negative side effect is now controlled by combining the *C. parvum* dose with ½ ml of Xylocaine (2%) before injecting patients (Israel and Halpern, 1972).

Chronic assay on rats confirms the results already published on the stimulating action of different organisms belonging to four main groups of anaerobic corynebacteria, especially *Propionibacterium avidum* (O'Neill *et al.*, 1973), on the reticuloendothelial system of different laboratory rodents (Halpern *et al.*, 1963; Stiffel *et al.*, 1966; Adlam and Scott, 1973). Again, the classical effects on RES organs (spleen, nodes, and liver) have already been described with precision by these authors. Classical hematological changes: an increase of leukocytes and polynuclears (Halpern *et al.*, 1963; Adlam, 1973) and a slight decrease of hemoglobin (Halpern *et al.*, 1963) are also confirmed in studies performed on rats.

However, the results of our limited experiment on monkeys, which was designed only as a toxicological study, may lead to questions about the RES stimulation in subhuman primates. Only once, in a pioneering work by Prévot *et al.* (1958), is a monkey study mentioned, just briefly reporting that the experimental infection by corynebacteria, regularly observed in rabbits with the specific histological lesions, could not be obtained with guinea pigs and monkeys. Under our conditions, even with repeated high doses of inactivated *C. parvum*, it was impossible to detect any macroscopic or microscopic signs of organ stimulation. It seems that this preliminary observation points to a need for further work with monkeys to see if the functional immunostimulation, as observed in laboratory rodents, can be reproduced in primates.

Summary

This work had very practical aims: to study different aspects of *C. parvum* toxicity in order to obtain a clear distinction between subtoxic and stimulant effects to develop reliable tests to check these potential toxic actions, and to control strictly different production batches.

In terms of acute toxicity, *C. parvum* generally does not lead to mortality; so, subacute toxicity can be measured, especially with the quantitative mouse weight-gain test. However, accurate sensitivity to toxicity is observed for some inbred mice, especially Balb/c, C_{57}Bl, and, at a lesser level, AKR. A researcher must be aware of this special sensitivity in order to design experimental protocols with these animal models.

Because of the mode of administration of *Corynebacterium*, careful observation of sensitization reactions must be made. We have described two tests for general-immediate or general-delayed specific sensitization.

Inflammation is a damageable side effect of *C. parvum* suspensions: a rabbit intradermal assay provides an accurate tool for comparing the inflammation effects of different lots.

Results observed in chronic toxicity assays on rats and monkeys are reported. *C. parvum* can be injected repeatedly, even in high doses, without toxicity, the limiting factor for this administration being local inflammation at the injection site.

Besides true toxic effects, the stimulation of reticuloendothelial organs observed in these long-term experiments is reported and discussed.

Acknowledgments

The authors would like to thank Mrs. M. Zayet and Mr. M. Musetescu for helpful comments, Dr. C. Stellmann and Mr. G. Beranger for statistical work. The expert assistance of Miss O. Barge and Miss M. Arpin-Gonnet for technical work and the assistance of Mrs. C. Cambet and Miss M. Saubin for secretarial work is gratefully acknowledged.

References

Adlam, C. (1973). Studies on the histamine sensitization produced in mice by *Corynebacterium parvum. J. Med. Microbiol.* **6**:527.

Adlam, C., and Scott, M. T. (1973). Lymphoreticular stimulatory properties of *Corynebacterium parvum* and related bacteria. *J. Med. Microbiol.* **6**:261.

Cummins, C. S., and Johnson, J. L. (1974). *Corynebacterium parvum:* a synonym for *Propionibacterium acnes? J. Gen. Microbiol.* **80**:433.

Currie, G. A., and Bagshawe, K. D. (1970). Active immunotherapy with *Corynebacterium parvum* and chemotherapy in murine fibrosarcomas. *Br. Med. J.* **1**:541.

Fisher, J. C., Grace, W. R., and Mannick, J. A. (1970). The effect of nonspecific immune stimulation with *Corynebacterium parvum* on patterns of tumor growth. *Cancer* **26**:1379.

Halpern, B. N., Prévot, A. R., Biozzi, G., Stiffel, C., Mouton, D., Morard, J. C., Bouthillier, Y., and Decreusefond, C. (1963). Stimulation de l'activité phagocytaire du système réticuloendothélial provoquée par *Corynebacterium parvum. J. Reticuloendothel. Soc.* **1**:77.

Halpern, B. N., Biozzi, G., Stiffel, C., and Mouton, D. (1966). Inhibition of tumor growth by administration of killed *Corynebacterium parvum. Nature (Lond.)* **212**:853.

Halpern, B. N., Fray, A., Crepin, Y., Platica, O., Sparros, L., Lorinet, A. M., and Rabourdin, A. (1973a). Action inhibitrice du *Corynebacterium parvum* sur le développement des tumeurs malignes syngénéiques et son mécanisme. *C. R. Acad. Sci.* **276**:1911.

Halpern, B., Fray, A., Crepin, Y., Platica, O., Lorinet, A. M., Rabourdin, A., Sparros, L., and Isac, R. (1973b). *Corynebacterium parvum,* a potent immunostimulant in experimental infections and in malignancies. *Immunopotentiation. Excerpta Med.* Sect. **18**:217.

Israel, L. and Halpern, B. N. (1972). Le *Corynebacterium parvum* dans les cancers avancés. Première évaluation de l'activité thérapeutique de cette immuno-stimuline. *Nouv. Press Med.* **1**:19.

Johnson, J. L. and Cummins, C. S. (1972). Cell-wall composition and deoxyribonucleic acid similarities among the anaerobic coryneforms, classical propionibacteria, and strains of *Arachnia propionica. J. Bacteriol.* **109**:1047.

Lamensans A., Stiffel, C., Mollier, M. F., Laurent, M., Mouton, D., and Biozzi, G. (1968). Effet protecteur de *Corynebacterium parvum* contre la leucémie greffée AKR. Relations avec l'activité catalasique hépatique et la fonction phagocytaire du système réticuloendothélial. *Rev. Fr. Etud. Clin. Biol.* **13**:773.

O'Neill, G. J., Henderson, D. C., and White, R. G. (1973). The role of anaerobic coryneforms on specific and nonspecific immunological reactions. I. Effect on particle clearance and humoral and cell-mediated immunological responses. *Immunology* **24**:977.

Prévot, A. R. and Courdurier, J. (1948). Recherches sur quatre espèces anaérobies strictes du genre *Corynebacterium: C. liquefaciens, C. diphtheroides, C. avidum, C. parvum. Ann. Inst. Pasteur, Paris* **76**:232.

Prévot, A. R. and Tardieux, P. (1953). Recherches sur le pouvoir pathogène des espèces anaérobies strictes du genre *Corynebacterium. Ann. Inst. Pasteur, Paris* **84**:879.

Prévot, A. R., Levaditi, J. C., Nazimoff, O., and Thouvenot, H. (1958). Circonstances d'apparition et évolution de la réticulose plasmodiale qui caractérise certaines formes de Corynébactériose expérimentale du lapin. *Ann. Inst. Pasteur, Paris,* **94**:405.

Stiffel, C., Mouton, D., Bouthillier, Y., Decreusefond, C., and Biozzi, G. (1966). Variabilité de la réponse du SRE à deux substances microbiennes selon l'espèce animale. *J. Reticuloendothel. Soc.* **3**:439.

White, R. G., O'Neill, G. J., Henderson, D. C., Carter, J., and Wilkinson, P. C. (1973). The adjuvant activity of "*Corynebacterium parvum*" in specific and nonspecific immunity. *Nonspecific Factors Influencing Host Resistance,* p. 285 (W. Braun and J. Ungar, Eds.), Karger, Basel.

Woodruff, M. F. A. and Dunbar, N. (1973). The effect of *Corynebacterium parvum* and other reticuloendothelial stimulants on transplanted tumours in mice. *Immunopotentiation. Excerpta Med.* Sect. **18**:287.

DISCUSSION

DIMITROV: What was the age of the C_{57} B1 and AKR mice?

ROUMIANTZEFF: I am unable to say the exact age because we were interested in comparing mice of the same weight. In our toxicity assays, we usually used mice weighing between 18 and 20 g. Perhaps there is a difference in the maturity of the different mice, but I cannot comment on it.

DIMITROV: This is an extremely important point when toxicity is being measured, because it is well known that AKR mice—after the age of six months—start to develop tumors and, with the large dose of *Corynebacterium parvum* used by Dr. Roumiantzeff, the tumor growth could be very rapid; in fact, all the mice died when high doses of *C. parvum* were used. I do not think that these mice are appropriate for toxicity studies. I do not agree that *C. parvum* is not toxic to mice.

WHITE: There was a reference by Dr. Roumiantzeff to inflammation at the local site. What about necrosis: how much necrosis is seen at the local site of injection of *C. parvum?*

ROUMIANTZEFF: We used three dose levels for the rat experiments. During any of the clinical examinations at any of the 27 injections, even with the high dosage of 2000 μg, we never saw any local or functional change. At autopsy, we examined the site histologically and were unable to find any specific lesion with the 200 μg or 800 μg doses. However, in the animals which had received the 2000 μg dose, there was a lot of degeneration and microabscesses. We found nothing in the monkeys, but the highest dose used in them was only 800 μg, equivalent to about 8 to 10 human doses.

PRÉVOT: I was very much interested by Dr. Roumiantzeff's presentation. I would like to make two remarks:

1. Dr. Roumiantzeff uses the term *"Corynebacterium"* for *parvum* and *"Propionibacterium"* for *avidum*. Both are very closely related species belonging to the genus *Corynebacterium anaerobium*, as I have shown in many publications. May I recall that *Propionibacterium* has been defined by Orla Janssen as a quite innocuous bacterium, propionic ferments being found widespread in the microbial world. In contrast, *Corynebacterium avidum* is highly pathogenic. We should not commit the error made by Cummings and others by calling it *"Propionibacterium."*

2. The error of including several species of *Corynebacterium anaerobium* into the genus *Propionibacterium* cannot be, at present, resolved definitively. We lack specific genotypic features, which were of great help in the definitive classification of other bacteria, such as *Salmonella*, of which 8000 genotypes are known today, many others being continuously discovered. I believe that in the near future such a classification may become possible when the active substances (reticulostimulins) are defined in the manner followed now by Professor Lederer.

ROUMIANTZEFF: If I used the term of *Propionibacterium*, it was for being understood by our English-speaking colleagues, who often referred to the Cummings and Johnson terminology. It was my intention to specify the equivalencies of *Corynebacterium* and *Propionibacterium*, admitted to by the English-speaking authors.

OETTGEN: Dr. Roumiantzeff has been referring to the human dose. Would he agree that we do not know what dose should be used in man?

ROUMIANTZEFF: I tried to indicate an equivalence between the dose used in animals and the usual human doses, as used by Professor Halpern and Professor Israel in France, which is about 4 mg. This is equivalent to about 70 μg/kg in animals. It may not mean anything of significance.

WANEBO: Please, could Dr. Roumiantzeff tell me again what was the maximum toxicity dose for the mouse and monkey? Secondly, was any toxicity observed in monkeys when they were given barbiturates or any other drugs—for example, to be anesthetized—as well as the *C. parvum?*

ROUMIANTZEFF: The monkeys were given light anesthesia at zero time and after eight weeks, in order to obtain biopsy material.

WANEBO: There was no unusual toxicity when they received the anesthetic? What kind of anesthetic was used?

ROUMIANTZEFF: Tranquilizers were given to keep the monkeys quiet; it was not a real anesthesia to put them to sleep. I know only the brand name, not the chemical composition.

WANEBO: There is a question of toxicity in the use of barbiturates in animals receiving *C. parvum*. Since this is relevant to human protocols, I wonder whether there is any toxicity with the use of these drugs with *C. parvum*.

GRIFFITH: Are the weights of vaccine expressed as wet or dry weights?

ROUMIANTZEFF: Dry weights of vaccine are used, after complete dialysis, to ensure that the material is pure.

ADLAM: I should like to concur about the tolerance of mice to *C. parvum* varying from mouse strain to mouse strain. For example, we have worked with a line of Balb/c mice which are extremely susceptible to *C parvum* injection, owing to their small adult body weight. Others working with Balb/c have found them able to tolerate large doses of *C. parvum*.

In our laboratory, we have been involved with many toxicity studies in both primates and small animals. I have, for example, repeatedly dosed rabbits intravenously (up to 16 injections, twice weekly) with 1.4 mg dry weight of organisms. These animals put on weight at a rate similar to uninjected control rabbits.

In answer to Dr. Wanebo's question concerning barbiturates, Mrs. B. Mosedale of our laboratory (manuscript in preparation) and Dr. J. Castro (*Eur. J. Canc.*, in press) have shown that mice which have received *C. parvum* are sensitized to barbiturates such as Nembutal (pentobarbitone). *C. parvum* treatment did not sensitize mice to ether. Barbiturate sensitizations may depend on the strain of mouse. Some studies that I carried out on histamine sensitization in mice using *C. parvum* showed that, whereas some mouse strains were highly sensitized to histamine challenge, other mouse strains remained resistant to histamine (*J. Med. Microbiol.* **6**:527, 1973).

JOLLÈS: Professor Prévot mentioned substances of low molecular weight isolated by Lederer's group from mycobacteria possessing immunostimulating properties. I would like to state that simultaneously, but independently, other groups isolated similar, if not identical substances. I would like to mention M. Hiu from Professor Mathé's department, a group working in Strasbourg, and also our own group. I believe that there is presently a general trend in research in which several different teams are engaged.

WRBA: I am not a bacteriologist, but I understand that we are dealing with different strains—for instance, with *Corynebacterium* from American tissue-type collection. Talking about human doses and toxicity, it is difficult to compare animal studies to humans when the animal strains display different toxicities. How can we make sure that we are talking about the same thing?

ROUMIANTZEFF: Perhaps I was not sufficiently precise; it is always the same strain, but different batches of vaccine were used. Our aim was to have a laboratory method by which the different activities and toxicities of these batches could be measured.

WRBA: Of course, I agree that such a method is needed. But will our results be comparable?

ROUMIANTZEFF: With a standardized test, if the conditions for production are the same—for instance, strain medium condition of culture, we hope to obtain measurements of acute toxicity and, more important, of other aspects of toxicity.

HALPERN: As a result of this discussion, I should like to stress that it is clear that the various strains of mice display different sensitivities to *C. parvum*. I have studied several strains, and there are differences among them. Dr. Roumiantzeff has shown the particular sensitivity of the C_{57} B1 strain, which we have also found from the beginning.

The data obtained in my laboratory also show some differences among the Corynebacteria obtained from the Pasteur Institute, the Institut Mérieux, and from Wellcome. The Wellcome strain, with which I have carried out only a limited number of experiments, appeared to be better tolerated; perhaps less toxic might be a more satisfactory way to express it. The animals were able to support higher doses of the Wellcome strain than of the Mérieux strain. These differences were of small magnitude, but they existed, and are difficult to explain. I hoped that some explanation might have been put forward during this discussion, but it has not.

There are also big differences among animal species. In this situation, the word "toxicity" does not have a real pharmacological meaning, because we are dealing with a biological substance, which is stimulating biological functions. It is puzzling that a stimulatory effect on biological functions may lead to illness and weakness, and sometimes to death. What are the mechanisms involved? This is an important question which has not been answered.

Part II
Toxicology, Pharmacology, Adjuvant Properties

3

The Nature
of the Active Principle
of *Corynebacterium parvum*

C. ADLAM, D. E. REID, and P. TORKINGTON

Before the start of our studies, it had already been established that lymphoreticular stimulatory activity, as measured by an increase in carbon clearance, was present in the cell walls of *Corynebacterium parvum* organisms, that this activity was stable to formalin and heat treatments, and that lysis of the organism with a specific phage destroyed activity (Prévot and Thouvenot, 1964; Prévot *et al.,* 1968). With this knowledge, we used both whole *C. parvum* organisms (Wellcome Number CN 6134) and their disrupted cell walls as starting materials for our purified sample. Our aim was to produce a material which could eventually be used as a clinical alternative to the whole organism. Therefore, on a weight-to-weight basis, no loss of activity or increase in toxicity could be tolerated in our sample.

The primary method for estimating the enhancement of lymphoreticular stimulatory activity used throughout the various purification procedures was the simple measure of an increase in weight of the spleen and liver following intravenous injection of the *C. parvum* material. We have accumulated considerable evidence showing that this measurement correlates with the other lymphoreticular stimulation parameters known for *C. parvum*, including adjuvant

C. ADLAM, D. E. REID, and P. TORKINGTON, Wellcome Research Laboratories, Langley Court, Beckenham, Kent, BR3 3BS, Great Britain.

action, histamine sensitization, and antitumor effects (Adlam and Scott, 1973; Adlam, 1973; Adlam, unpublished results).

The extraction procedure used in the present work was based on the phenol/water method of Westphal and Jann (1964), as modified by Wheat (1966) to retain cell-wall mucopeptide.

When the *C. parvum* cell walls produced by the mild mechanical disintegration method of Novotny (1964) were extracted with phenol/water at 68°C and the resultant mixture centrifuged at 8000*g*, phase separation resulted. A colorless aqueous phase lay on top of an interface of white particulate material. Beneath the interface, the phenolic layer was brown in color and contained protein and lipid components extracted from the cells. Under the phenolic phase, a pellet was seen at the base of the centrifuge container. On dialyzing the different phases, active material was recovered only from the interface. The pellet, originally under the phenol phase, assumed a rubbery consistency and was clearly a mixture of cell walls and DNA, since treatment with desoxyribonuclease successfully broke down the material so that it could be easily resuspended. Brown waxy material was recovered on dialyzing the phenol phase, but possessed no activity, nor did the freeze-dried aqueous phase material which was produced either before or after dialysis. Table I shows the results of an experiment in which the lymphoreticular stimulatory activity of the interface fraction (fraction 4) was measured by determining its effect on spleen and liver weight. The antitumor effect of the same material is shown in Fig. 1; the tumor used was the allogenic Sarcoma 180 T/G (Sartorelli *et al.,* 1966).

Table I. Spleen and Liver Weight-Increasing Abilities of Cell Wall Disintegrated, Phenol/Water Extract of *C. parvum* CN 6134[a]

	Spleen weight, mg	Liver weight, mg
Saline	102 ± 5	1058 ± 32
Whole organisms	363 ± 20	2230 ± 71
Phenol/water extract of broken organisms (fraction 4)	250 ± 30	1744 ± 96

[a]1.4 mg dry weight of *C. parvum* material was injected into groups of 10 W-Swiss female mice, weighing 16–20 g. Animals were sacrificed 10 days after injection, and their spleens and livers were excised and weighed. Results are given as mg of mean organ weight per 20-g mouse with the standard errors shown.

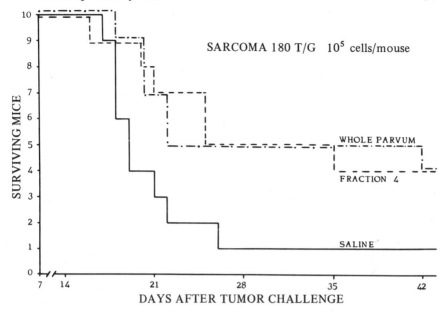

Fig. 1. Antitumor effect of interface material resulting from phenol/water extraction of disrupted *C. parvum* cell walls: Groups of 10 W-Swiss mice received 10^5 Sarcoma 180 T/G cells intraperitoneally; 24 h later, they were intravenously injected with either saline, whole *C. parvum* cells (1.4 mg/mouse), or fraction 4 (interface material, 1.4 mg/mouse) respectively. Deaths of individual mice were recorded for 40 days.

Infrared spectroscopy showed the active interface material to consist of two-thirds carbohydrate and one-third peptide, with negligible lipid. A very small amount of a third component, probably nucleic acid, was also present in these fractions. Approximately 60% of the starting material could be accounted for in the interface layer.

Although this method was an extremely convenient one for obtaining relatively pure "glycopeptide," results among the experiments varied, and even under the very mildest disruption procedures used (Table I), some activity was always lost as a result of the initial disintegration step. This loss of activity may reflect the size of the cell-wall fragments released on disintegration: the smaller the particles, the less the activity seen. This, however, remains a subject in need of further study.

On reverting to whole *C. parvum* cells as starting material, it was noted that little interface material resulted after phenol/water extraction. In this case, all activity was centrifuged to the bottom of the centrifuge tube at 8000g. Electron microscopy showed that considerable numbers of organisms still had cytoplasmic contents, and nucleic acids were still present within their cell walls; this was

Table II. Spleen and Liver Weight-Increasing Abilities of Whole
C. parvum Cells (CN 6134) Extracted with Phenol/Water and
Subjected to the Further Purification Procedures Shown[a]

	Spleen weight, mg	Liver weight, mg
Saline	122 ± 8	1109 ± 29
Whole organisms	441 ± 61	2374 ± 70
Phenol-extracted	588 ± 69	3034 ± 300
Lipid-solvent-extracted	446 ± 58	2655 ± 231
Pronase digested	521 ± 64	2708 ± 277
RNase/DNase digested	516 ± 71	2851 ± 156
10% TCA digested	431 ± 91	2217 ± 206

[a]1.4 mg dry-weight of *C. parvum* material was injected into groups of 10
W-Swiss female mice, weighing 16–20 g. Animals were sacrificed 10 days
after injection, and their spleens and livers were excized and weighed.
Results are given as mg of mean organ weight per 20-g mouse with the
standard errors shown.

in marked contrast to the electron micrographs of broken cell interface material,
where little cytoplasmic contamination was seen.

It was therefore desirable to develop methods for removing, either chemically or enzymatically, the unwanted cytoplasmic materials from the cells after
phenol extraction; studies to find the best method are still being carried out.
Table II summarizes the steps used so far in preparing *C. parvum* material and
shows that the activity of the various extracts (as measured by the increase in
weight of the spleens and livers of mice receiving the various extracts) is
comparable. Little activity has, therefore, been lost as a result of these sequential
manipulations. Electron microscopy of the TCA-extracted material revealed that
most of the cytoplasmic material had been removed. It is therefore the opinion
of the authors that the lymphoreticular stimulatory activity of *C. parvum* may
be isolated from the whole organism and represents the "murein" glycopeptide
of the cell wall.

Studies are now in progress to further analyze the active material chemically
and to ascertain how many of the lymphoreticular stimulatory properties,
inherent in the whole organism, are present in the extracted material.

References

Adlam, C. (1973). Studies on the histamine sensitization produced in mice by *Corynebacterium parvum. J. Med. Microbiol.* **6**:527.

Adlam, C. and Scott, M. T. (1973). Lymphoreticular stimulatory properties of *Corynebacterium parvum* and related bacteria. *J. Med. Microbiol.* **6**:261.

Novotny, P. (1964). A simple rotary disintegrator for microorganisms and animal tissues. *Nature, (Lond.)* **202**:364.

Prévot, A. R. and Thouvenot, H. (1964). Inhibition de la synthèse de la réticulostimuline chez les souches lysogènes de Corynébactéries anaérobies. *C.R. Acad. Sci.* **259**:1447.

Prévot, A. R., Nguyen-Dang, T., and Thouvenot, H. (1968). Influence des parois cellulaires du *Corynebacterium parvum* (souche 936 B) sur le système réticulo-endothèlial de la souris. *C.R. Acad. Sci.* **267**:1061.

Sartorelli, A. C., Fischer, D. S., and Downs, W. G. (1966). Use of Sarcoma 180 T/G to prepare hyperimmune ascitic fluid in the mouse. *J. Immunol.* **96**:676.

Westphal, O. and Jann, K. (1964). *Methods in Carbohydrate Chemistry,* Vol. V, p. 83, (R. L. Whistler and M. L. Wolfrom, eds.), Academic Press, New York and London.

Wheat, R. W. (1966). *Methods in Enzymology,* Vol. VIII, p. 60, (E. F. Neufeld and V. Ginsburg, eds.), Academic Press, New York and London.

4

Study on Soluble Substances Extracted from *Corynebacterium parvum*

P. JOLLÈS, D. MIGLIORE-SAMOUR,
M. KORONTZIS, F. FLOC'H,
R. MARAL, and G. H. WERNER

Abstract

Immunopotentiating water-soluble substances were obtained from delipidated cells of *Corynebacterium parvum* (strain Prévot). The immunostimulant and adjuvant activities of a crude water-soluble extract and of a low molecular-weight purified fraction were demonstrated by different techniques.

Introduction

This communication deals with preliminary data concerning the preparation and certain biological properties of water-soluble substances isolated from *Corynebacterium parvum* (strain Prévot). The aim of our investigations is the

---

P. JOLLÈS, D. MIGLIORE-SAMOUR, and M. KORONTZIS, Laboratory of Proteins, University of Paris V, 45 rue des Saints-Pères, Paris, France. F. FLOC'H, R. MARAL, and G. H. WERNER, Laboratoires de Recherches, Société des Usines Chimiques, Rhône-Poulenc, Vitry-sur-Seine, France.

purification of adjuvant-active compounds (immunostimulants) devoid of side effects. In the preparation of these compounds, we have tried to make use of the experience gained over many years in the course of our studies of mycobacterial immunostimulants (Jollès and Paraf, 1973).

In the case of mycobacteria, adjuvant activity was first related to insoluble substances (Jollès and Paraf, 1973). Among them we may name cell walls from human, as well as from nonhuman, mycobacterial cells and also a chloroform-extractable, ether-soluble glycolipid fraction from human strains, called wax D (White *et al.*, 1958, 1964), which contains a nitrogen moiety and possesses the same adjuvant activity as the killed mycobacteria used in Freund's complete adjuvant. We studied the chemical structure of this nitrogen-containing part in detail and demonstrated a close relationship between the peptidoglycan of an active wax D and the material which constitutes the backbone of mycobacterial, as well as other, cell walls (Migliore and Jollès, 1968, 1969).

Mycobacterial cell walls and wax D had a number of undesirable side effects, such as an arthritis-inducing ability (Waksmann *et al.*, 1960), which limited the possible applications of these insoluble adjuvants. For this reason, we tried to obtain simpler adjuvant-active compounds, particularly hydrosoluble substances. In our first series of experiments, we were able to demonstrate that these substances did not have several of the side effects encountered with the insoluble substances.

We worked out two preparation procedures (Jollès *et al.*, 1968; Migliore-Samour and Jollès, 1972). Both were simple techniques which did not need the preparation of complicated intermediary products, such as cell walls, nor the addition of enzymes. High-molecular-weight (Migliore-Samour and Jollès, 1972) and low-molecular-weight (Migliore-Samour and Jollès, 1973) water-soluble active substances were obtained; the smallest one was a heptapeptide-tetrasaccharide without neutral sugars (Werner *et al.*, 1974).

Results

Purification of Water-Soluble Substances from *C. parvum*

We applied the purification procedures which we had worked out for mycobacteria to *C. parvum*. A first preparation procedure allowed us to obtain hydrosoluble compounds in which the sugars were acetylated. The acetylation of delipidated cells was performed with a mixture of pyridine and acetic anhydride at 28°C over a period of 48 h. The fraction which remained alcohol-soluble was dried and subjected to extraction by water. The compounds which were soluble in alcohol and water were subjected to further purification on Biogel P-10 with 0.01 N acetic acid as eluent (Jollès *et al.*, 1968; Migliore-Samour and Jollès, 1973).

A second preparation procedure of hydrosoluble adjuvants was worked out

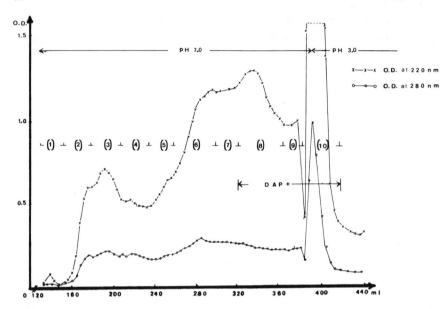

Fig. 1. Chromatogram on DEAE-cellulose (75 cm × 2.5 cm), 0.05 M veronal–HCl buffer (*p*H 7) of S_{70} fraction from delipidated cells of *Corynebacterium parvum* (strain Prévot). Eluent: 0.05 M sodium citrate buffer (*p*H 3.0).

in which the sugars remained unchanged (Migliore-Samour and Jollès, 1972). We thus obtained adjuvants which may be called "native type." In this brief communication we have chosen to discuss only this type of compound.

Bacterial residues from which the lipids had been removed were ground and homogenized in water with an Ultra-Turrax. After stirring and centrifugation, the supernatant was treated several times with different amounts of ammonium sulfate, centrifuged, and lyophilized. The supernatant obtained after the addition of $(NH_4)_2SO_4$ until 70% saturation (S_{70}) was attained was already quite active. The biological properties of this crude water-soluble extract will be discussed later.

Further purification of this extract was achieved by chromatography on DEAE-cellulose equilibrated with a 0.05 M veronal–HCl buffer (*p*H 7) and eluted with a 0.05 M sodium citrate buffer (*p*H 3) or by filtration on Biogel P-10 with 0.01 N acetic acid as eluent. The fractions were monitored at 220 and 280 nm. Each fraction was submitted to amino acid and amino sugar analyses. Figure 1 shows a chromatogram on DEAE-cellulose; the fractions containing DAP, and thus the bacterial peptidoglycan, namely fractions 8–10, were biologically active. The molecular weight of fraction 8 was about 6000, and that of fraction 10 about 4000, but even smaller active substances could be obtained; their detailed structure is under investigation.

Biological Activities of Water-Soluble Substances from *C. parvum*

The biological activities which we shall briefly report are those of the crude water-soluble material and those of the more purified extract obtained by DEAE-cellulose chromatography.

These two kinds of substances were examined from the viewpoint of the following activities:

1. Adjuvant effect on the production of delayed-type hypersensitivity to ovalbumin in the guinea pig [immunized with 1 mg of ovalbumin in Freund's incomplete adjuvant (FIA), containing, in addition, 0.5 mg of the substance under test].
2. Adjuvant effect on the production of antibodies to influenza virus in the rabbit (2 intramuscular injections, 3 weeks apart, with the B/Mass./3/66 strain in FIA containing 1.0 mg of the substance under test).
3. Stimulating effect on antibody-producing cells in mouse spleen. We followed the technique of Jerne and Nordin (1963); the compounds were intravenously administered at a dose of 25 mg/kg on days 0, 1, and 2 after immunization of RP-XXI male mice with sheep red blood cells; the animals were killed on day 3.
4. Stimulating effect on colloidal carbon clearance in the mouse, following the technique of Halpern *et al.* (1951); CD-1 female mice were treated with 25 mg/kg i.v. of the substance under test on day 0; the injection of colloidal carbon was performed on day 2.

In most of these tests, the activity of the water-soluble substances extracted from *C. parvum* was compared with that of killed whole bacterial cells from the same species (kindly supplied by the Mérieux Institute) and with that of killed whole bacterial cells of *Mycobacterium tuberculosis* (H_{37} Ra strain).

Table I gives the results of such a comparison. The figures relating to Jerne's technique are the ratios of the average number of plaques in the spleens of control mice to the average number of plaques in the spleens of treated animals. In the carbon clearance test, the activity is expressed as the ratio of rate of clearance (K value) in treated animals to controls. The index of adjuvant activity on hypersensitivity to ovalbumin is the ratio of the surface of the 48-h erythematous reaction in the guinea pigs immunized with the antigen plus the substance under test to that of the same reaction in animals injected with ovalbumin in FIA. Finally, the index of adjuvant activity on the production of anti-influenza virus antibodies is the ratio of the hemagglutination-inhibiting titers in sera of rabbits immunized with the antigen plus the substance under test to the corresponding titers in rabbits immunized with antigen plus FIA.

From these results it may be concluded that:

(a) Both the crude and purified water-soluble substances from *C. parvum* enhance the appearance of antibody-producing cells in mouse spleen

Table I. Summary of Activities Using Various Immunological Techniques[a]

| Preparation | Mouse spleen PFC (Jerne) | Carbon clearance (mouse) | Hypersensitivity to | | Anti-influenza antibodies (rabbit) + FIA |
			ovalbumin (guinea pig) + FIA	ABA-tyrosine (guinea pig) + FIA	
Crude water-soluble extract	0.46	3.23	25.6	89	10
Purified water-soluble substance	0.28	3.03	4.8	N.D.	4
Corynebacterium parvum, whole cells	0.74 (i.p.)	4.2	32.4	N.D.	N.D.
FCA (H_{37}Ra)	0.56[b] (s.c.)	N.D.	38.5	91	4

[a]PFC: plaque-forming cells; FIA: Freund's incomplete adjuvant; ABA-tyrosine: azobenzarsonate-acetyl-L-tyrosine; FCA: Freund's complete adjuvant; N.D.: not determined.
[b]*Mycobacterium phlei.*

more efficiently than the whole microbial cells from the same species, and the more purified substance is more active than the crude one.

(b) Carbon clearance by the reticuloendothelial system of the mouse is stimulated by the two water-soluble substances almost as well as by whole *C. parvum* cells.

(c) Adjuvant effect on the production of hypersensitivity to ovalbumin in the guinea pig (and also to azobenzarsonate-acetyl-L-tyrosine in the same species) is seen with the crude water-soluble starting material to a degree which is quite similar to that of whole mycobacterial cells and that of killed whole *C. parvum* cells, but such an activity has practically disappeared from the more purified substance.

(d) The crude water-soluble starting material exerts a striking adjuvant effect on the production of antibodies to influenza virus in the rabbit, while the more purified substance does the same to a lesser degree, comparable, however, with that of Freund's complete adjuvant (H_{37}Ra).

Passing mention may finally be made of the activity of the less purified water-soluble substance from *C. parvum,* in comparison with the activity of killed whole bacterial cells from the same species, on the infection of adult CD-1 mice with encephalomyocarditis (EMC) virus and adult Balb/c mice with the "plasma variant" of Moloney sarcoma virus. Figure 2 shows the cumulative mortality curves of mice which were injected intravenously, 2 h before EMC virus inoculation (s.c.), with various doses of the crude water-soluble starting material from *C. parvum*. The results of a similar experiment performed with killed whole *C. parvum* cells are also shown. Partial, but dose-dependent, protection against this virus infection was seen in both experiments, but the water-soluble material appeared to be more active than the bacterial cells; it must be noted, however, that with the latter, optimal activity in this experimental system was seen when the mice were injected 6 days before infection.

Figure 3 gives the results of a comparative study of the effects of the crude water-soluble material and of *C. parvum* whole cells on the splenomegaly induced with Balb/c mice by the Moloney sarcoma virus. In both cases, the substances were injected i.v. (at a 1.5 mg/kg dose for the extract and a 20 mg/kg dose for the whole cells) 4 days before inoculation with the virus. No further treatment was performed, and spleen weight was determined 21 days after virus inoculation. The water-soluble substance showed significant activity in reducing virus-induced splenomegaly, while the *C. parvum* cell suspension had no effect.

We may conclude from these preliminary data that, in several experimental systems, crude or even purified water-soluble substances extracted from *C. parvum* exert an immunostimulating effect which is as marked as, and in some instances higher than, that of a suspension of whole cells from this organism. Such findings may, in the future, have implications in the therapeutic use of these types of preparations.

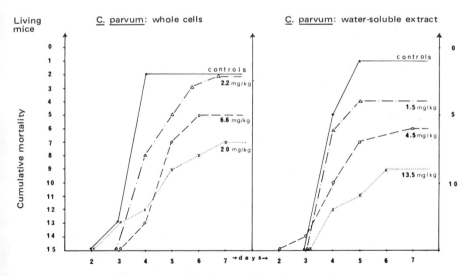

Fig. 2 Effect of *Corynebacterium parvum* whole cells and of crude water-soluble material on EMC virus infection of CD-1 mice.

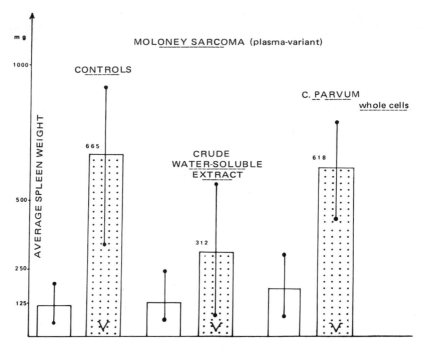

Fig. 3. Effect of *Corynebacterium parvum* whole cells and of crude water-soluble material on infection of Balb/c mice with Moloney sarcoma virus ("plasma variant" strain).

References

Halpern, B. N., Biozzi, G., Mene, G., and Benaceraf, B. (1951). Etude quantitative de l'activité granulopexique du système réticuloendothelial par l'injection intraveineuse d'encre de chine chez les diverses espèces animales. I. Méthodes d'étude quantitative de l'activité granulopexique du système réticuloendothelial par injection intraveineuse des particules de carbone de dimensions connues. *Ann. Inst. Pasteur, Paris* **80**:582–604.

Jerne, N. K. and Nordin, A. A. (1963). Plaque formation in agar by single antibody-producing cells. *Science* **140**:405.

Jollès, P. and Paraf, A. (1973). *Chemical and Biological Basis of Adjuvants*, Springer Verlag, Berlin.

Jollès, P., Migliore, D., and Bonhomme, F. (1968). Wax D, peptidoglycolipid of *Mycobacterium tuberculosis:* further purification and study of an adjuvant arthritis-inhibiting subfraction. *Immunology* **14**:159–163.

Migliore, D. and Jollès, P. (1968). Contribution to the study of the structure of adjuvant-active waxes D from mycobacteria: Isolation of a peptidocylcan. *FEBS Lett.* **1**:7–9.

Migliore, D. and Jollès, P. (1969). Sur la structure chimique de la partie azotée des cires D, peptidoglycolipides des mycobactéries. *C. R. Acad. Sci.* **269 D**:2268–2271.

Migliore-Samour, D. and Jollès, P. (1972). A hydrosoluble adjuvant-active mycobacterial "polysaccharide-peptidoglycan." Preparation by a simple extraction technique of the bacterial cells (strain Peurois). *FEBS Lett.* **25**:301–304.

Migliore-Samour, D. and Jollès, P. (1973). Hydrosoluble adjuvant-active mycobacterial fractions of low molecular weight. *FEBS Lett.* 35:317–321.

Waksmann, B. H., Pearson, C. M., and Sharp, J. J. (1960). Studies of arthritis and other lesions induced in rats by injection of mycobacterial adjuvant II. Evidence that the disease is a disseminated immunologic response to exogenous antigen. *J. Immunol.* 85:403–447.

Werner, G. H., Maral, F., Floc'h, F., Migliore-Samour, D., and Jollès, P. (1974). Activites biologiques des adjuvants hydrosolubles de faible poids moleculaire extraits de *Mycobacterium tuberculosis* var. *hominis*. *C. R. Acad. Sci.* 278 D:789–792.

White, R. G., Bernstock, L., Johns, R. G., and Lederer, E. (1958). The influence of components of *M. tuberculosis* and other mycobacteria upon antibody production to ovalbumin. *Immunology* 1:54–66.

White, R. G., Jollès, P., Samour, D., and Lederer, E. (1964). Correlation of adjuvant activity and chemical structure of wax D fractions of mycobacteria. *Immunology* 7:158–171.

5

Results Obtained in Our Adjuvant Screening Model with *Corynebacterium parvum* and *Corynebacterium granulosum**

G. MATHÉ, OLGA HALLE-PANNENKO, and J. L. AMIEL

Abstract

Corynebacterium parvum and three preparations of *Corynebacterium granulosum* have been shown by one or several previous experiments to be able to stimulate immune responses. These agents were submitted to a screening battery, the object of which was to detect "systemic adjuvants of immunity" useful in cancer immunotherapy. The tests of this battery are: (a) the hemolytic plaque-forming cell test (Jerne), which produces an immune reaction requiring thymus-

G. MATHÉ, OLGA HALLE-PANNENKO, and J. L. AMIEL, Institut de Cancérologie et d'Immunogénétique, INSERM et Association Claude-Bernard, Hôpital Paul-Brousse, 14–16, Avenue Paul-Vaillant Couturier, 94800 Villejuif, France.

*This work was supported by grants from the Institut National de la Santé et de la Recherche Médicale, Contract 71,5.414.1, and by the Centre National de la Recherche Scientifique, Contract 519.908.

derived and bone marrow-derived lymphocyte cooperation; (b) the graft-versus-host reaction which produces an immune reaction involving only thymus-derived lymphocytes; and (c) the immunoprophylaxis of three murine tumors, a leukemia (L1210), and two solid tumors (Lewis' tumor and ICIG CI$_1$).

Materials and Methods

Three tumors were chosen for the immunoprophylaxis tests: L1210 leukemia—a leukemia in which almost all the malignant cells are "in the cycle," with no quiescent cells—and two tumors not growing so quickly, with quiescent cells, Lewis lung tumor and ICIG CI$_1$ solid tumor—a tumor recently induced with dimethylbenzanthracene in our institute. Lewis tumor and ICIG CI$_1$ are susceptible to enhancement.

The tests of activity in the three tumor systems were preceded by screening for immunological activity in two nontumorous systems. After preliminary experiments (Mathé *et al.*, 1971), the following were chosen: (a) the hemolytic plaque-forming cell test (Jerne *et al.*, 1963), because it is simple and inexpensive and because it enabled us to study the dose factor, the time factor, and the route-of-administration factor; and (b) the graft-versus-host reaction, in which the adjuvant candidate is administered to the donors because it is a reaction that involves only T lymphocytes (Stutman and Good, 1969), while the Jerne test involves T and B lymphocytes (Claman *et al.*, 1966). Finally, this last test enabled us to detect a possible immuno-inhibition as well as an immunostimulation in response to cell-surface antigens.

In summary, this battery can answer these important questions: Is a given agent an immuno-adjuvant or an immuno-inhibitor, or both, depending on time and route factors? Is it influencing a pure T-lymphocyte reaction? Does it induce a growth-retarding effect or a growth-enhancing effect, or both, depending on various factors, such as the route of administration and the variety of tumor?

For all tests, the same animals, DBA/2 × C$_{57}$Bl/6 F$_1$ pathogen-free mice, three months of age, were used. The tumors were from parental origin.

For the hemolytic plaque-forming cell test, 192 mice were used for each product. They were randomized into 32 experimental groups, each comprising six animals. These 32 groups were randomized in four series, which, for evident technical reasons, were submitted to the test on different days. The agents were injected by four routes, i.v., i.p., s.c., and i.d. They were administered once, either 14, 5, or 2.5 days before the day of the administration of the sheep red cells, on day 0 (the same day as antigen administration), or 1, 2, or 3 days after the sheep red cells had been administered. The plaques were counted 4 days after the i.p. injection of sheep red cells. For the statistical analysis of the results, the Student-Fisher test was used.

For the graft-versus-host reaction, 40 mice were used for each product. They were randomized into five experimental groups. The DBA/2 × C$_{57}$Bl/6 F$_1$ recipients were irradiated with 500 rads (225 kV, 12 mA, 0.2 Ci, D=50 cm).

Table I. *Corynebacterium* Preparations Submitted to the Screening Tests

Agents	Obtained from	Composition	Doses per mouse[a]
C. parvum	Institut Pasteur	Suspension of dead bacterias	400 μg
C. granulosum A	Institut Pasteur	Killed bacilli	400 μg
C. granulosum B	Institut Pasteur	Membranes treated by phenol in the cold	100 μg
C. granulosum C	Institut Pasteur	Membranes prepared by mechanical action	100 μg

[a]Determined by preliminary studies.

They were given i.v. injections of 10^7 bone-marrow and 2.5×10^7 lymph-node cells of C_{57} B1/6 mice, which were normal for the control group and which had been treated either i.v., i.p., s.c., or i.d. with one of the adjuvant candidates at the doses indicated in Table I. This treatment was administered to the donors 60 h before the sacrifice. The mortality of the recipients was studied and compared to that of controls. This is a test that we established in 1960 (Mathé and Amiel, 1960). For the statistic analysis of the results, the Wilcoxon test was used.

For the immunoprophylaxis of L1210 leukemia, Lewis tumor, and ICIG CI_1, 40 mice were used for each tumor and each product. They were randomized into five experimental groups. The product was injected 2.5 days before the administration of the tumor cells. The same four routes of administration as mentioned for the other tests were used. The mortality of the animals was recorded, and the cumulative mortality curve was established. The different experimental groups were compared with controls. The Student-Fisher test was used to statistically evaluate L1210 leukemia (all animals died within a few days) and the nonparametric Wilcoxon's test was used for the two other tumors (mortality is more spread out).

The great number of groups that we had to study forced us to randomize not only the animals, but the different experimental protocols as well. Each experiment comprised controls, so that the curves for the controls are multiple, and they may differ slightly from one experiment to another.

To express the results, the following index (I) was calculated.

For the hemolytic plaque-forming cell (Jerne):

$$I = \frac{\bar{N}_{TM}}{\bar{\bar{N}}_C}$$

where $\bar{N}_{TM}$ is the mean number of plaque-forming cells per spleen of the tested mice and $\bar{N}_C$ is the mean number of plaque-forming cells per spleen of the controls.

For graft-versus-host reaction and the tumors:

$$I = \frac{\overline{S}_{TM}}{\overline{S}_C}$$

where $\overline{S}_{TM}$ is the median of survivals of experimental animals, and $\overline{S}_C$ is the median of survival of the controls.

Each group that produced a significant result was the object of a repetition of the same experiment, increasing the probability that a given positive result was due to the material studied and not appreciably influenced by the animals and the ecological conditions of the laboratory. The final significance of the result, given as S+, was calculated using the results of both experiments.

The degree of immunomodification found in each group of animals may not be in perfect correlation with the degree of statistical significance of the result. The former indicates the pharmacological effect in the experiments and the latter (statistical significance) depends on the variability in each group.

C. parvum and *C. granulosum* preparation methods have been published by Raynaud *et al.* (1972).

Results

With the Jerne hemolytic plaque-forming cell test, *C. parvum* induced only immunostimulation when given i.v. 14 days before the administration of sheep red cells and on days 0, 2, and 3, when given i.p. 5 and 2.5 days before sheep red cells, and when given s.c. on day 1 (Table II). *C. granulosum* A (killed bacillus) induced only immunostimulation when given i.v. 14 days before, i.p. 5 and 2.5

Table II. Hemolytic Plaque-Forming Cell Test (Jerne), Effect of *C. parvum* (400 µg/mouse) on PFC/Spleen

Days[a]	i.v.		i.p.		i.d.		s.c.	
−14	I[b] = 1.5	S[c] = 1%	I = 1.1	NS[c]	I = 0.75 NS		I = 0.75	NS
− 5	I = 1.1	NS	I = 1.2	S = 5%	I = 0.75 NS		I = 1.1	NS
− 2.5	I = 1.1	NS	I = 1.3	S = 1%	I = 0.8 NS		I = 1.1	NS
0	I = 1.6	S = 2%	I = 1.1	NS	I = 1.1 NS		I = 0.75	NS
+ 1	I = 1.1	NS	I = 1.1	NS	I = 1.1 NS		I = 1.8	S = 2%
+ 2	I = 2	S = 1%	I = 1.1	NS	I = 1.1 NS		I = 1.1	NS
+ 3	I = 1.8	S = 2%	I = 1.1	NS	I = 1.02 NS		I = 1.1	NS

[a]Before (−) and after (+) the injection of sheep red cells.
[b]$I = \overline{N}_{TM}/\overline{N}_C$.
[c]Statistics: Student-Fisher test. S = significant. NS = nonsignificant.

Table III. Hemolytic Plaque-Forming Cell Test (Jerne), Effect of *C. granulosum* A (400 μg/mouse) on PFC/Spleen

	Route			
Days[a]	i.v.	i.p.	i.d.	s.c.
−14	I^b = 1.7 S^c = 1%	I = 1.01 NS^c	I = 1.1 NS	I = 1.19 S = 5%
− 5	I = 1.1 NS	I = 1.2 S = 5%	I = 1.1 NS	I = 0.54 NS
− 2.5	I = 1.1 NS	I = 1.2 S = 2%	I = 1.1 NS	I = 1 NS
0	I = 0.75 NS	I = 1.01 NS	I = 1.1 NS	I = 1.32 S = 5%
+ 1	I = 0.8 NS	I = 0.85 NS	I = 1.09 NS	I = 1 NS
+ 2	I = 1 NS	I = 1.1 NS	I = 0.9 NS	I = 1 NS
+ 3	I = 1.1 NS	I = 0.75 NS	I = 0.75 NS	I = 1.1 NS

[a]Before (−) and after (+) the injection of sheep red cells.
[b]$I = \bar{N}_{TM}/\bar{N}_C$.
[c]Statistics: Student-Fisher test. S = significant. NS = nonsignificant.

days before, and s.c. 14 days before sheep red cells were administered, and s.c. on day 0 (Table III). *C. granulosum* B (membranes treated with phenol in the cold) was an immunostimulant only when given i.v. 14 days before sheep red cells and on day 2, when given i.p. 5 and 2.5 days before sheep red cells and on days 0 and 3, and when given s.c. on days 0, 2, and 3 (Table IV). *C. granulosum* C (membranes prepared by mechanical action) was only immunostimulating and

Table IV. Hemolytic Plaque-Forming Cell Test (Jerne), Effect of *C. granulosum* B (100 μg/mouse) on PFC/Spleen

	Route			
Days[a]	i.v.	i.p.	i.d.	s.c.
−14	I^b = 1.75 S^c = 5%	I = 1.1 NS^c	I = 0.75 NS	I = 1.1 NS
− 5	I = 0.75 NS	I = 1.5 S = 5%	I = 0.75 NS	I = 1.1 NS
− 2.5	I = 0.90 NS	I = 1.5 S = 5%	I = 0.8 NS	I = 1.1 NS
0	I = 0.75 NS	I = 1.7 S = 1%	I = 1.1 NS	I = 3 S = 2%
+ 1	I = 1.2 NS	I = 1.1 NS	I = 1.1 NS	I = 1.1 NS
+ 2	I = 1.75 S = 1%	I = 1.1 NS	I = 1.1 NS	I = 3 S = 5%
+ 3	I = 1.1 NS	I = 1.5 S = 5%	I = 1.1 NS	I = 3.8 S = 2%

[a]Before (−) and after (+) the injection of sheep red cells.
[b]$I = \bar{N}_{TM}/\bar{N}_C$.
[c]Statistics: Student-Fisher test. S = significant. NS = nonsignificant.

Table V. Hemolytic Plaque-Forming Cell Test (Jerne), Effect of *C. granulosum* C (100 μg/mouse) on PFC/Spleen

	Route			
Days[a]	i.v.	i.p.	i.d.	s.c.
−14	I[b] = 1.06 NS[c]	I = 0.75 NS	I = 0.80 NS	I = 0.82 NS
− 5	I = 2.01 S[c] = 1%	I = 0.87 NS	I = 0.93 NS	I = 0.81 NS
− 2.5	I = 1.10 NS	I = 1.10 NS	I = 0.80 NS	I = 1.10 NS
0	I = 0.75 NS	I = 0.75 NS	I = 0.82 NS	I = 1.10 NS
+ 1	I = 0.80 NS	I = 1.06 NS	I = 1.01 NS	I = 1.10 NS
+ 2	I = 0.83 NS	I = 0.75 NS	I = 0.94 NS	I = 1.10 NS
+ 3	I = 1.03 NS	I = 0.90 NS	I = 0.76 NS	I = 1.10 NS

[a]Before (−) and after (+) the injection of sheep red cells.
[b]$I = \bar{N}_{TM}/\bar{N}_C$.
[c]Statistics: Student-Fisher test. S = significant. NS = nonsignificant.

exerted its effect only when given i.v. 5 days before the administration of sheep red cells (Table V).

The graft-versus-host reaction test showed two kinds of results. Mortality was either unaffected or accelerated, as with *C. granulosum* A injected i.v. and *C. granulosum* B injected s.c., or it was delayed, as with *C. granulosum* C injected i.v. and *C. granulosum* C injected i.p. (Table VI).

The L1210 leukemia mortality was delayed with *C. parvum* i.v., *C. granulosum* A i.v., i.p., and s.c., *C. granulosum* C i.v. and i.p. (Table VII).

Lewis' solid tumor mortality was delayed with *C. parvum* i.v., *C. granulosum* A i.v., *C. granulosum* B i.v., and *C. granulosum* C s.c. (Table VIII).

ICIG CI$_1$ solid tumor mortality was not affected (Table IX).

Discussion

Our results confirm the immunostimulation by preparations of *C. parvum* or *C. granulosum*. One important point is that with these products, no immunodepression on any of the three tumors occurred.

Our results show the importance of several factors in the immunostimulation by corynebacteria products. For the route of administration, no general rule can be made; its effect is variable, at least with these agents. The time factor appeared to be important for the results of the Jerne test. It was generally considered that such systemic adjuvants could work only if administered before the antigen. Our previous experimental research on adjuvants of immunity showed that this concept was incorrect (Mathé, 1968; Mathé *et al.*, 1969), and the present work definitely confirms that this is false. With the Jerne test, *C.*

Table VI. Effect of Corynebacteria (Injected on Day −2.5) on GVH Lethality, Summary of Results

"SIA"	Route							
	i.v.		i.p.		i.d.		s.c.	
C. parvum	$I^a = 0.85$	NS	$I = 1.30$	NS	$I = 1.28$	NS	$I = 1.30$	NS
C. granulosum A	$I = 0.80$	$S^b = 4\%$	$I = 1.20$	NS	$I = 1.30$	NS	$I = 1.20$	NS
C. granulosum B	$I = 1.35$	$S = 2\%$	$I = 1$	NS	$I = 1.20$	NS	$I = 0.07$	$S = 2\%$
C. granulosum C	$I = 1$	NS	$I = 1.80$	$S = 1\%$	$I = 1.15$	NS	$I = 1$	NS

$^a I = \bar{S}_{TM}/\bar{S}_C.$
^{b}Statistics: nonparametric text of Wilcoxon. S = significant. NS = nonsignificant.

Table VII. Effect of Corynebacteria (Injected on Day −2.5) for Immunoprophylaxis of L 1210 Leukemia, Summary of Results

"SIA"	Route			
	i.v.	i.p.	i.d.	s.c.
C. parvum	$I^a = 1.15$ $S^b = 1\%$	$I = 1$ NS^b	$I = 1$ NS	$I = 1$ NS
C. granulosum A	$I = 1.2$ $S = 1\%$	$I = 1.4$ $S = 5\%$	$I = 1$ NS	$I = 1.15$ $S = 2\%$
C. granulosum B	$I = 1.09$ NS	$I = 1.10$ NS	$I = 1$ NS	$I = 1$ NS
C. granulosum C	$I = 1.2$ $S = 1\%$	$I = 1.2$ $S = 5\%$	$I = 1$ NS	$I = 1$ NS

$^a I = \bar{S}_{TM}/\bar{S}_C$.
^{b}Statistics: Student-Fisher test. S = significant. NS = nonsignificant.

Table VIII. Effect of Corynebacteria (Injected on Day −2.5) for Immunoprophylaxis of Lewis Tumor, Summary of Results

"SIA"	Route			
	i.v.	i.p.	i.d.	s.c.
C. parvum	I^a = 1.2 S^b = 2%	I = 1 NS	I = 0.9 NS	I = 0.9 NS
C. granulosum A	I = 1.2 S = 2%	I = 1.1 NS	I = 1 NS	I = 1.1 NS
C. granulosum B	I = 1.2 S = 1%	I = 1.1 NS	I = 0.9 NS	I = 1.1 NS
C. granulosum C	I = 1.1 NS	I = 1 NS	I = 1 NS	I = 1.8 S = 2%

$^a I = \bar{S}_{TM}/\bar{S}_C$.
^{b}Statistics: nonparametric test of Wilcoxon. S = significant. NS = nonsignificant.

Table IX. Effect of Corynebacteria (Injected on Day −2.5) for Immunoprophylaxis of ICIG C11, Summary of Results

"SIA"	\multicolumn{8}{c}{Route}
	i.v.		i.p.		i.d.		s.c.	
C. parvum	$I^a = 1$	NS^b	$I = 1.07$	NS	$I = 0.77$	NS	$I = 0.95$	NS
C. granulosum A	$I = 1.09$	NS	$I = 1.01$	NS	$I = 0.75$	NS	$I = 0.91$	NS
C. granulosum B	$I = 1.06$	NS	$I = 0.83$	NS	$I = 0.81$	NS	$I = 1$	NS
C. granulosum C	$I = 1$	NS	$I = 0.92$	NS	$I = 0.81$	NS	$I = 0.90$	NS

$^a I = \bar{S}_{TM}/\bar{S}_C$.

^{b}Statistics: nonparametric test of Wilcoxon. NS = nonsignificant.

parvum and *C. granulosum* B were able to increase the number of hemolytic plaque-forming cell test, even when administered after the sheep red cells. Another important factor that must be considered is the physicochemical characterization of the agent. Important differences were observed in the effects of the different preparations of *C. granulosum*.

These are some of the factors that may play an important role in systemic adjuvants of immunity pharmacokinetics and that, if not considered, may cause tests to be misinterpreted. Hence, there is a necessity for a screening battery comprised of several tests and taking several factors into account.

References

Claman, H. N., Chaperon, A. E., and Triplett, K. (1966). Thymus marrow-cell combination. Synergism in antibody production. *Proc. Soc. Exp. Biol. Med.* 122:1167.

Jerne, N. K., Nordin, A. A., and Henry, C. C. (1963). The agar-plaque technique for recognizing antibody-producing cells. In: *Cell-Bound Antibodies, Vol. 1*, p. 109, Wistar Institute, Philadelphia.

Mathé, G. (1968). Immunothérapie active de la leucémie L1210 appliquée après la greffe tumorale. *Rev. Fr. Et. Clin. Biol.* 13:881.

Mathé, G. and Amiel, J. L. (1960). Aspects histologiques des lésions induites dans les organes hématopoïétiques par l'injection à des hybrides F_1 irradiés de cellules ganglionnaires d'une des lignées parentales. *Rev. Fr. Etud. Clin. Biol.* 5:20.

Mathé, G., Pouillart, P., and Lapeyraque, F. (1969). Active immunotherapy of L1210 leukaemia applied after the graft of tumour cells. *Br. J. Cancer* 23:814.

Mathé, G., Hayat, M., Amiel, J. L., and Hiu, I. J. (1971). Systemic immunity adjuvants and their use in cancer treatment. *Proc. Am. Assoc. Cancer Res.* 12 (abst. 128):32.

Mathé, G., Kamel, M., Dezfulian, M., Halle-Pamenko, O., and Bourut, C. (1973). An experimental screening for "systemic adjuvants of immunity" applicable in cancer immunotherapy. *Cancer Res.* 33:1987.

Raynaud, M., Kouznetzova, B., Bizzini, B., and Chermann, J. C. (1972). Etude de l'effet immunostimulant de diverses espèces de Corynébactéries anaérobies et de leur fraction. *Ann. Inst. Pasteur,* 122:695.

Stutman, O. and Good, R. A. (1969). Absence of synergism between thymus and bone marrow in graft-versus-host reaction. *Proc. Soc. Exp. Biol. Med.* 130:848.

6

Analysis of the *Corynebacterium parvum* Adjuvant Effects at the Cellular and Subcellular Levels

EDITH WIENER

Introduction

Systemic pretreatment of mice with *Corynebacterium parvum* vaccine (CP) exerts a powerful adjuvant effect on antibody production against various T-cell-dependent (Biozzi *et al.*, 1966) and -independent (Howard *et al.*, 1973a) antigens. Previous work has provided evidence that this involves stimulation of B cells at a time when cell-mediated immunity, but not helper, activities of T cells are inhibited. It has been suggested that this adjuvant action of CP on B cells, like the suppressive effect on T cells, is mediated via activated macrophages (Howard *et al.*, 1973b).

We have recently been attempting to further localize the adjuvant effect of CP at the cellular and subcellular levels. Our main approach has been to see whether activation of macrophages is an important causal factor and, if so, in what way these activated cells might modify the immune response.

EDITH WIENER, Department of Experimental Immunobiology, Wellcome Research Laboratories, Beckenham, Kent BR3 3BS, England.

Methods and Results

For tackling the first problem, we employed the modified Marbrook system (Diener and Armstrong, 1967) for the *in vitro* production of antibody against sheep erythrocytes (SRBC) by CBAT6T6 mouse spleen cells. The cells were cultured in RPMI medium buffered with Hepes buffer and bicarbonate, containing 5% fetal calf serum. Figure 1 shows the IgM response against various numbers of sheep red blood cells by spleen cells from mice pretreated with CP (Wellcome strain CN 6134, batch PX289, 350 μg, i.v.) at day −7 compared to that by controls. Antibody production by the CP-treated spleen cells was augmented, and this effect was more pronounced with low antigen concentrations. This result reflects the adjuvant effect of CP *in vivo,* which is also greater with subimmunogenic doses of antigen (Howard *et al.,* 1973b).

The *in vitro* immune response to SRBC is dependent on the presence of an optimal number of macrophages in the culture (Shortman *et al.,* 1970; Feldman and Palmer, 1971). This requirement makes it possible to study the relative efficacy of CP and normal macrophages in antibody production. To this end, normal spleen cells were depleted of macrophages by filtration through a glass-bead column (Shortman *et al.,* 1971), which greatly reduces their ability to

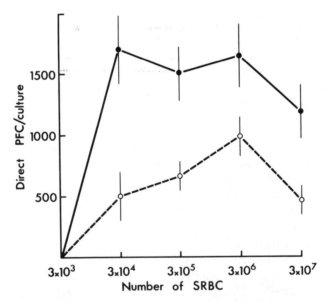

Fig. 1. The *in vitro* immune response by CP-treated and control spleen cells to various numbers of SRBC. 350 μg CP was injected i.v. 7 days prior to spleen-cell harvest. Antibody formation was assayed as direct plaque-forming cells (PFC) according to Cunningham and Szenberg (1968). CP: ●——●; Control: ○– – –○. Mean ± standard error ($n = 6$).

Table I. The Relative Efficiency of CP-Treated and Normal
Peritoneal Cells (PC) in Partially Reconstituting the *in Vivo*
Immune Response of Macrophage (Mϕ)-Depleted Normal
Spleen Cells to 3×10^6 SRBC[a]

Cells in culture	Direct PFC/culture ($\pm$ S.E.)
Normal spleen cells	1880 ± 40
Normal Mϕ-depleted spleen cells	230 ± 110
Normal Mϕ-depleted spleen cells + CP-treated PC (10^5)	720 ± 120
Normal Mϕ-depleted spleen cells + CP-treated nonadherent PC (10^5)	80 ± 80
Normal Mϕ-depleted spleen cells + normal PC (10^5)	120 ± 60

[a]350 μg CP was injected i.v. 7 days prior to PC harvest. Antibody
formation was assayed as direct plaque-forming cells (PFC) according to Cunningham and Szenberg (1968). Mean $\pm$ standard error (n
= 3).

mount an antibody response to SRBC. The spleen cells were then enriched with
macrophage-containing peritoneal cells from CP-treated and normal animals, and
the cell mixtures were cultured with the antigen. Table I illustrates the result of
such an experiment. IgM production by the unfractionated spleen cells was
lowered considerably by removal of the macrophages. The addition of 10^5
peritoneal cells from CP-treated mice partially restored the immune response,
whereas the addition of the same number of cells from normal mice failed to do
so. Furthermore, nonadherent cells from the peritoneum of CP-treated mice did
not restore responsiveness. This result implies that macrophages from CP-treated
animals are much more efficient than normal in promoting the immune response
to SRBC and that they are important mediators of the adjuvant effect.

The second question we asked ourselves was in which way are CP-stimulated
macrophages different from normal ones with regard to their role in antibody
formation. To clarify this problem we studied their *in vitro* handling of the
antigen, keyhole limpet hemocyanin (KLH), to which antibody production *in
vivo* is stimulated by the adjuvant. For the assessment of antigen handling, we
employed KLH labeled with ^{125}I and relatively pure macrophage populations
(Wiener and Curelaru, 1973), obtained by the culture of peritoneal cells from

mice pretreated with CP at day −7 and controls. Antigen uptake was initially slightly slower by the CP macrophages, but after 1 h, both kinds of macrophages showed similar KLH contents.

The next step in antigen handling, its degradation, was estimated in terms of TCA-soluble radioactivity appearing in the cells and in the medium after the exposure of macrophages to the labeled antigen (Wiener and Curelaru, 1973). Figure 2 shows that KLH was degraded to a lesser extent in the CP-treated macrophages (judged by the level of TCA-soluble counts), although the rates of antigen digestion expressed by the slope of the curves were similar in CP and normal cells.

The reduction in [^{125}I]-KLH degradation by CP-activated macrophages could be due to lower levels of lysosomal enzymes. This is unlikely, however, as the specific activities of several acid hydrolases were found to be similar in CP-treated and normal peritoneal macrophages. Alternatively, the lesser degree of antigen digestion in the CP macrophages could be the result of a modified distribution of KLH between the lysosomal compartment and the cellular membrane, where protein digestion does not take place (Unanue et al., 1969).

Hence, we studied membrane-bound KLH (in terms of trypsin-removable radioactivity) (Wiener and Bandieri, 1975) after exposure of the cells to the antigen. We could demonstrate that immediately following exposure to antigen, the CP cells had 3–4 times more membrane-bound KLH than normal macro-phages. Subsequently, the amount of antigen on the surface of the adjuvant-

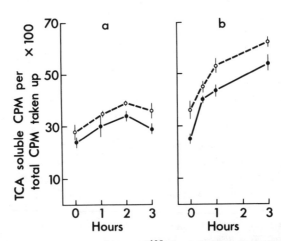

Fig. 2. The intracellular digestion of [^{125}I]-KLH after its uptake by cultured CP-treated and control peritoneal macrophages. 350 μg CP was injected i.v. 7 days prior to peritoneal-cell harvest. (a) macrophages cultured for 2 h; (b) mac-rophages cultured for 24 h. The macrophages were exposed to 0.6 μg [^{125}I]-KLH/ml for 1 h at 37°C. CP: ●———●; Controls: ○− − −○. Mean ± standard error (n = 3).

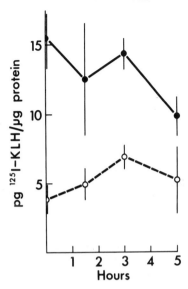

Fig. 3. Membrane-bound [^{125}I]-KLH after its uptake by cultured CP-treated and control peritoneal macrophages. 350 μg CP was injected i.v. 7 days prior to peritoneal-cell harvest. The macrophages had been cultured for 24 h. They were exposed to 0.6 μg [^{125}I]-KLH/ml for 1 h at 37°C. CP: ●——●; Controls: ○– – –○. Mean ± standard error ($n = 3$).

treated cells declined somewhat, but after 5 h was still twice that present on normal macrophages (Fig. 3).

We have been able to confirm that it is this greater proportion of KLH bound to the outer membrane of CP-activated macrophages which determines their lesser degree of antigen digestion. CP-treated and normal macrophages were treated with trypsin (Unanue et al., 1969) after exposure to ^{125}I-labeled KLH, so as to remove any antigen from the outer membrane. Antigen degradation was then followed in trypsin-treated and untreated cells derived from the same source. The previously observed difference in the extent of KLH degradation by CP-activated and normal cells was obliterated by trypsinization of the antigen-containing macrophages (Fig. 4).

Discussion

The present observations suggest that the adjuvant effect of CP is at least partially mediated via activated macrophages on whose surface the presentation of small amounts of antigen to potential antibody-forming cells is intensified.

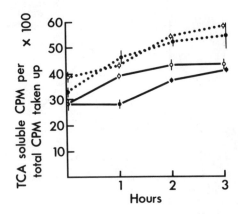

Fig. 4. The intracellular digestion of $[^{125}I]$-KLH after its uptake by cultured CP-treated and control macrophages, and subsequent trypsin treatment of the cells. 350 µg CP was injected i.v. 7 days prior to peritoneal-cell harvest. The macrophages had been cultured for 2 h. They were exposed to 0.6 µg $[^{125}I]$-KLH/ml for 1 h at 37° C. Untreated cells: CP, ●——●; Controls, ○——○. Trypsin-treated cells: CP, ●— —●; Controls ○— —○. Mean ± standard errors ($n = 3$).

The greater binding of antigen to the surface of CP-stimulated macrophages possibly involves distinct membrane sites, whose nature and generation are problems which remain to be solved. Further studies, now in progress, may reveal whether macrophage-activation by CP influences the immune response by mechanisms other than antigen presentation alone.

Summary

The role of macrophages in the adjuvant action of *C. parvum* (CP) was studied in cultures of CBAT6T6 spleen cells during antibody formation against sheep erythrocytes (SRBC). IgM production by spleen cells derived from mice pretreated with CP at day −7 was significantly higher than that by the corresponding control cells. The effect was most marked with a subimmunogenic dose of antigen. Moreover, adherent peritoneal cells from the CP-treated mice were much more efficient than controls in restoring IgM formation of normal macrophage-depleted spleen cells. Handling of the antigen, keyhold limpet hemocyanin, labeled with ^{125}I by cultured peritoneal macrophages from the same CP-treated mice was modified. In these cells, $[^{125}I]$-KLH was degraded to a lesser extent than in normal macrophages due to a higher degree of antigen binding to the cell surface. The results suggest that the adjuvant effect of *C. parvum* is at least partially mediated via activated macrophages, on whose surface the presentation of small amounts of antigen to potential antibody-forming cells is intensified.

References

Biozzi, G., Stiffel, C., Mouton, D., Liacopoulos-Briot, M., Decreusefond, C., and Bouthillier, Y. (1966). Etude du phenomene de l'immuno-cyto-adherence au cours de l'immunisation. *Ann. Inst. Pasteur, Paris* **110**:7.

Cunningham, A. and Szenberg, A. (1968). Further improvements on the plaque technique for detecting single antibody forming cells. *Immunology* **14**:599.

Diener, E. and Armstrong, W. P. (1967). Induction of antibody formation and tolerance *in vitro* to a purified protein antigen. *Lancet* **2**:1281.

Feldman, M. and Palmer, J. (1971). The requirement for macrophages in the immune response *in vitro*. *Cell. Immunol.* **2**:399.

Howard, J. G., Christie, G. H., and Scott, M. T. (1973a). Biological effects of *Corynebacterium parvum*. IV. Adjuvant and inhibitory activities on B lymphocytes. *Cell. Immunol.* **7**:290.

Howard, J. G., Scott, M. T., and Christie, G. H. (1973b). Cellular mechanisms underlying the adjuvant activity of *Corynebacterium parvum:* interactions of activated macrophages with T and B lymphocytes. Immunopotentiation, *Vol. 18*, p. 101, Ciba Found. Symp. (J. W. Wolstenholme and J. Knight, Eds.), Associated Scientific Publishers, Amsterdam.

Shortman, K., Diener, E., Russel, P. J., and Armstrong, W. D. (1970). The role of nonlymphoid accessory cells in the immune response. *J. Exp. Med.* **131**:461.

Shortman, K., Williams, N., Jackson, H., Russel, P., Byrt, P., and Diener, E. (1971). The separation of different cell classes from lymphoid organs. IV. The separation of lymphocytes from phagocytes on glass-bead columns and its effect on subpopulations of lymphocytes and antibody-forming cells. *J. Cell Biol.* **48**:566.

Unanue, E. R., Cerottini, J. C., and Bedford, M. (1969). Persistence of antigen on the surface of macrophages. *Nature (Lond.)* **222**:1193.

Wiener, E., and Bandieri, A. (1975). Differences in antigen handling by peritoneal macrophages from the Biozzi high and low responder lines of mice. *Eur. J. Immunol.* **4**:457.

Wiener, E. and Curelaru, Z. (1973). The incomplete digestion of proteins taken up by macrophages. *J. Reticuloendothel. Soc.* **13**:210.

DISCUSSION

PARAF: One of the main problems is to understand at what level the adjuvants are active. This problem cannot be solved at present, but at least we can try to develop a system in which questions such as "are adjuvants active at the cell membrane level?" are asked.

The enzymatic activities of the cell membranes have been studied in normal and transformed 3T3 cells. In culture during cell growth, there is a certain amount of enzymatic activities, such as ATPase, amino acid influx, glucose influx, and so on [D. O. Foster and A. B. Pardee (1969). *J. Biol. Chem.* **244**:2675; B. M. Sefton and H. Rubin (1971). *Proc. Natl. Acad. Sci.* **68**:3154; S. K. Bose and B. O. Zlotnick (1973). *Proc. Natl. Acad. Sci.* **70**:2374]. But, as soon as normal cells susceptible to contact inhibition come into contact, there is a sharp reduction in enzymatic activity. With transformed cells, however, even though there is contact between cells, no change in cell-membrane activity is observed.

Working with plasmacytoma cells, we have developed a system where it is possible to isolate purified cell membranes. This work was done by L. Lelièvre [(1973). *Biochim. Biophys. Acta* **291**:662–670; L. Lelièvre and A. Paraf (1973). **291**:671–679], who found that if such membranes are isolated from contact-inhibited cells, there is a 95% drop in the enzymatic activity when compared to membranes isolated from growing cells.

With such purified cell membranes, it is possible to check whether, according to the dose used, there is enhancement or lowering of the enzymatic activities. The cell membranes were purified in such a way as to separate two sorts of vesicles [A. Zachowski and A. Paraf (1974). *Biochem. Biophys. Res. Commun.* **57**:787]: (a) the right-side-out vesicles isolated on a polymer of Concanavalin A and (b) the inside-out vesicles.

It is interesting to note that the "inside-out" vesicles, which are known to have no exposed sites for fixation of concanavalin A, show no change in the

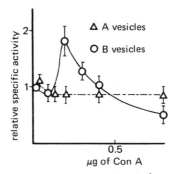

Fig. 1. **Modulation of the 5′-nucle-otidase activity by adding various amounts of Con A to A or B vesicles.** (Kinetics are linear up to the end of the test: 30 min).

enzymatic activity, irrespective of the dose of concanavalin A of the 5′-nucleotidase. The right side-out vesicles show a 50–100% enhancement in enzymatic activity with a very small amount of concanavalin A—between 0.1 and 0.3 μg/ml for 40 μg of purified vesicles. However, if the concentration of concanavalin A is raised to 0.5–1 μg/ml, there is a sharp decline in the enzyme activity.

This experiment could serve as a model for studying other adjuvants, i.e., there are probably other so-called adjuvants which enhance enzymatic activity in such a way that cells are just ready to divide. An increased immune response would then be expected from these cells. On the other hand, other types of adjuvants can be expected to lower the enzymatic activity, and, in this sense, such substances would inhibit the immune response.

FELDMAN: My comment is to Dr. Wiener's presentation. It has been shown that antigens which are thymus-independant are also macrophage-independent. Therefore, it might be of interest to check whether *Corynebacterium parvum* has an effect under these conditions.

Furthermore, when antigens produce antibodies in the absence of the thymus, they will never make IgG. I would like to know whether any distinction was made with regard to those antibodies: which antibodies are involved, IgM or IgG?

WIENER: We measured IgG response by the ordinary method, but have not been able to detect any—not in the primary response, anyway. We are now searching for it more carefully.

With regard to the antigens being macrophage-independent, this has not yet been proven; it is a controversial matter.

ADLAM: I was extremely interested in the presentation by Dr. Werner, because if they have obtained a soluble extract of *C. parvum* which works in these various systems, this is a great advance. I have three questions: First, what were the comparative doses of the whole organism and the water-soluble extract which were used? Second, what was the route of injection of the *C. parvum*? Third, did the water-soluble extract have any antitumor action?

WERNER: First, the doses varied from one experiment to another. Let us consider, for instance the example of Moloney sarcoma. The water-soluble crude extract was injected at a dose of 1.5 mg/kg i.v., four days before the i.p. injection of the virus, while the whole cells were injected at a dose of 25 mg/kg i.v., at the same time. In this particular system, about 20 times less of the water-soluble substance was injected than of the whole cells.

In other systems, such as the production of hypersensitivity to ovalbumin in the guinea pig, we worked on a equal-weight basis—that is, 0.5 mg of either the soluble substances or of the whole cells was injected with Freund's incomplete adjuvant.

With regard to the route of injection, in the EMC experiments, both the water-soluble extract and the whole cells were injected intravenously 2 h prior to virus inoculation, the virus itself being injected subcutaneously.

We have not yet investigated whether the water-soluble extract has anti-tumor activity, although this is going to be done. All that has been seen so far is its effect on the Moloney sarcoma virus-induced splenomegaly.

DESBORDES: Numerous experiments are carried out with a view to studying lipidic germs (especially the Corynebacteria), their importance and their value as inducers of a nonspecific immunity.

In collaboration with A. M. Levy, Mrs. Mauss, and Mrs. Lindenman from the Centre International de l'Enfance, Paris, we studied the response of mouse parathymic nodes to an intraperitoneal injection of *Corynebacterium*. The 8-week-old mouse was injected with 0.250 mg (in a constant volume of 0.25 ml). We took samples from the nodes 24 and 48 h, 5 days, and, finally, 15 days later.

The results were as follows:

(a) 3 hours later, there was no distinct immunological response.

(b) 24 hours later, there was a marked inflammatory reaction. Veins were noticeably dilated in the paracortical region and there was afflux of lymphocytes in the blood—node directions. Lymphocytic blast cells were seen in the cortical and even paracortical regions.

(c) 48 hours later, the volume of the node had increased considerably. The cortical region was quite visible, and many blast cells could be seen in the cortical folliculi. Large lymphocytic basophile cells appeared. The para-cortical region was greater than the cortical region.

(d) 5 days later, hypertrophy of the node was evidenced. Hyperplasia of the paracortical regions, which seemed to contain few lymphocytes, had occurred. Postcapillary veins were dilated; their walls allowed for the penetration of many lymphocytes. Numerous reticulated cells could be found in the paracortical region, whereas in the cortical region, lymphocytes were abundant; in the medullary sinus, blastic cells and hyperbasophil cells could be distinctly located.

(e) 15 days later there was evidence of a very large node. The cortical region was extremely developed. Numerous light areas appeared in the hypertrophied tissues. Nevertheless, the paracortical area was full of lymphoid cells. The vein net was blocked with an accumulation of lymphocytes in the blood—node directions.

In conclusion, the i.p. injection of *C. parvum* resulted in obvious stimulation of the mouse parathymic node. This reaction may be divided into 3 stages: (1) during the 4 days following the injection, lymphocytic retention in the cortical region occurred; (2) from the 6th day onward, there was an intense influx of basophilic lymphocytes from the circulating blood; (3) on the 15th day, the cortical region was expanded. The paracortical region is likely to play an important part in the mobilization of T lymphocytes.

PETIT: D. Jollès, what is known about the chemical composition of the crude water-soluble extract in fraction 6 of the *C. parvum* which Dr. Werner tested for biological activities?

JOLLÈS: When chromatographed on DEAE-cellulose, I have shown that all the low-molecular-weight soluble substances, ranging in molecular weight from 6000 to 3000 or 4000, are present. We have now further purified each of these fractions. Fraction 6, about which Dr. Werner has spoken, has a molecular weight of 6000 and contains a peptidoglycan, alanine, glutamic acid, diaminopimelic acid, and so on. This particular fraction still contains 40% natural sugars. Of course, there are other fractions—such as the corresponding mycobacterial fraction—which have no natural sugars.

MCBRIDE: Toward the end of the growth cycle of *C. parvum* there is a soluble antigen produced which is an acidic polysaccharide, with a molecular weight somewhere about 100,000—150,000. It contains galactose, N-acetylglucosamine, and so on, and a small proportion—up to about 10%—of amino acids. This polysaccharide, or polysaccharide plus peptide, is strongly antigenic and is a major component of the cell wall of *C. parvum*.

It is possible to bind this antigen onto red cells directly, without any intermediary. It seems that at least part of the antigen—the soluble part—can bind to red cells of various types.

Is it known whether the substances obtained by Dr. Adlam and Dr. Jollès are antigenic, whether they can react with cell membranes in any way, and can the speakers comment on whether these substances are peculiar to *C. parvum* and whether they have done any other bacterial controls in their systems?

ADLAM: I do not know anything about the 100,000 molecular-weight polysaccharide produced at the end of the growth phase. I have not worked with this sort of material. My only comment is that if *C. parvum* is grown too long, it lyses and loses its activity. Our material is probably the backbone of the cell wall—as was shown on the electron micrographs. This is not to say that the material described by Dr. McBride could not be extracted from our material, nor that there several fractions could not be isolated from *C. parvum* (as there are for BCG) with a variety of properties.

MCBRIDE: Is it antigenic?

ADLAM: It is definitely antigenic.

SACHS: From what we heard this morning about different strains of mice having varying susceptibilities to the effects of the bacterium, it is clear that there is a genetic basis for susceptibility. Clearly, people may obtain completely different results depending on the type of tumor and strain of mice used. The use of *C. parvum* extracts in humans may also have different results on each subject, depending on the genetic constitution of the person being dealt with. Has anybody any information about the genetic basis of the susceptibility and whether one or two genes are involved? The latter could be checked by means of breeding experiments. This is extremely important, not only for studying immunotherapy with this compound, but also for every type of chemotherapy. What is known about the genetic basis, and to what extent are researchers ensuring that if they say something works, or does not work, they are using it against the same genetic background?

DIMITROV: Dr. Amiel, did you demonstrate that BCG, *C. parvum* and the fraction of *C. granulosum* had exactly the same action on Lewis lung tumor?

AMIEL: I cannot say that they are the same. The results were statistically significant, as compared to the control group. For the tests of the tumors we used only one adjuvant, and the most significant results were living BCG for the three types of tumors. After living BCG, the most constant results were obtained with the *Corynebacterium*, either *parvum* or *granulosum*. With these two types of compounds, we had few immunodepressive results. This is not true with the extracts of BCG. It may be interesting to know whether or not the soluble extract of the *Corynebacterium* will have an immunodepressive effect on some tumors.

There is no longer any question that whole-organism preparations of BCG or *Corynebacterium* are able to stop the progression of some tumors. They can be used as a reference to find out whether other products warrant use in clinical trials.

It is important to know whether the mechanism of action of BCG—which is certainly very complicated—on macrophages, B cells, and T cells involves a rapid action on the thymus, and, also, whether there is any similarity in the induction of granuloma in liver with BCG and *Corynebacterium*. Another problem is to find out whether an additive therapeutic effect results from administering BCG and *Corynebacterium* together. There is insufficient evidence from both mice and human trials to answer this question definitively. However, there are indications suggesting that the effect can be additive.

DIMITROV: When were the vaccines injected?

AMIEL: As I showed on the slides, we tried several different days before the test for each product. For most tests, the best time was two weeks prior to the antigen challenge; this is true for sheep red blood cells and for the tumor. However, we still had positive results, both with BCG and *Corynebacterium*, if the vaccines were given two or five days before the challenge, or even one, two, or three days after the challenge.

The classical idea that the adjuvant will be effective only if given before the antigens is not entirely true. Evidently, the mechanism is the same, but if the antigen challenge by the tumor leaves sufficient delay, then the stimulus by *Corynebacterium* or BCG can give results. The effect also depends on the number of tumor cells injected.

DIMITROV: This is one of the most important tumors for evaluation of the tumor-remission studies, and I think we must discuss this subject later. There is some controversy concerning Dr. Amiel's results.

WHISNANT: I should like to comment on two points: first, Dr. Sachs's important comment about genetic variability. Many of the variations seen in toxicity, such as were shown earlier today, may be explained by genetic variability in strains of mice. Dr. Sheldon Woolf, from the National Institutes of Health, has reported that strains of mice have marked susceptibility to endotoxin which is clearly segregable on a genetic basis. Those of us who are doing this kind of work should keep the genetics in mind. Second, Dr. Feldman commented about T-independent antigens. Are T-independent responses also macrophage-independent?

FELDMAN: So far, all T-independent antigens which have been tested were found to be macrophage-independent too. However, in all these cases, only IgM antibodies were formed, and there was no formation of IgG.

WHISNANT: In that light, could Dr. Feldman explain Dr. James Howard's results about enhancement of any pneumococcal responses to *C. parvum?*

FELDMAN: Instead of attempting an explanation, I think it would be better to do some experiments.

PARAF: There is a lot of controversy about the time interval which should occur between inoculation of the adjuvant and injection of different types of tumor cells or viruses. I must emphasize that we could be faced with two completely different mechanisms.

Most people are talking about an immune response, in other words, the specific activity of antibodies or specific T cells. We know the kinetics of such a response. There is another possibility, however. Seven years ago, together with Dr. Jollès, we showed that there could be interferon synthesis. In this case, when the adjuvant is injected, there can be a low synthesis of interferon, but as soon as the virus is injected, there can be an enormous amount of interferon within a few hours—not only in cells, but also in the blood stream. It is well-known now that interferon acts not only on virus multiplication, but also on cell multiplication.

Has anybody tried to separate immune response completely from interferon synthesis in these trials, looking all the time at the injection of adjuvant versus the transformed cells or viruses?

WANEBO: Could Dr. Amiel comment on the immune depression—or what he interpreted as such—in his experiments with *C. parvum?* Was this related to timing?

AMIEL: When I said "immune depression" in these tests, I did not mean to imply that I understood the mechanism of action. As has been shown for other systems, it is possible that there is a stimulation of some immune reaction; I will not talk about "blocking antibodies" because everything is too easily explained in that way today, but it is possible that there is an enhancement phenomenon. Perhaps there is a better way of expressing it than by the phrase "immune depression." I do not want to use "immune depression," except for the therapist's point of view, whether in mice or men.

With BCG, and probably also *Corynebacterium,* there is a strong stimulation of macrophages, with nonspecific cytotoxicity of macrophages. This action takes place even if the adjuvant is given after the antigenic stimulus. After stimulation with BCG or *Corynebacterium,* very positive results are found in mice when macrophages are tested *in vitro.* In fact, the first reaction in the thymus to BCG—and the same will probably be true for *Corynebacterium—*

starts 2 h after injection. Thus, if it is given two days after the inoculation of the tumor cells, which will kill the mice within 12 days, it is not surprising that there is an effect on the growth of the tumor. We are a little too fascinated by the fact that the product is given two days before, or one day after, the antigenic stimulus. In some systems it does not matter very much.

ATTIÉ: Has anyone with experience of immunotherapy in animals bearing tumors observed cases of facilitation with extremely rapid growth of the tumor after immunotherapy?

HALPERN: Data on this matter will be given later.

Part III
Corynebacterium parvum in Microbial Immunity

7

Stimulating Effect of *Corynebacterium parvum* and *C. parvum* Extract on the Macrophage Activities against *Salmonella typhimurium* and *Listeria monocytogenes*

ROBERT M. FAUVE

It was shown ten years ago by Halpern *et al.* (1964) that *Corynebacterium parvum* is a powerful stimulant of the reticuloendothelial system. Since then, enhanced resistance against tumor invasion in animals and man and against bacterial infections have been documented (Adlam *et al.*, 1972; Halpern *et al.*, 1973). It is well-known that the outcome of a bacterial infection depends not only on the ingestive capacity of phagocytic cells, but also on their bactericidal capacity. In the present report, we will consider the increase of bacterial killing by macrophages from mice treated with *C. parvum,* and it will be shown that a phospholipid extract from *C. parvum* can stimulate not only the ingestive capacity of spleen and liver macrophages, but also their bactericidal efficiency.

ROBERT M. FAUVE, Unité d'Immunophysiologie Cellulaire, Département de Biologie Moléculaire, Institut Pasteur, Paris, France

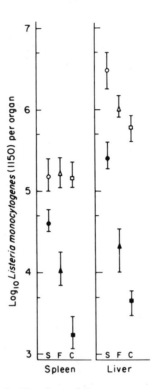

Fig. 1. Number of *L. monocytoge-nes* (1150) found in the spleen and the liver 15 min (white symbols) and 3 h (black symbols) after infection in mice treated with either saline (S), formalin (F), or *C. parvum* (C).

C. parvum is very often used in the form of a suspension in formalin. Since formalin is known to induce a strong inflammatory reaction after injection, we first investigated the possible adjuvant effect of formalin in the stimulation of macrophages in comparison with a heat-killed suspension of *C. parvum*. Three groups of 10 mice were injected intravenously with 0.5 ml of one of three solutions: S, pyrogen-free saline; F, pyrogen-free saline containing 2% of formalin; and C, pyrogen-free saline containing 200 µg of heat-killed *C. parvum* strain 936B from the Pasteur Institute. Four days later, all mice were infected intravenously with 9×10^6 *Listeria monocytogenes* strain 1150 (Fauve and Hevin, 1971). Five mice in each group were bled by cervical section 15 and 180 min later. Bacterial counts were performed on liver and spleen homogenates. The results are summarized in Fig. 1. The number of bacteria found in the spleens of the three groups were about the same 15 minutes after infection.

In contrast, 3 h later, bacterial count was about four times higher in S than in F and five times higher in F than in C. In the liver of these mice, 15 minutes after infection, there were twice as many bacteria in S as in F and nearly as many bacteria in F as in C. Three hours later, the number of bacteria in the S group was ten times greater than in F and five times greater in F than in C. These results showed that formalin injected intravenously into mice is able to increase the bactericidal capacity of liver and spleen macrophages four days later. The following experiments were therefore undertaken with heat-killed *C. parvum*.

In order to follow the increased bactericidal capacity of spleen and liver macrophages, mice were injected subcutaneously with 0.2 ml of pyrogen-free saline containing 200 μg of *C. parvum*. Control mice received 0.2 ml of pyrogen-free saline subcutaneously. Immediately and 4, 7, 10, and 14 days after treatment, 6 mice of each group were intravenously infected with 8×10^6 *L. monocytogenes* strain 1150. Fifteen minutes and three hours later, mice were killed by cervical section. Bacterial counts were performed on spleen and liver homogenates. The bactericidal capacity of spleen and liver macrophages from treated mice was evaluated as a percentage by means of the formula:

$$\frac{N_e(15) - N_e(3h)}{N_t(15) - N_t(3h)} \times 100$$

where $N_e(15)$ and $N_e(3h)$ are the numbers of bacteria found in a given organ from treated mice 15 min and 3 h after infection, respectively, and $N_t(15)$ and $N_t(3h)$ are the corresponding numbers of bacteria found in the organs from control mice. The results are summarized in Fig. 2. The percentage of increase in

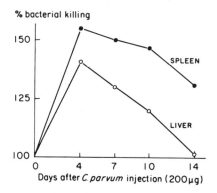

Fig. 2. Increase of bacterial killing of *L. monocytogenes* in the spleen and the liver of mice previously injected with 200 μg of *C. parvum*.

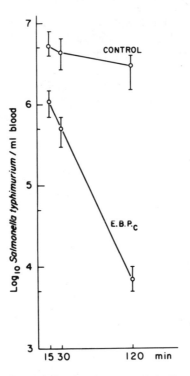

Fig. 3. Blood clearance of *S. typhimurium* in mice injected with saline (control) or with 1 mg of EBP$_c$ 18 h before the injection of 7×10^6 *Salmonella*.

bactericidal capacity of the liver macrophages, in comparison with controls, was 42, 30, 20, and 2% on the 4th, 7th, 10th, and 14th day after treatment, respectively. On the same days, the increase in the bactericidal killing was even greater: 60, 50, 45, and 32% in the spleen.

Such an increased bactericidal capacity may be induced by some constituent(s) of *C. parvum*. Since phospholipids are known to have a very high turnover in macrophages, we tested a crude phospholipid extract of *C. parvum* on mice. This phospholipid extract (EBP$_c$) was obtained by the method of Folch (Fauve and Hevin, 1974), not only to investigate the bacterial killing by macrophages, but also to study their ingestive capacity.

The uptake of virulent, smooth bacteria was tested with *Salmonella typhimurium* C$_5$ (LD$_{50}$ = 200) and *Klebsiella pneumoniae* (LD$_{50}$ = 60). Mice injected intravenously, either with pyrogen-free saline alone or saline containing 1 mg of EBP$_c$ were infected 18 h later, either with 3×10^5 *K. pneumoniae* or with 7×10^6 *S. typhimurium*. At the times indicated in Fig. 3 (*K. pneumoniae*) and Fig. 4 (*S. typhimurium*), the mice were bled from the axillary vein, and bacterial counts were performed on 0.5 ml of blood after suitable dilution and plating on nutrient agar. In contrast with saline-treated mice, EBP_c-treated mice were able to clear bacteria very efficiently, and at the end of the experiment, the bacterial count was smaller than in the controls by a factor of nearly 1000. This difference can be explained either by a bactericidal effect of EBP_c, by the occurrence of opsonins in treated animals, or by an activation of the ingestive capacity of spleen and liver macrophages. Since we have shown (Fauve and Hevin, 1974) that phospholipid extracts from other bacteria, such as *S. typhimurium* and *L. monocytogenes*, are devoid of bactericidal activity and do not induce increased opsonic or bactericidal activities in the serum of mice, it seems reasonable to conclude that such increased bacterial clearance is the result of an activation of the macrophage ingestive capacity.

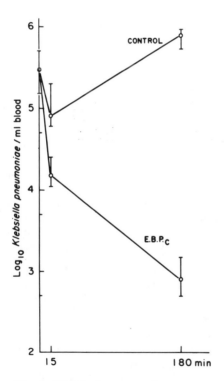

Fig. 4. Blood clearance of *K. pneumoniae* in mice injected with saline (control) or with 1 mg of EBP_c 18 h before the injection of 3×10^5 *Klebsiella*.

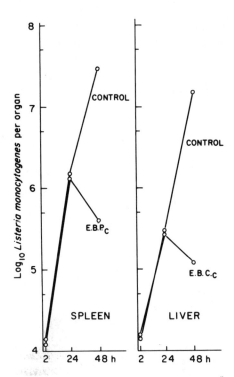

Fig. 5. Fate of an inoculum of 4×10^5 *Listeria* in the liver and spleen of mice injected with saline (control) or with 1 mg of EBP_c 15 h before infection.

Since it has been shown that mice treated with EBP are much more resistant to infection by *L. monocytogenes, S. typhimurium,* and *Yersinia pestis* (Fauve and Hevin, 1974), and—recently—*Pseudomonas aeruginosa,* we tested the action of EBP_c on virulent *L. monocytogenes.* For this purpose, three groups of 4 mice were injected intravenously with 1 mg of EBP_c and three other groups with saline. Fifteen hours later, mice from all groups were injected with 4×10^5 *Listeria* ($LD_{50} = 2.5 \times 10^5$). Bacterial counts of livers and spleens were performed 2, 24, and 48 h after infection. As shown in Fig. 5, the slopes of bacterial growth in the spleen and liver are the same during the first 24 h. In contrast, 48 h later, nearly 100 times fewer bacteria are found in treated mice than in controls.

As noted previously (Fauve and Hevin, 1974), it has been shown that lipid extracts from mycobacteria can increase the resistance of mice against bacterial infection. However, we are not aware of reports showing that phospholipid extract from *C. parvum* can increase the ingestive and bactericidal capacity of liver and spleen macrophages. This stimulating effect has always been observed without any evidence of liver and spleen hypertrophy. Furthermore, we did not find any thymus aplasia following EBP$_c$ injection. These observations lead us to conclude that this phospholipid extract does not reproduce all the known biological effects of *C. parvum,* since it is well-established that the injection of this bacteria induces an increase in spleen and liver weight. Nevertheless, it is interesting that EBP$_c$ can produce *in vivo* the well-known stimulating effect of *C. parvum* on the reticuloendothelial system. From present investigations, we have established by using chromatography that most, if not all, the activity of EBP is present in one fraction, which is a phospholipid with a low molecular weight.

It is too early to describe the mechanism of action of this fraction; however, it seems that this phospholipid does not act through T lymphocytes. Indeed, we have recently found that EBP is able to stimulate nude mice. In contrast, it was found that EBP extracted from *S. typhimurium,* which is a better source than *C. parvum,* is able to increase the thymidine incorporation in B lymphocytes (Marchal and Fauve, 1973). It does not seem that the activation of macrophages requires the participation of B lymphocytes and their multiplication, since we have recently found that EBP can protect heavily irradiated mice against a 50 LD$_{50}$ dose of *K. pneumoniae.*

References

Adlam, C., Broughton, E. S., and Scott, M. T. (1972). Enhanced resistance of mice to infection with bacteria following pretreatment with *Corynebacterium parvum. Nat. New Biol.* 235:219–220.

Fauve, R. M. and Hevin, M. B. (1971). Pouvoir bactéricide des macrophages spléniques et hépatiques de souris envers *Listeria monocytogens.* Influence du traitement préalable des animaux par des glucocorticoïdes, une endotoxine, *Corynebacterium parvum* et l'acide polyinosinique, Polycytidylique (Poly : I.C.). *Ann. Inst. Pasteur, Paris* 120:399–411.

Fauve, R. M. and Hevin, M. B. (1974). Immunostimulation with bacterial phospholipid extracts. *Proc. Natl. Acad. Sci. USA* 71:573–577.

Halpern, B. N., Prévot, A. R., Biozzi, G., Stiffel, C., and Mouton, D. (1964). Stimulation de l'activité phagocytaire du système réticuloendothélial provoquée par *Corynebacterium parvum. J. Reticuloendothel. Soc.* 1:77–96.

Halpern, B. N., Fray, A., Crepin, Y., Platiga, O., Lorinet, A. M., Rabourdin, A., Sparros, L., and Isac, R. (1973). *Corynebacterium parvum,* a potent immunostimulant in experimental infections and in malignancies. In: *Immunopotentiation,* pp. 217–234, Ciba Foundation Symposium, Association of Scientific Publishers, Amsterdam.

Marchal, G. and Fauve, R. M. (1973). Action d'un extrait bactérien phospholipidique (EBP) sur les lymphocytes spléniques de souris. *C. R. Acad. Sci.* 277:2581–2584.

Metchnikoff, E. (1901). *L'Immunité dans les Maladies Infectieuses,* pp. 315–340, Masson and Cie.

8

Antiviral Properties of *Corynebacterium parvum*

ITALINA CERUTTI

Abstract

In *in vivo* and *in vitro* experiments, we observed that the peritoneal exudates from mice treated with *Corynebacterium parvum* contain a factor which inhibits vesicular stomatitis virus and encephalomyocarditis virus. This inhibitor does not seem to possess the usual biological properties attributed to interferon.

Introduction

Treatment of mice with *C. parvum* increases their resistance to tumor grafts (Halpern and Israel, 1971; Halpern *et al.*, 1973a; Halpern *et al.*, 1973b) and bacterial infection (Adlam *et al.*, 1972). This antitumoral and antibacterial action cannot be entirely explained by the stimulating effect of *C. parvum* on the reticuloendothelial cell system (RES). Different substances, such as lipids, hormones, or microbial extracts, may provoke an increase of phagocytosis without, however, improving the animals' resistance to tumor spread or bacterial invasion (Old *et al.*, 1961). On the other hand, previous studies have shown that interferon (the antiviral effects of which are well known) inhibits tumor development (Atanasiu and Chany, 1960; Gresser *et al.*, 1967). It was, therefore, of interest to investigate whether or not the injection of *C. parvum* in the mouse

ITALIANA CERUTTI, Institut National de la Santé et de la Recherche Médicale, U. 43 de Recherches sur les Infections Virales, Hôpital St. Vincent-de-Paul, 74 Avenue Denfert-Rochereau, 75014 Paris, France would increase the resistance of the animal to viral infection. If so, the resistance provoked by *C. parvum* could perhaps be explained by interferon induced by this microorganism.

Materials and Methods

Animals

Inbred male Swiss and C_{57} Bl/6 mice, 8–10 weeks old, were obtained from the C.N.R.S. (Orleans, France); male IC mice, 8–10 weeks old, were obtained from the Institut du Cancer (Villejuif, France).

Cell Line

Mouse L-929 cells, routinely propagated in the laboratory, were used in all the experiments.

Bacteria

Anaerobic *C. parvum*, inactivated by heat and formalin (0.002%), was supplied by Dr. Halpern (Institut d'Immunobiologie, Paris, France) and injected (0.1 ml/mouse) intraperitoneally and intravenously at 250 µg, 500 µg, or 1000 µg (dry weight germ) doses.

Viruses

Newcastle disease virus (NDV), Kansas strain (10^9 egg ID/50), (used to induce interferon synthesis) was injected (0.1 ml/mouse) intraperitoneally and intravenously.

Encephalomyocarditis virus (EMC), used as a challenge virus, was injected (0.5 ml/mouse) intraperitoneally and intravenously at a concentration of 200 LD_{50}. The lethal effect of this virus produced a flaccid paralysis which appeared 4 days after inoculation.

Vesicular stomatitis virus (VSV) was employed as a challenge virus at the multiplicity of infection (MOI) = 0.1 PFU/cell.

Antiviral Factor

This factor, present in the mouse peritoneal exudates, was obtained as follows: C_{57} Bl/6 mice were treated intraperitoneally with *C. parvum* (500 µg). Forty-eight hours later, the exudates were collected after washing of the peritoneal cavity with Eagle's medium (MEM) (1 ml/mouse). After centrifugation at 2000 rpm for 10 min, the *p*H of the supernatant containing the antiviral factor was adjusted to *p*H 7.4.

Interferon Induction and Assay

Swiss, C_{57}Bl/6, and IC mice were treated intravenously by NDV or *C. parvum* (500 µg). Blood samples were taken by cardiac tapping. The antiviral activity of the sera was assayed using L cells which were infected after a 24-h incubation period by VSV. The interferon titer is expressed as the reverse of the dilution which protects 50% of the cells.

$C_{57}Bl/6$ macrophages were collected after washing of the peritoneum with 1 ml of MEM.

Actinomycin D

Actinomycin D (purchased from Merck, Sharp, and Dohme) was employed at a concentration of 1 μg/ml (which inhibits 90% of [^{3}H] uridine incorporation in cellular RNA).

Results

The Action of *C. parvum* on the Lethal Effect of EMC in Mice

C. parvum was injected in Swiss mice at concentrations of 250 μg, 500 μg, or 1000 μg. The protection against the lethal effect of EMC was compared to that of interferon synthesis induced by NDV. *C. parvum* and NDV were injected intraperitoneally and 2 or 7 days later, were followed by an injection of EMC. The percentage of survival was calculated after a 1-month observation period of groups of 30 mice per experimental series. As shown in Fig. 1, the survival obtained in the groups under bacterial treatment (C, D, E) clearly shows an increased resistance of the animals against the lethal effect of the virus. For a dose of 500 μg, approximately 50% of the animals were protected, while 95% died in the control group (group A). The decrease of protection observed for a dose of 1000 μg was probably due to a toxic effect of *C. parvum*.

Action of *C. parvum* on VSV Replication

An antiviral action was also found in the centrifuged supernatant of the peritoneal exudates of Swiss mice treated with 500 μg of *C. parvum* (injected intraperitoneally). The supernatant of the exudates in contact with L cells, and simultaneously with VSV, inhibited viral multiplication. The inhibitory action of this factor was maximal when mouse peritoneal exudates were taken 48 h after stimulation by *C. parvum* (Fig. 2). Moreover, the antiviral effect of the exudates increased when a suspension of spleen cells (from syngenic animals) was injected in the peritoneum prior to *C. parvum* injection.

In further experiments we explored the possibility that this antiviral action of *C. parvum* could be due to interferon.

Induction of Interferon Synthesis by *C. parvum*

The appearance of interferon in the serum of mice after treatment with *C. parvum* (500 μg/0.1 ml/mouse, live or inactivated by using either heat or formalin) was studied. NDV was used as a reference (Fig. 3). Three different mice strains were employed: $C_{57}Bl/6$, Swiss, and IC, known for their capacity to produce interferon at different levels after viral induction. Serum samples

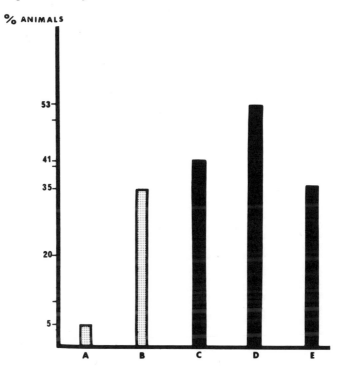

Fig. 1. Decrease of the lethal effect in groups of Swiss mice treated with *C. parvum* or **NDV** and infected with **EMC**. Percentage of survival after a 1-month observation period. A: Control EMC; B: NDV + EMC; C: *C. parvum*, 250 μg/0.1 ml + EMC; D: *C. parvum*, 500 μg/0.1 ml + EMC; E: *C. parvum*, 1000 μg/0.1 ml + EMC.

were taken between 2 and 24 h after bacterial treatment. No detectable amount of viral inhibitory material was found after assay in cell cultures, using VSV as the challenge virus.

The presence of interferon was also explored locally in peritoneal cells in the following manner: (a) either peritoneal macrophage cells from normal Swiss mice were incubated for 24 h at 37°C and infected with 500 μg of *C. parvum*, or (b) treated with 500 μg of *C. parvum* and resuspended in MEM after centrifugation. In the cell samples taken between 2 and 24 h, no inhibitor similar to interferon was identified.

Properties of the Antiviral Factor Diffusing from *C. parvum*-Induced Macrophages

The antiviral factor isolated in the centrifuged supernatant of mice exudates treated with *C. parvum* can be distinguished from interferon in two different ways: (1) The biological activity of interferon is destroyed after heating at 56°C for 30 min. The factor present in the supernatant is resistant to the same treatment. (2) Interferon activity needs the integrity of cell-protein synthesis. Treatment of the cells by actinomycin D, before or at the same time as interferon, prevents the establishment of the antiviral state. The same treatment does not affect the antiviral action of the inhibitor.

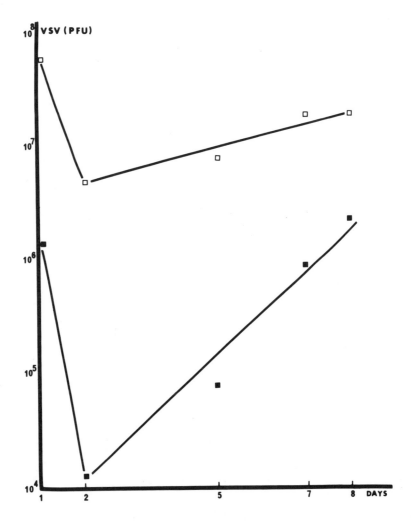

Fig. 2. **Antiviral effect of peritoneal exudates on L cells.** □ Treated with formalin (0.002%); ■ treated with *C. parvum* (500 μg). VSV yield is expressed in PFU/ml.

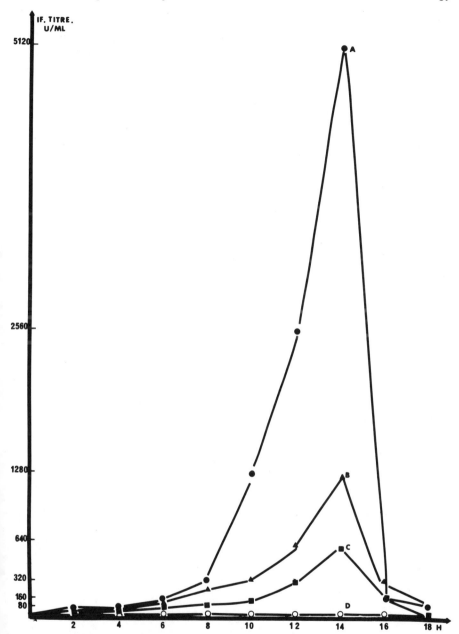

Fig. 3. Interferon eliminated in the serum of groups of mice injected with NDV. ● A: C₅₇Bl/6; ▲ B: Swiss, ■ C: IC; ○ D: the same mice strains as A, B, C, but inoculated with *C. parvum,* showing no detectable amount of interferon appearing in the serum.

Discussion and Conclusion

In the peritoneal exudates of mice injected with *C. parvum,* a factor possessing inhibitory properties on viral multiplication was isolated. Interferon was not detected in the serum in the peritoneal exudates of mice, nor in the supernatant of cultured macrophages. This inhibitor seems to be different from interferon in its thermoresistance at pH 7.4 (in contrast to the thermolability of interferon) and its mode of action. The antiviral effect of the latter is not inhibited after treatment of the cells with actinomycin D. The inhibitor is liberated in the supernatant late when compared to interferon (24 h). A maximal effect is obtained 48 h after stimulation of the mice.

Injection of normal spleen cells from syngenic animals into the peritoneum prior to *C. parvum* increases the amount of inhibitor liberated in the exudates.

It would be of interest to draw a parallel between the well-known antitumoral effect and the antiviral effect of *C. parvum* presented here. This problem cannot be answered at present and will be the subject of future investigations.

Acknowledgment

The author thanks Drs. B. Halpern, C. Chany, and P. Bouquet for their valuable advice, and C. Girard for her help with the manuscript.

References

Adlam, C., Broughton, E. S., and Scott, M. T. (1972). Enhanced resistance of mice to infection with bacteria after treatment with *C. parvum. Nat. New Biol.* **235:**219.

Atanasiu, P. and Chany, C. (1960). Action d'un interféron provenant de cellules malignes l'infection expérimentale du hamster nouveau-né par le virus du polyome. *C.R. Acad. Sci., Paris* **251:**1687.

Gresser, I., Falcoff, R., Fontaine-Brouty-Boye, D., Zajdela, F., Coppey, J., and Falcoff, E. (1967). Interferon and murine leukemia. IV. Further studies on the efficacy of interferon preparations administered after inoculation of Friend virus. *Proc. Soc. Exp. Biol. Med.* **126:**791.

Halpern, B. and Israel, L. (1971). Etude de l'action d'une immunostimuline associée aux Corynébactéries anaérobies dans les néoplasies expérimentales et humaines. *C.R. Acad. Sci., Paris* **273:**2186.

Halpern, B., Fray, A., Crepin, Y., Platica, O., Lorinet, A. M., Rabourdin, A., Sparros, L., and Isac, R. (1973a). *Corynebacterium parvum, a Potent Immunostimulant in Experimental Infections and in Malignancies.* Ciba Foundation Symposium, London.

Halpern, B., Fray, A., Crepin, Y., Platica, O., Sparros, L., Lorinet, A. M., and Rabourdin, A. (1973b). Action inhibitrice du *Corynebacterium parvum* sur le développement des tumeurs malignes syngéniques et son mécanisme. *C.R. Acad. Sci., Paris* **276:**1911.

Old, L. J., Benacerraf, B., Clarke, D. A., Carswell, E. A., and Stockert, E. (1961). The role of the reticuloendothelial system in the host reaction to neoplasia. *Cancer Res.* **21:**1281.

9

The Effects of
Corynebacterium parvum
Suspension
on the Response to
Tetanus Toxoid

P. A. KNIGHT and R. N. LUCKEN

Abstract

The effects of *Corynebacterium parvum* suspension on the immune response of mice to tetanus toxoid were examined using toxin challenges and passive hemagglutination. The responses measured by toxin challenge were reduced as a result of the administration of *C. parvum* under all the circumstances investigated.

The effects of *C. parvum* on the antibody response, as measured by passive hemagglutination, were more varied. When given with, or before, a single dose of toxoid, *C. parvum* caused a slight increase in the response seen at 7 days and a slight decrease in the response seen at 21 days after the administration of the toxoid.

When given with, or before, the first of two doses of toxoid, *C. parvum*

P. A. KNIGHT and R. N. LUCKEN, Department of Bacteriology, Wellcome Research Laboratories, Beckenham, Kent, England.

reduced the titer measurable 14 days after the second dose, but increased the titer if given with, or before, the second dose of toxoid. The treatment of hemagglutination assays with 2-mercaptoethanol did not materially alter the pattern of effects produced by *C. parvum*.

Introduction

Suspensions of *C. parvum* possess a wide variety of immunological and pharmacological properties. These properties include the ability to sensitize mice to histamine (Adlam *et al.*, 1973), the inhibition of tumor growth (Halpern *et al.*, 1966), the prolongation of the survival of allografts (Castro, 1973), the suppression of T cells (Scott, 1972), and the potentiation of the immune response to sheep erythrocytes (Neveu *et al.*, 1964), bacterial antigens (Gall, 1972), as well as nonspecific resistance to infection (Adlam *et al.*, 1973).

Bacterial toxoids are strong, thymus-dependent, soluble antigens that evoke a protective response that is entirely humoral. These toxoids are susceptible to the action of a wide range of adjuvants, many of which are relatively ineffective with many other antigens (Gall, 1972). *C. parvum* suspension was found by Gall to have no detectable effects upon the protective response to a small dose of diphtheria toxoid in guinea pigs.

Since the assay method employed by Gall was designed to measure only large effects, it was decided to examine the effects of *C. parvum* on mice receiving a range of doses of toxoid. Doses were chosen so that small changes in the immune response to toxoid, resulting from the treatment with *C. parvum*, could be quantitated.

Materials and Methods

C. parvum vaccine, lot CA 126, contained 0.84 mg (dry weight) of the bacteria per 0.2 ml dose and had an opacity of Brown's tube 60. The material had been shown to be active in liver and spleen weight gain, tumor repression, adjuvant activity, and histamine-sensitization assays.

Antigen

Purified tetanus toxoid (10 Lf/ml, approx. 100 I.I.U/ml) was always given subcutaneously. Both toxoid and *C. parvum* suspension was prepared at the Wellcome Research Laboratories.

Mice

Normal, outbred, Swiss albino mice, weighing 18–22 g, were obtained from Evans Corner, Carshalton, Surrey, U.K. and Oxford Laboratory Animals Centre, Bicester, Oxon, U. K.

Challenge Tests

Groups of at least 20 mice were randomly allocated between *C. parvum* treatments and toxoid doses. The animals were challenged subcutaneously with 100 LD$_{50}$ of tetanus toxin 28 days after the administration of a single dose of toxin, or 14 days after the second dose where a two-dose regime was employed.

Animals were observed for 5 days after challenge, and probit analysis was performed on the proportion of survivors to calculate the dose of toxoid required to protect 50% of the mice (the PD$_{50}$) under each *C. parvum* treatment. The effect of each *C. parvum* treatment was summarized as the interaction factor obtained by dividing the PD$_{50}$ for toxoid in the absence of *C. parvum* treatment by that obtained with the *C. parvum* treatment. Five mice were randomly selected from each treatment group and were tail bled 7 and 21 days after a single dose of toxoid or 14 days after the second of 2 doses. The resulting sera were individually titrated for tetanus antibody by passive hemagglutination in plastic hemagglutination trays, using a modification of the method of Fulthorpe (1962). The sera were adsorbed by incubation with a mixture of hydroquinone-formalized sheep erythrocytes (Fulthorpe *et al.*, 1963) and hyflosupercell to prevent nonspecific agglutination. Parallel titrations were performed on the sera in the presence of 0.01 M 2-mercaptoethanol.

Results

The effect of *C. parvum* treatment on the protective response to toxoid is shown in Table I. The proportion of mice protected by the toxoid was significantly reduced by *C. parvum* under each of the circumstances tested, but was most marked when the *C. parvum* was given intravenously 4 days before the toxoid, when it resulted in a 30-fold increase in the dose of toxoid required to protect the mice. There was no evidence of a nonspecific protection against challenge by *C. parvum* in unimmunized mice.

The hemagglutinating antibody response at 7 days was too low to measure in the majority of groups, but animals receiving 3 Lf of toxoid produced marginally higher titers when treated with *C. parvum* (Fig. 1). The effect of the *C. parvum* was most marked when it was given subcutaneously 4 days before the toxoid, when the difference from the toxoid only control was significant ($P < 0.05$). Sera obtained 21 days after the toxoid (Fig. 1) did not show any enhanced response in the *C. parvum*-treated groups, but reflected the diminished response already seen in the challenge results. Treatment of the sera with 2-mercaptoethanol failed to alter the relative titers of *C. parvum*-treated and untreated animals at either interval (Fig. 2).

When two doses of toxoid (separated by an interval of 28 days) were used to protect mice against toxin challenge, the response was reduced (Table II). The reduction was most marked and attained significance when the *C. parvum* was given intravenously 4 days before, or simultaneously with, the first dose of

Table I. Effect of *C. parvum* on the Protective Value of a Single Dose of Plain Tetanus Toxoid Given at Day 4

		Proportion of mice surviving 100 LD_{50} challenge at day 32			
			C. parvum treatment		
Toxoid dose (Lf)	Day:	0	0	4	No
	Route:	i.v.	s.c.	i.v.	*C. parvum*
3		10/19	17/20	11/19	21/21
1		5/20	12/20	17/25	19/20
0.33		5/22	8/19	5/20	19/22
0.11		1/20	8/19	2/20	8/20
none		–	–	0/20	–
PD_{50} for tetanus toxoid (Lf)		2.47	0.37	0.98	0.08
Interaction factor		0.032	0.212	0.082	1
(95% Fiducial limits)		(0.008–0.086)	(0.074–0.509)	(0.025–0.199)	

Table II. Effect of C. parvum on the Protective Value of Two Doses[a] of Plain Tetanus Toxoid

| | Proportion of mice surviving 100 LD_{50} challenge at day 46 | | | | |
| | C. parvum treatment (0.2 ml i.v.) | | | | |
Toxoid dose (Lf)	Day: 0	4	28	32	No C. parvum
0.032	0/20	2/18	5/20	11/19	9/21
0.016	3/21	2/20	2/20	0/19	4/19
0.008	0/20	0/19	1/19	0/19	0/20
PD_{50} for tetanus toxoid (Lf)	0.095	0.084	0.061	0.042	0.041
Interaction factor	0.43	0.49	0.72	0.98	1
(95% Fiducial limits)	(0.16–0.84)	(0.19–0.92)	(0.35–1.31)	(0.53–1.95)	

[a]Toxoid given subcutaneously at days 4 and 32.

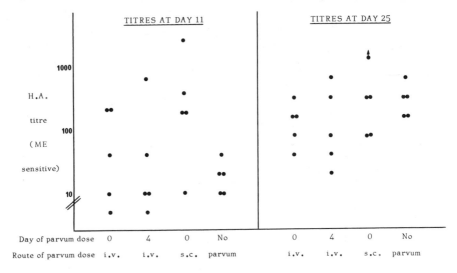

Fig. 1. Effect of *C. parvum* suspension on the hemagglutinating-antibody response to 3 Lf of tetanus toxoid given at day 4.

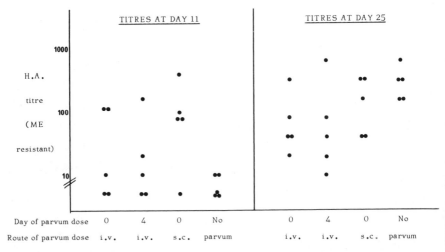

Fig. 2. Effect of *C. parvum* suspension on the hemagglutinating-antibody response to 3 Lf of tetanus toxoid given at day 4 (mercaptoethanol-resistant antibody).

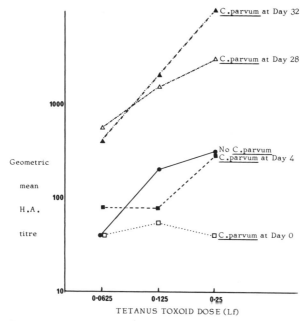

Fig. 3. Effect of *C. parvum* suspension on the titer of antibody elicited by 2 doses of tetanus toxoid at days 4 and 32.

toxoid. The effect was smaller and nonsignificant when the *C. parvum* dose was associated with the second dose of toxoid.

In a parallel experiment in which slightly larger doses of toxoid were used and the animals were bled instead of challenged, the administration of *C. parvum* 4 days before the first dose of toxoid significantly depressed the hemagglutinating-antibody response in parallel with the results seen in the challenge experiment (Fig. 3). *C. parvum* given simultaneously with the first dose produced a marginal, nonsignificant depression, but when given before—or at the same time—as the second dose of toxoid, it produced a large increase in response which was highly significant. The data presented in Fig. 4 show that the increase in antibody was mercaptoethanol-resistant and that the large increase of apparent immunogenity of the toxoid (interaction factors of 7.2 for *C. parvum* given 4 days before the second dose of toxoid and 11.4 when given at the same time) were therefore IgG, despite the negative response measured by challenge.

Discussion

It is clear from the above results that *C. parvum* depresses, rather than potentiates, the antitoxic response to tetanus toxoid and that hemagglutinating-antibody levels are similarly affected when the interval between the *C. parvum*

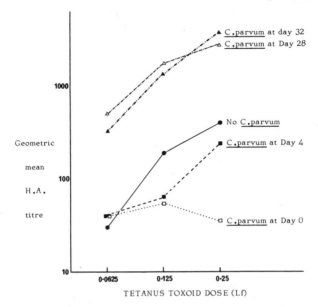

Fig. 4. Effect of *C. parvum* suspension on the titer of mercaptoethanol-resistant antibody elicited by 2 doses of tetanus toxoid at days 4 and 32.

treatment and bleeding or challenge is a long one. At the same time, *C. parvum* given to previously immunized animals with a second dose of toxoid causes an increase in the mercaptoethanol-resistant antibody response to the toxoid, in contrast to the antitoxic response measured at the same time. Mercaptoethanol-resistant hemagglutinating antibody and protection are generally closely correlated in antitetanus sera, although instances of failure to correlate have been reported (Sheffield and Perkins, 1967).

The failure of hemagglutinating antibody to protect might be attributable to one of three causes: (1) the *C. parvum* treatment might result in an increased susceptibility of the mice to tetanus toxin; (2) the increased response may have been confined to a nonantitoxic subclass of IgG; or (3) it may have been directed to a part of the toxoid molecule that was not associated with protection or to an accessory antigen.

Another peculiarity of the effect of *C. parvum* on toxoid is the apparent adjuvant effect associated with the second dose of toxoid, but not with the first. The effects of a very wide range of adjuvants have been examined with tetanus toxoid, none of which have exerted more than a minimal effect when given with the second dose of toxoid.

The total effect of *C. parvum* on the response to tetanus toxoid represents a balance between depression of long-term responses and the depression of basal immunity, possibly due to T-cell suppression and increased short-term hemagglutinating antibody responses, particularly in animals with pre-existing basal immunity.

Acknowledgments

The authors wish to acknowledge the excellent technical assistance of Mrs. V. Sullivan.

References

Adlam, C., Broughton, E. S., and Scott, M. T. (1973). Enhanced resistance of mice following pretreatment with *Corynebacterium parvum*. *Nat. New Biol.* **235**:219.

Castro, J. E. (1973). *Symposium on Immunopotentiation,* p. 116, Ciba Symposium Series 19.

Fulthorpe, A. J. (1962). Multiple diphtheria antigen–antibody systems investigated by passive-hemagglutination techniques and other methods. *Immunology* **5**:30–45.

Fulthorpe, A. J., Parke, J. A. C., Tovey, J. E., and Monkton, J. C. (1963). Pregnancy diagnosis by a one-stage passive-hemagglutination method. *Br. Med. J.* 1049–1054.

Gall, D. (1972). Adjuvants and different immune systems. *Report and Proceedings of Alhydrogel Symposium on Vaccine Adjuvants, London, 1971.* Superfos, Copenhagen.

Halpern, B. N., Biozzi, G., Stiffel, C., and Mouton, D. (1966). Inhibition of tumor growth by administration of killed *Corynebacterium parvum*. *Nature (Lond.)* **212**:853.

Neveu, T., Bronellec, A., and Biozzi, G. (1964). Propriétés adjuvantes de *Corynebacterium parvum* sur la production d'anticorps et sur l'induction de l'hypersensibilité retardee envers les protéines conjugées. *Ann. Inst. Pasteur, Paris* **106**:771–777.

Scott, M. T. (1972). Biological effects of the adjuvant *Corynebacterium parvum*. I. Inhibition of PHA, mixed lymphocyte, and G.V.H. reactivity. *Cell Immunol.* **5**:459–468.

Sheffield, F. and Perkins, F. T. (1967). The response of guinea pigs to the diphtheria toxoid component of combined antigens of different formulations. Int. Symp. Combined Vaccines Marburg/L Symp. Ser. *Immunobiol. Standard* **7**:121. Karger, Basel.

DISCUSSION

DAVIES: When corynebacteria were injected twice, was there a far better effect on the second occasion, in relation, for example, to the capacity to clear *Salmonella?*

FAUVE: Whole cells or extract?

DAVIES: Whole cells would do.

FAUVE: I only used one injection with whole cells.

DAVIES: How can you be absolutely sure that an alteration in the distribution of the organisms did not occur? The curves show clearly that there is an alteration in the number of the organisms present—which is assumed to be a bactericidal effect. How is it possible to be sure that under abnormal circumstances, the distribution of *Listeria* is exactly the same as under normal circumstances?

FAUVE: We can be sure that we did not have an alteration in the distribution of the bacteria following EBP treatment since in a comparative study, we made bacterial cultures on all organ homogenates and on whole blood.

DAVIES: The result in the nude-mouse experiments is interesting. It is said—perhaps correctly—that when nude mice are injected with certain compounds, there is some demonstration of T-cell function. I am not sure whether this is absolutely true; if so, this would somewhat flaw Dr. Fauve's argument that there was no T-cell function in the activation of the macrophages because nude mice were used.

FAUVE: I agree with Dr. Davies, that in some conditions there is some demonstration of T-cell function in nude mice. Nevertheless, antitheta serum does not inhibit the mitogenic effect of EBP, and irradiation still allows the protection against *L. monocytogenes.*

MC BRIDE: Does Dr. Fauve's *C. parvum* extract induce splenomegaly in normal mice and nude mice?

FAUVE: That is an interesting question. I forgot to mention that we have been unable so far to find any splenomegaly—any hepatomegaly—or any thymus aplasia, nor did EBP treatment increase the sensitivity of mice to endotoxin. This led me to conclude that this phospholipid—which has some interesting aspects—is certainly not responsible for the many known effects of *C. parvum*.

PARAF: Is the phospholipid active on cells in culture?

FAUVE: On peritoneal macrophage it is almost inactive, but I have insufficient data to give any statistics.

We have now isolated the active phospholipid which is responsible for most of the activities. This was not mentioned earlier because the phospholipid was not isolated from *C. parvum*. To our great surprise, it was active on spleen macrophage, but apparently not on peritoneal macrophage. There are still some technical points to be solved, so I cannot say categorically that it is not active on the latter, but we are sure that it acts on spleen macrophage *in vitro*.

WHITE: How was the bacteria extracted to obtain the phospholipid?

FAUVE: By the well-known method of Folch [(1957). *J. Biol. Chem.* **226**:497–509].

ADLAM: Have any other phospholipids been tried, for example, nonbacterial phospholipids such as lecithin? Do these nonbacterial phospholipids have any effect on the clearance of the organisms?

FAUVE: As I said previously, this active extract was obtained from other bacteria. Among some known phospholipids, lecithin—for instance—is not active on either the clearance or the bacterial effect of macrophages against *L. monocytogenes*.

WERNER: I was asking Dr. Cerutti about two matters: First, the timing of treatment before the infection. She replied that the first injection was given seven days and the second, two days, before EMC virus infection.

My second question was whether the activity of the supernatant from the stimulated macrophages (or the peritoneal fluid from the treated mice) was also seen when it was tested against VSV virus on cells not of mouse origin. Dr. Cerutti answered that, so far, she has exclusively tested that activity on L cells and mouse embryo cells. The active factor is distinguished from interferon by the fact that it is thermostable and not sensitive to actinomycin inhibition.

CHANY: The virus employed in these experiments is the encephalomyocarditis virus. One tissue-culture infectious unit of this strain kills the animal. Thus, the results observed here are remarkable because of the difficulty—even with large quantities of interferon—the mice had in obtaining protection against this virus. It is likely that the inhibitor detected in the peritoneal exudate does not oppose the integrity of cellular protein synthesis. The mechanism of the antiviral effect obtained here is apparently unknown.

BOMFORD: Has Dr. Cerutti tested the peritoneal factor for antiviral activity by putting it on peritoneal macrophages? I wonder whether it is a substance which would activate macrophages rather than have any interferon activity?

CERUTTI: I have not tested this extract on macrophages. I was mainly interested in interferon activity, and other biological aspects were somewhat neglected.

CHERMAN: Did you study the effect of *C. parvum* on other viruses?

CERUTTI: In animals experiments we used only EMC virus because, as Professor Chany said, this virus is very pathogenic for the mice and the mortality rate is high. This motivated the selection of EMC for the present experiments. In L-cell culture, however, VSV was assayed along with EMC virus. The replication of both viruses was strongly impaired by the peritoneal exudate.

CHERMAN: Have you tried to inject the peritoneal exudate *in vivo* after the EMC virus inoculation as prophylactic treatment?

CERUTTI: I have not made this type of assays, since originally we thought that *C. parvum* could act through the interferon mechanism.

WHITE: Is there any evidence that the *C. parvum*-treated animal catabolizes the toxoid? In other words, does the half-life of the toxoid decrease in the *C. parvum*-treated mice?

KNIGHT: We have, at present, no data on the effect of *C. parvum* on the response to toxoid given by the intravenous route.

HALPERN: Does Dr. Knight know anything about the fate of the toxoid injected intravenously, or by another route: how long it persists in the blood and whether it is picked up by some of the reticuloendothelial cells? What happens to this substance in the organism when injected by means of a rapidly absorbing route?

KNIGHT: In these experiments, the toxoid was always given subcutaneously. When it is given as a fluid, as this was, we do not think that it persists recognizably for very long; of course, we were giving extremely small doses. It may be a different matter intravenously. Our impression is that there is a considerable difference between what happens to a toxoid which is administered intravenously and one which is injected subcutaneously. We have no data, at present, on the intravenous route.

WHISNANT: Can Dr. Knight shed some light on pertussis vaccine as an adjuvant.

I believe that it is peculiar in its effect on secondary versus primary immunization? There are other similarities between *C. parvum* and pertussis.

KNIGHT: But of course, that would not necessarily conflict with the situation that we have seen with *C. parvum,* where the increase is confined to the hemagglutinating-antibody response. There is no evidence of any increase in the protective response.

HALPERN: If I remember correctly, Dr. Adlam has published a paper in which he showed that *C. parvum* protects mice against a considerable dose of pertussis bacteria.

KNIGHT: I do not think that there is any evidence of a reflection in tetanus of the protective effects which we see in pertussis. This antitoxic immunity goes on without the help of any cellular systems.

WILKINSON: This sounds like an unusual adjuvant effect in which the adjuvant acts after the antigen has been recognized and responded to, in other words, on the second dose. Does Dr. Knight know whether the time at which a second dose is given is important? Must it be a short time after the primary response, or can it be left for a long time and still have the same effect?

KNIGHT: All of our two-dose experiments involved a 28-day interval between the first and second dose of toxoid, and we would regard this as a moderately long interval. We have no experience with longer or shorter intervals.

Part IV
Action of
Corynebacterium on the
Immune Cell System

10

In Vivo Effects of Lymphocytes Sensitized *in Vitro* against Tumor Cells

A. J. TREVES, I. R. COHEN, and M. FELDMAN

Experiments are reported on immunotherapy of lethal lung metastasis by lymphocytes sensitized *in culture* against a syngenic tumor. We used the Lewis lung carcinoma (3LL) which had originated in a $C_{57}Bl$ mouse. $C_{57}Bl$ mice were footpad inoculated with tumor cells. Seven days later, the tumor-bearing leg was amputated, and the animals were inoculated with syngenic lymphocytes which had been sensitized on monolayers of 3LL-tumor cells. The sensitized lymphocytes significantly reduced the development of lethal lung metastasis of the 3LL-tumor cells.

Tumor-specific antigens (TSA) have been demonstrated in almost all tumors in which they have been carefully sought (Klein, 1971). However, the immunogenicity of TSA was generally found to be significantly lower than that of other cell-surface immunogens, such as the H-2 antigens in mice or the HLA in man. Hence, by ordinary procedures of immunization against autologous or syngenic tumors, only a low level of immune resistance to tumor growth was achieved. Furthermore, syngenic immunization with tumor cells evokes both antibody production and cell-mediated immunity (CMI). It is the latter response which seems to be responsible for host resistance to tumor progression. Antibodies, on

A. J. TREVES, I. R. COHEN, and M. FELDMAN, Department of Cell Biology, The Weizmann Institute of Science, Rehovot, Israel.

the other hand, may exert a blocking effect on host resistance, i.e., an enhancing effect on tumor growth. It seemed, therefore, that if cell-mediated immunity was evoked by tumor cells in the absence of antibodies, this should result in a more effective host resistance to tumor progression.

In our laboratory, we developed a system for the *in vitro* induction of cell-mediated immunity (Feldman *et al.*, 1972). Lymphocytes cultured on xenogenic or allogenic fibroblasts became sensitized against the cell-surface antigens of the fibroblasts and manifested the capacity to lyse specific target cells syngenic to the sensitizing fibroblasts. No antibody production by the sensitized lymphocytes could be detected, and, in fact, lymphocytes sensitized in culture did not manifest any measurable intracellular synthesis of immunoglobulins. Lymphocytes could thus be made to undergo sensitization in culture and manifest an immune response which was of a "pure" cell-mediated type. Furthermore, lymphocytes sensitized in culture inflicted an extent of cell-mediated lysis significantly greater than the lytic effect produced by equal populations of lymphocytes sensitized *in vivo* (Berke *et al.*, 1971). Lymphocytes allosensitized in culture, when inoculated into mice syngenic with the lymphocytes, conferred on the recipients a state of adoptive immunity manifested by the prevention of growth of tumors from an H-2 phenotype identical to the fibroblasts against which the lymphocytes were sensitized (Cohen *et al.*, 1971a). This *in vitro* system of sensitization was found to have two additional properties: It could respond to relatively weak immunogens which *in vivo* were incapable of evoking an immune response (Berke *et al.*, 1971), and it could be used for inducing autosensitization (Cohen *et al.*, 1971b; Cohen and Wekerle, 1973). In the latter case, lymphocytes could recognize *in vitro* and react against autologous cell-surface antigens. This recognition, however, was prevented if the lymphocytes were pre-incubated with autologous serum. Lymphocytes autosensitized *in vitro* and then inoculated into syngenic recipients elicited an autoimmune reaction (Cohen *et al.*, 1971b; Orgad and Cohen, 1974). Hence, lymphocytes are prevented from reacting against autologous antigens due to the blocking effect of some specific serum factors (possibly soluble antigens, which under normal conditions are shed off cells); yet, once sensitized *in vitro*, they are no longer blockable by such factors.

It therefore seemed to us that such an *in vitro* system which (1) permits the induction of a CMI in the absence of antibody, (2) elicits a reaction which is more intense than the parallel reaction induced *in vivo*, and (3) can react against self-antigens could be applied in experiments aimed at sensitization against tumor-specific antigens.

We, therefore, sensitized lymphocytes against a syngenic tumor with the aim of testing the effect of such lymphocytes on the prevention of tumor growth *in vivo*. Since the problem of human cancer is in the prevention of metastasis following surgical or radiotherapeutic removal of the primary tumor, we chose a mouse tumor which, unlike most mouse tumors, produces a high incidence of

Table I. The Effect of *in Vitro*-Sensitized Lymphocytes on Tumor Metastases

Experiment No.	Number of lymphocytes injected ($\times 10^6$)	Percentage of surviving mice treated with lymphocytes			
		Anti-3LL	Antifibroblasts	Unsensitized	None
1	14	82 (14/17)	—	35 (6/17)	53 (9/17)
2	4	50 (7/14)	17 (2/14)	14 (2/14)	—
3	8	100 (4/4)	—	—	20 (1/5)
4	17	67 (8/12)	46 (6/13)	46 (6/13)	40 (4/10)
5	8.5	85 (11/13)	—	—	56 (9/16)
6	9	58 (7/12)	—	—	33 (4/12)
7[a]	14	50 (8/16)	—	—	33 (6/18)
8[a]	14	67 (4/6)	50 (5/10)	—	36 (4/11)
Total survival		67 (63/94)[b]	35 (13/37)	32 (14/44)	42 (37/89)

[a] Lymphocytes were obtained from mice bearing 3LL tumors.
[b] $P < 0.0025$ compared to each of the control groups (χ^2 test).

lung metastases following intramuscular or subcutaneous grafting. We used the Lewis lung carcinoma (3LL) which originated in a $C_{57}Bl$ mouse. 10^6 3LL cells were injected into the right, hind footpad. Six or 7 days later, a local tumor growth was observed, and the leg was amputated. Two days following surgery, the mice were injected intravenously with 10^6 spleen cells which had been sensitized in culture against monolayers of irradiated 3LL tumor cells. Control mice were injected after surgery with unsensitized lymphocytes or with lymphocytes sensitized against syngenic or foreign fibroblasts. Prevention of lethal lung metastases and survival served as an assay for immunotherapy. The results of eight independent experiments are summarized in Table I. In each experiment, mice injected with lymphocytes sensitized *in vitro* against 3LL cells were protected against the development of lung metastasis in comparison with mice injected with unsensitized lymphocytes or with lymphocytes sensitized against rat or mouse fibroblasts and with uninjected mice ($P < 0.01$). Protection was achieved with sensitized lymphocytes obtained either from normal or from tumor-bearing animals. Thus, lymphocytes sensitized *in vitro* against tumor cells were effective in mediating immunotherapy against the progression of lethal tumor metastasis.

The significance of the results suggests a new approach toward tumor immunotherapy, based on the *in vitro* sensitization of lymphocytes against tumor cells and followed by the inoculation of the lymphocytes into the tumor-bearing organism. However, these results invite further studies in which immunopotentiators should be tested both *in vitro* and *in vivo*. The system of sensitization in cell culture used in this immunotherapeutic model was found in previous studies to involve the sensitization of T lymphocytes (Altman *et al.*, 1973). Yet, this seemed to be dependent on the participation of macrophages (Lonai and Feldman, 1971). Hence, the *in vitro* application of either adjuvants which act directly on T cells or adjuvants which activate macrophages might augment the antitumor effect. Furthermore, although the specific *in vitro* sensitization seems to be based on T lymphocytes, the effect of lymphocytes which kill or prevent the growth of tumor cells *in vivo* need not be the progeny of the *in vitro*-sensitized cells. Thus, lymphocytes sensitized in culture were shown to recruit other T lymphocytes to act as specific effector lymphocytes (Treves and Cohen; 1973). These *in vitro*-sensitized lymphocytes may confer on macrophages cytotoxic or cytostatic properties (Evans *et al.*, 1972). The *in vivo* development of effectors in response to signals of lymphocytes sensitized *in vitro* might be affected by immunopotentiators applied to the recipient organism.

References

Altman, A., Cohen, I. R., and Feldman, M. (1973). Normal T-cell receptors for alloantigens. *Cell. Immunol.* 7:134.

Berke, G., Clark, W. R., and Feldman, M. (1971). *In vitro* induction of a heterograft reaction. Immunological parameters of the sensitization of rat lymphocytes against mouse cells *in vitro*. *Transplantation* 12:237.

Cohen, I. R. and Wekerle, H. (1973). Regulation of autosensitization: the immune activation and specific inhibition of self-recognizing thymus-derived lymphocytes. *J. Exp. Med.* 137:224.

Cohen, I. R., Globerson, A., and Feldman, M. (1971a). Rejection of tumor allografts by mouse spleen sensitized *in vitro*. *J. Exp. Med.* 133:821.

Cohen, I. R., Globerson, A., and Feldman, M. (1971b). Autosensitization *in vitro*. *J. Exp. Med.* 133:834.

Evans, R., Grant, C. K., Cox, H., Steele, K., and Alexander, P. (1972). Thymus-derived lymphocytes produce an immunologically specific macrophage-arming factor. *J. Exp. Med.* 136:1318.

Feldman, M., Cohen, I. R., and Wekerle, H. (1972). T-cell mediated immunity *in vitro:* an analysis of antigen recognition and target-cell lysis. *Transplant. Rev.* 12:57.

Klein, G. (1971). Immunological studies in a human tumor. *Isr. J. Med. Sci.* 7:111.

Lonai, P. and Feldman, M. (1971). Studies on the effect of macrophages in an *in vitro* graft-reactions system. *Immunology* 21:861.

Orgad, S. and Cohen, I. R. (1974). Autoimmune encephalomyelitis: Activation of thymus lymphocytes against syngeneic brain antigens *in vitro*. *Science* 183:1083.

Treves, A. J. and Cohen, I. R. (1973). Recruitment of effector T lymphocytes against a tumor allograft by T lymphocytes sensitized *in vitro*. *J. Natl. Cancer Inst.* 51:1919.

11

The Action of Local Injections of *Corynebacterium parvum* in Facilitating the Extravasation of Activated Lymphoid Cells

J. G. HALL and A. R. MOORE

Abstract

Lymph-borne immunoblasts were obtained by collecting thoracic duct lymph from rats stimulated antigenically with *Corynebacterium parvum,* BCG and *Brucella abortus.* The immunoblasts were labeled by *in vitro* incubation with [^{125}I]-UDR. After being washed, they were injected intravenously into syngenic rats. These recipients had received intradermal injections of various antigens a few days previous to immunoblast injection. The entry of the labeled immunoblasts into these intradermal injection sites was monitored by counting the radioactivity that accumulated in the sites 24 h after injection.

It was found that only the cutaneous sites of injection of BCG or *C. parvum* attracted significant numbers of immunoblasts and that the immunological specificity of the injected cells played no demonstrable role in guiding them to their destination. It was concluded that local injections of *C. parvum* or BCG

J. G. HALL, Institute for Cancer Research, Royal Marsden Hospital, Chester Beatty Research Center, Clifton Avenue, Belmont, Sutton, Surrey, U.K. and A. R. MOORE, Division of Tumour Immunology, Chester Beatty Research Institute, Institute of Cancer Research, Royal Cancer Hospital, Downs Road, Sutton, Surrey, U.K.

bring about a change in the local capillaries that causes lymphoid cells to extravasate in increased numbers.

Introduction

It is generally accepted that the immunological rejection of antigenic tumors is effected to a large extent by the complex mechanisms of cell-mediated immunity. In the case of solid tumors or allografts, the rejection process is usually heralded by a local infiltrate of mononuclear cells which have extravasated from the blood. Unfortunately, the total destruction of established, syngenic tumors by immunological processes is a rare event. One of the paradoxes of experimental tumor immunology is that in tumor-bearing animals, it is often possible to demonstrate an abundance of cytotoxic lymphocytes and/or macrophages in the spleen, the lymph nodes, and the blood, and yet the tumor continues to grow until it kills its host. Cytotoxic cells can only kill tumor cells by first making contact with them, and, clearly, the only cytotoxic cells that can do this are those which extravasate from the blood and enter the tumor tissue. In an immediate sense, cytotoxic cells which are confined to the lymphoid organs are redundant. It seems proper, therefore, to concentrate our attention on freely circulating lymphoid cells and to try and find out what makes them leave the blood vessels and attack their target tissue, be it tumor or allograft.

The simple view that a specifically sensitized lymphoid cell is automatically endowed with the ability to "home," like a guided missile, onto its target has not been borne out by *in vivo* experiments (Najarian and Feldman, 1962; Billingham *et al.*, 1962; Prendergast, 1964; Hall, 1967; Moore and Hall, 1973), although, occasionally, more optimistic results have been claimed (Lance and Cooper, 1972). However, it is generally true to say that when specifically sensitized, syngenic lymphocytes are injected intravenously into animals bearing a tumor or an allograft, only a very small percentage of the injected cells actually succeed in penetrating to the target. The numbers that do penetrate are too small by several orders of magnitude to achieve the ratios of killer cells to target cells needed for the usual *in vitro* cytotoxic assays.

It is against this background that we sought to find a means of encouraging lymphoid cells to leave the blood vessels at sites where they may be needed. For practical reasons, we restricted our attention to one class of lymphoid cell, the lymph-borne immunoblast (Hall, 1971). These cells may be collected in the thoracic duct lymph of rats after antigenic stimulation of the caudal somatic lymph nodes (Delorme *et al.*, 1969). They take up precursors of DNA with avidity and can thus be easily labeled with $[^{125}I]$iodo deoxyuridine. Their normal distribution pattern after intravenous injection into syngenic recipients has been thoroughly established (Hall *et al.*, 1972; Halstead and Hall, 1972) and can be easily monitored by counting the γ-emission from small pieces of recipient tissue. It is not our purpose here to suggest that such cells are necessarily implicated in tumor rejection, although there is considerable support for such a view (Alexander and Hall, 1970). We are merely using them as a model system, because we know a good deal about them. It has already been established that the immunological specificity of immunoblasts plays little, if any, role in guiding them to their destination and that a special property of the capillary wall must mediate their extravasation (Moore and Hall, 1972; 1973). The specific question we set out to answer is whether or not this property can be induced in capillaries by local injections of bacterial products, etc., i.e., can practical therapeutic means be used to encourage immunoblasts to extravasate.

Experimental Procedures

Adult, male, hooded rats, weighing about 200 g, were taken from our own barrier-maintained colony as required.

Donor rats received 8 s.c. injections of antigen (usually either *Corynebacterium parvum* or *Brucella abortus*) in the hindquarter region to stimulate the caudal, somatic lymph nodes. Four days later, their thoracic ducts were cannulated, and the lymph was collected for 60 h in consecutive 8–12 h periods. The washed lymph cells were incubated for 1 h *in vitro* in TC 199 containing $[^{125}I]$-UDR at a concentration of 0.5 μCi/ml. After being washed, the cells were intravenously injected into syngenic recipient rats at a dose of $1-5 \times 10^7$ total cells, of which about 10% were labeled immunoblasts, containing about 10^5 cpm of cell-bound radioactivity. Usually, each recipient had two rows of 4 skin lesions, approximately 5 mm in diameter, along its ventral abdominal wall on either side of the midline. The lesions had been prepared 3–4 days previously by intradermally injecting suspensions of antigens or turpentine or by applying dinitrochlorobenzene in acetone, or a heated copper spatula, to the skin. Control sites were prepared by an i.d. injection of normal saline. The recipients were killed 15 h after receiving the injections of labeled cells. Circular pieces of shorn skin, with a radius of 5 mm from the center of each lesion, were excised, rinsed in saline, fixed in 10% formalin–saline for 1 h, blotted dry, and weighed. The γ-emission from each specimen was counted in a Packard 3002 scintillation spectrometer. The results were corrected for background noise and expressed as cpm per gram. Samples with counting rates less than two standard deviations above the means of replicate blanks were scored as having no activity.

The *C. parvum* used in this study was a killed suspension prepared by the Wellcome Laboratories (batch EZ 174). The BCG (Glaxo) was a standard, dried vaccine containing viable organisms. Precise experimental details have been published elsewhere (Moore and Hall, 1973).

Results

In this study, 100 donor rats and a similar number of recipient rats were used and 400 skin lesions were examined, only some of which are recorded here. The salient findings are presented in Table I.

Table I. The Specific Radioactivities of Various Skin Lesions in the Abdominal Wall of Rats 15 h After Receiving an i.v. Injection of Syngenic Thoracic Duct Lymph Cells Labeled with [^{125}I]-UDR *in Vitro*

Number and type of lesion	Mean specific activity, cpm/g[a]
60 Control, saline injection sites	50 (10–120)
30 *Corynebacterium parvum* injection sites	330 (150–640)
10 BCG injection sites	320 (200–580)
14 *Brucella abortus* injection sites	150 (10–300)
5 *Bordetella pertussis* injection sites	120 (50–250)
17 SRBC injection sites	100 (20–220)
5 Primary DNCB application sites	30 (20–40)
5 Secondary DNCB application sites	40 (30–50)
11 Turpentine injection sites	75 (50–150)
6 Thermal injury sites	50 (20–100)

[a]Minimum and maximum values are shown in parentheses.

It can be seen that the only lesions that contained substantial levels of radioactivity that did not overlap the control valves were the sites of injection of *C. parvum* or BCG. It was concluded that of the materials tested, only these two organisms were undeniably able to facilitate the extravasation of immunoblasts. The effects of injecting *Bordetella pertussis, B. abortus,* or SRBC were significant, but bearing in mind the variance of the controls, they must be regarded as marginal.

It must be noted that even the *C. parvum* and BCG lesions never contained more than 1% of the injected dose of radioactivity, as in previous studies (Hall *et al.,* 1972). The bulk of the injected activity could be found in the lamina propria of the small gut.

Discussion

It is clear that the skin lesions which resulted from injections of *C. parvum* or BCG had an attraction for immunoblasts, but the mechanism involved is unknown, except in so far as immunologically specific factors are unlikely to be involved (Moore and Hall, 1973). Nonetheless, some special conditions are necessary if immunoblasts are to extravasate locally. The results showed that immunoblasts did not participate indiscriminately in all cellular exudates. For example, they were conspicuously absent from the sites of acute inflammation caused by turpentine injections, thermal injury, or the primary application of DNCB—even though these lesions were the sites of grossly increased capillary permeability that could be demonstrated by the extravasation of Evans blue. In this they differ from certain types of small lymphocytes that can participate in acute reactions (Koster and McGregor, 1970). Similarly, the immunoblasts did not enter the sites of DTH reactions, such as those that result from applying a small challenging dose of DNCB to previously sensitized animals, even though these sites were detectably indurated. This finding has been confirmed by an autoradiographic study of DTH lesions in the skin of sheep which, so far, has not yielded evidence of a particularly marked extravasation of immunoblasts (Hall, unpublished observations). Apparently factors related to the particular properties of *C. parvum* and BCG are more important than particular properties of various types of immune reactions. Both *C. parvum* and BCG are known to be stimulants of the RES and have both been successfully used as conventional adjuvants and in the "nonspecific immunotherapy" of tumors. Indeed, this is the basis for this meeting. It is tempting to believe that these properties are not unrelated to the phenomenon of immunoblast extravasation. One may speculate that the activation of macrophages caused by these organisms and the events of granuloma formation may release factors which interact with the local capillaries, causing them to permit the extravasation of immunoblasts. This may be a further factor in the regression of experimental tumors that can follow the intralesional injection of this class of organism (Bartlett *et al.*, 1972).

References

Alexander, P. and Hall, J. G. (1970). The role of immunoblasts in host resistance and immunotherapy of primary sarcomata. *Adv. Cancer Res.* **13**:1.

Bartlett, G. L., Zbar, B., and Rapp, H. J. (1972). Suppression of murine tumor growth by immune reaction to BCG strain of *Mycobacterium bovis. J. Natl. Cancer Inst.* **48**:245.

Billingham, R. E., Silvers, W. K., and Wilson, D. B. (1962). The adoptive transfer of transplantation immunity by means of blood-borne cells. *Lancet* **1**:512.

Delorme, E. J., Hodgett, J., Hall, J. G., and Alexander, P. (1969). The significance of large basophilic cells in lymph following antigenic challenge. *Proc. Roy. Soc. B.* **174**:229.

Hall, J. G. (1967). Studies of cells in the afferent and efferent lymph of nodes draining the sites of skin homografts. *J. Exp. Med.* **125**:737.

Hall, J. G. (1971). The lymph-borne cells of the immune response: A review. *The Scientific Basis of Medicine*, p. 39, University of London, The Athlone Press,

Hall, J. G., Parry, D. M., and Smith, M. E. (1972). The distribution and differentiation of lymph-borne immunoblasts after intravenous injection into syngenic recipients. *Cell Tissue Kinet.* **5**:269.

Halstead, T. and Hall, J. G. (1972). The homing of lymph-borne immunoblasts to the small gut of neonatal rats. *Transplantation* **14**:339.

Koster, F. and McGregor, D. D. (1970). Rat thoracic duct lymphocytes: types that participate in inflammation. *Science* **167**:1137.

Lance, E. M. and Cooper, S. (1972). Homing of specifically sensitized lymphocytes to allografts of skin. *Cell. Immunol.* **5**:66.

Moore, A. R. and Hall, J. G. (1972). Evidence for a primary association between immunoblasts and the small gut. *Nature (Lond.)* **239**:161.

Moore, A. R. and Hall, J. G. (1973). Nonspecific entry of thoracic duct immunoblasts into intradermal foci of antigens. *Cell. Immunol.* **8**:112.

Najarian, J. S. and Feldman, J. D. (1962). Passive transfer of transplantation immunity. *J. Exp. Med.* **115**:1083.

Prendergast, R. A. (1964). Cellular specificity in the homograft reaction. *J. Exp. Med.* **119**:377.

12

Kinetics of Proliferation of Bone-Marrow Cell Lines after Injections of Immunostimulant Bacteria

L. TOUJAS, L. DAZORD, and J. GUELFI

Abstract

The splenomegaly which was induced by the inoculation of *Corynebacterium granulosum* or *Brucella abortus* into irradiated and cell-reconstituted mice was found to be dependent on the presence of bone-marrow cells. The kinetics of proliferation in the spleen of the bone-marrow-derived cell lines was studied in normal mice. The curve of the number of splenic stem cells looked biphasic: a drop was measured at 24 h after bacterial injection, followed by an increase first measured at 48 h after injection. Certain blastic precursor cells (erythroblasts, megakaryocytes) were elevated from day 5. The peak value of the total cell count was reached on day 10. In contrast, the lymphocyte precursors in the spleen—as evaluated by the count of spontaneous rosette-forming cells—were never enhanced.

Introduction

The intravenous injection into the mouse of 500 µg of inactivated *Corynebacterium parvum* (Prévot *et al.*, 1963), *Corynebacterium granulosum* (Toujas *et*

L. TOUJAS, L. DAZORD, and J. GUELFI, Laboratoire de Recherche du Centre Regional de Lutte contre le Cancer, Pontchaillou, Rennes, France.

al., 1973b), or even inactivated *Brucella abortus* (Toujas *et al.*, 1972b) produces an important hepatosplenic hyperplasia, reaching a maximum in about ten days. At this time, the liver weight will have doubled and the spleen weight will have increased by six or seven times.

Similar injections of Corynebacteria (Amiel *et al.*, 1969; Toujas *et al.*, 1973b) or, under certain conditions, of *Brucella* (Toujas *et al.*, 1973a) enhance the immune response against sheep red blood cells (SRBC). The number of spleen cells synthesizing hemolytic antibodies is increased, and this immuno-stimulation reaches its maximum efficiency when SRBC are given about 5 days after the bacteria.

The question arises whether a particular event taking place on the fifth day of spleen-cell proliferation can explain the elevation of immune response. In the present work we show (1) that cells developing in the spleen are of bone-marrow origin, (2) that on the fifth day, there is an increase in the spleen of certain precursors of mature cells (erythrocyte or platelet precursors), and (3) that this process does not apply to precursors of immunocompetent cells which recognize the antigen, since the number of spontaneous rosette-forming cells tends to decrease after injection of the immunostimulant.

Materials and Methods

Mice

Female (C_{57}Bl/6 × DBA2) F_1 hybrids or female CBA, AKR, C_3H were purchased from CNRS Orléans.

Bacteria

C. granulosum and *B. abortus* were kindly supplied by Prof. Raynaud and Prof. Pilet, respectively. Heat-inactivated bacterial suspensions were injected intravenously at a rate of 500 μg (dry weight) per mouse.

Irradiation–Cell-Reconstitution Experiments

Mice were irradiated as previously described (Toujas *et al.*, 1972a) and then reconstituted by 3 × 10^6–5 × 10^6 bone-marrow cells and/or an equal number of thymus cells. The experiments shown in Table I were carried out with hybrid mice, those of Table II and Fig. 1 with CBA mice reconstituted by bone-marrow cells from previously thymectomized, irradiated, and reconstituted isologous mice.

Evaluation of Immune Responses

The direct technique of plaque-forming cells (PFC) of Jerne and Nordin (1963) was used as before (Toujas *et al.*, 1972b). Anti-*Brucella* agglutinins were titrated by Wright's method.

Table I. Spleen Weight (mg) of Mice Lethally Irradiated and Reconstituted on Day 0 by Bone-Marrow and/or Thymus Cells[a]

| | Cell reconstitution | | | |
	None	5×10^6 thymus cells	5×10^6 bone-marrow cells	5×10^6 thymus and 5×10^6 bone-marrow cells
Saline	34.85 ± 6.57	41.6 ± 7.07	84.25 ± 8.89	107 ± 20.85
C. granulosum (500 μg i.v.)	—	—	373 ± 84	352 ± 44
B. abortus (500 μg i.v.)	52.28 ± 13.7	39.33 ± 8.35	355.8 ± 21.32	439 ± 91.5

[a]C. granulosum or B. abortus was injected on day 2; spleens were removed and weighed on day 12.

Table II. Number of PFC per Spleen Four Days after Intravenous Injection of 250 × 10⁶ SRBC[a]

	T+B	B
Controls	33,750 (6875–106,250)	1625 (0–6250)
B. abortus (500 μg i.v., 5 days before SRBC)	24,350 (21,875–27,500)	4375 (1250–10,625)

[a]Six-week-old mice were thymectomized (B) or not thymectomized (T+B), irradiated, bone-marrow-reconstituted, and introduced to the experiment after 30 days (4 mice per group).

Colony-Forming Units (CFU)

Till and McCulloch's (1961) technique was used as before (Toujas *et al.*, 1972a). Briefly, this consists of injecting given fractions of bone marrow or spleen from mice of a given experiment into other lethally irradiated mice. The CFU on the spleen of irradiated mice were counted after 8–10 days.

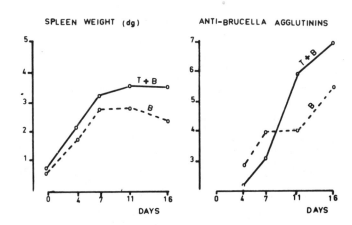

Fig. 1. Spleen weight and anti-agglutinin response in mice thymectomized (B) or not (T + B) on day 0, irradiated and bone marrow reconstituted after 7 days, and put into the experiment after 30 days. 500 μg B. abortus was injected on day 0.

Radioactively Labeled Iron ^{59}Fe Uptake

A 0.025 μg dose of [^{59}Fe] citrate was intraperitoneally injected 6 h before sampling bone marrow and spleen. The radioactivity was counted in a well counter for γ-radiation.

Spontaneous Rosette-Forming Cells (sRFC)

The number of spleen cells rosetting with SRBC was determined according to the technique of Bach and Dardenne (1971). In some experiments an antitheta serum was used. It was raised in AKR mice by weekly intraperitoneal injections of 5×10^7 C_3H thymus cells for seven weeks.

Results and Discussion

Role of Bone-Marrow Cells in the Production of Splenic Hypertrophy

Table I shows that the reconstitution of lethally irradiated mice by bone-marrow cells is necessary and sufficient to permit the splenomegaly induced by *C. granulosum* or *B. abortus* to appear. The addition of thymus cells did not significantly alter the results. It is interesting to note that $3 \times 10^6 - 5 \times 10^6$ bone-marrow cells were sufficient to induce a splenomegaly comparable to that obtained in normal animals.

The experiments described in Fig. 1 gave similar results, but in this case, a different procedure was used in which the mice were introduced into the experiment 30 days after thymectomy, irradiation, and cell reconstitution. The nonthymic dependence of *Brucella* antigens is also confirmed since anti-*Brucella* agglutinins were similarly elevated with or without thymectomy. However, thymectomy was clearly effective, as shown by a difference in PFC response to SRBC between the two groups of mice (Table II).

Kinetics of Bone-Marrow Cell Lines Proliferation

The proliferation in the spleen of cells of bone-marrow origin was investigated in normal mice injected with inactivated bacteria. Three stages in this cellular proliferation were tentatively identified: stem cells, evaluated by the CFU technique; mature cells, roughly measured by total nucleated cell count; and intermediate cells, identified as ^{59}Fe-incorporating precursors of erythrocytes or as megakaryocytes, precursors of platelets, measured by the number of giant cells per square centimeter of spleen histological section.

The results were roughly similar for *C. granulosum* and *B. abortus* (Fig. 2, Table III): (a) In the bone marrow, although the number of nucleated cells and the percentage of ^{59}Fe uptake fell sharply, the CFU content either remained unaffected or increased. This marrow, poor in cellularity, was, in fact, very active and produced stem cells which—at least during the first days—did not develop locally. (b) In the spleen, the CFU number showed a decrease after 24 h. This can be interpreted as a differentiation to more mature cells. After 48 h, a

Table III. Variations of Three Parameters of Bone-Marrow Cell Proliferation: Stem Cells (CFU), Erythroblasts ([59]Fe Uptake), and Total Nucleated Cell Content[a]

		Days after injection of *C. granulosum*						
	Controls	1	2	4	5	6	8	10
Bone marrow								
CFU	1590	—	1475	—	1642	—	—	1110
	± 78	—	± 30	—	± 31	—	—	± 134
Percentage of ^{59}Fe uptake	3.74		2.14		0.43			
	± 0.29	—	± 0.13	—	± 0.14	—	—	—
Total nucleated cell count ($\times 10^6$)	8.03	—	5.00	4.26	—	4.34	8.77	8.08
Spleen								
CFU	1168	560	2496		4000			4000
	± 72	± 68	± 146	—		—	—	
Percentage of ^{59}Fe uptake	8.75		2.70		24.70			23 75
	± 1.38	—	± 0.11	—	± 1.45	—	—	± 3.35
Total nucleated cell count ($\times 10^6$)	130	—	200	247	—	293	376	510

[a]500 μg *C. granulosum* was injected i.v. on day 0. The values given refer to the whole spleen or to a femoral bone marrow.

Table IV. Number of Giant Cells (Megakaryocytes?) per cm^2 of Spleen Histological Section at Different Times after Injection of 500 μg of *B. abortus*

Days after *B. abortus*	Number of giant cells/cm^2
0 (controls)	250
1	194
2	285
4	654
6	1254
10	2237

significant increase took place due to a local proliferation of splenic CFU or, more likely, due to a migration from the bone marrow. The curve of ^{59}Fe uptake in the spleen looked like that of CFU, first decreasing and then increasing, but there was a certain shift between the two curves. The rise of CFU was first recorded at 48 h, but that of ^{59}Fe uptake at about the 5th day—as if 3–4 days were the time necessary for a stem cell to become an erythroblast. The fifth

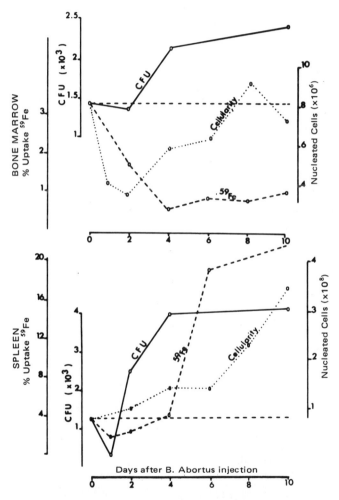

Fig. 2. Variations of three parameters of bone-marrow cell proliferation: stem cells (CFU), erythroblasts (^{59}Fe uptake), total nucleated cells content. 500 μg *B. abortus* was injected i.v. on day 0. The values given refer to the whole spleen or to a total femoral bone marrow.

Table V. Number of sRFC per 6000 Spleen Cells after Injection of *C. granulosum*

		Days after injection of *C. granulosum*						
	Controls	1	2	5	6	7	8	10
sRFC (+4°C)	7.0	4.3	3.0	3.0	1.8	2.25	2.0	1.6
sRFC after incubation at 37°C	5.5	4.3	–	2.8	–	2.3	–	–
sRFC after antitheta-serum treatment at +4°C	4.5	–	1.8	–	0.9	–	1.0	–

day was still remarkable for a sudden rise in the number of megakaryocytes per square centimeter of spleen (Table IV).

The important point seems to be that at a time when the animals were more reactive to the antigen, there was an elevation in the number of precursor cells for erythrocytes and platelets. It was also shown by cytological examination of spleen smears that polymorphonuclear precursors, characterized in the mouse by their annular nucleus, had also increased.

Influence of Immunostimulant Bacteria on the Number of Spontaneous Rosette-Forming Cells

The numeration of sRFC in the mouse spleen seems to be a convenient technique to evaluate the number of precursors of immunocompetent cells to the antigen SRBC.

Tables V and VI show that the injection of *C. granulosum* or *B. abortus* definitely did not provoke an increase in the number of sRFC per 6000 spleen cells, but, rather, induced a decrease in the number of sRFC. The absolute number of sRFC per whole spleen was also diminished. The incubation of cells at 37°C before rosette formation eliminated adherent cells, but did not greatly alter the overall results. The technique of incubation with antitheta serum did not seem to eliminate adherent cells. The antitheta-resistant cells were also decreased after bacterial injections.

Thus, although certain precursor cells of bone-marrow origin increased their number many times in the spleen after injection of *C. granulosum* or *B. abortus,* there was no parallel increase of precursors of immunocompetent cells. Our technique for evaluating immunocompetent-cell precursors may be imperfect since the target cells for the antigen would be a minor part of sRFC (Biozzi and Stiffel, 1972). Perhaps it is necessary to look elsewhere rather than to the

Table VI. Number of sRFC in the Spleen after Injection of *B. abortus*

| | Controls | Days after injection of *B. abortus* | | | |
		1	2	4	8
Number of sRFC per 6000 spleen cells	4.8	0.9	1.0	1.2	1.0
Number of sRFC in the whole spleen	74,500	17,500	25,000	32,000	43,500

increase of precursors of immunocompetent cells for the explanation of the immunostimulation seen on day 5. Other bone-marrow precursors, particularly macrophages, could play an important part. This decrease in the number of precursors of immunocompetent cells may be compared with the observation of Paraskevas *et al.* (1972), who showed a similar decrease after antigenic stimulation.

References

Amiel J. L., Litwin, J., and Berardet, M. (1969). Essais d'immunothérapie active non spécifique par *Corynebacterium parvum* formolé. *Rev. Eur. Etud. Clin. Biol.* 14:909.

Bach, J. F. and Dardenne, M. (1971). Activities of immunosuppressive agents *in vitro*. I. Rosette inhibition by azathioprine. *Rev. Eur. Etud. Clin. Biol.* 16:770.

Biozzi, G. and Stiffel, C. (1972). *Dynamique de la Réponse Immunologique* (Paul Bordet, Ed.), Flammarion, Paris, France.

Jerne, N. K. and Nordin, A. A. (1963). Plaque formations in agar by simple antibody-producing cells. *Science* 140:405.

Paraskevas, F., Ork, K. B., and Lee, S. I. (1972). Cell-surface associated gammaglobulins in lymphocyte-III changes of gammaglobulin-carrying lymphocytes during primary response. *J. Immunol.* 109:1254–1261.

Prévot, A. R., Halpern, B., Biozzi, G., Stiffel, C., Mouton, D., Morard, J. C., Bouthillier, Y., and Decreusefond, C. (1963). Stimulation du système réticulo-endothélial (SRE) par les corps microbiens tués de *Corynebacterium parvum*. *C. R. Acad. Sci. (Paris)* 257:13–17.

Till, J. E. and McCulloch, A. (1961). A direct measurement of the radiation sensitivity of normal mouse bone-marrow cells. *Radiat. Res.* 14:213.

Toujas, L., Dazord, L., Le Garrec, Y., and Sabolovic, D. (1972a). Modifications du nombre d'unités formatrices de colonies spléniques par des bacteries induisant l'immunostimulation non spécifique. *Experientia (Basel)* 28:1223–1224.

Toujas, L., Sabolovic, D., Dazord, L., Le Garrec, Y., Toujas, J. P., Guelfi, J., and Pilet, C. (1972b). The mechanism of immunostimulation induced by inactivated *Brucella abortus*. *Rev. Eur. Etud. Clin. Biol.* 17:267.

Toujas, L., Dazord, L., and Guelfi, J. (1973a). Augmentation des propriétés immunostimulantes de *Brucella abortus* inactivée par l'utilisation conjuguée d'un antisérum spécifique. *C. R. Acad. Sci. (Paris)* 276:433–436.

Toujas, L., Dazord, L., Martin, A., and Guelfi, J. (1973b). Simultaneous stimulation of plaque-forming cells and depression of cellular immunity to sheep erythrocytes after adjuvant treatment. *Biomed. Express (Paris)* 19:503–505.

DISCUSSION

MILAS: I would like to make several comments about the effect of treatment with *Corynebacterium parvum* or *Corynebacterium granulosum* on the function of T lymphocytes. This issue seems to be important, particularly in view of the widely-held belief that T cells play a major role in the destruction of tumor cells. Dr. Toujas has just presented evidence that a marked proliferation of cells occurs in the spleen of mice treated with *C. parvum*. We have observed a similar phenomenon with both *C. parvum* and *C. granulosum*. However, histological analysis of such spleens revealed that this takes place in the red pulp and is mostly a result of proliferation of macrophagelike cells and hematopoietic cells. In contrast, the white pulp is often reduced; in some instances it has almost completely disappeared. The questions arise: what happened to the lymphocytes, in particular to T cells? Is *C. granulosum* or *C. parvum* toxic for these cells, or has a redistribution of these cells taken place in the animals?

Spleen cells (as well as lymph node and peripheral blood lymphocytes) from mice treated with *C. granulosum* responded to *in vitro* stimulation by PHA less than the cells from normal mice, and their reactivity was not restored by removal of adherent cells. *C. granulosum*-treated mice tolerated allogenic skin grafts much longer than normal mice, suggesting that the number of functions of the T cells might indeed be decreased by this treatment. Woodruff *et al.*, [(1973). *Proc. Roy. Soc., London, B* **184**:97; (1973). *Immunopotentiation,* CIBA Symposium **18**:287] have already reported that mice do not need to have T cells in order to mount an antitumor response when treated with *C. parvum*. These observations may somewhat change our present thinking about the processes underlying the immunological resistance to tumors. Is, then, the role of other cells—for example macrophages—in antitumor resistance more important than was previously thought?

DAVIES: In the last three papers we heard accounts of very different experiments. The first, as Dr. Feldman told us, did not have anything to do with *C. parvum;* the second showed us one of the manifestations of the activity of *C. parvum;* the third showed a different effect of *C. parvum.* In discussing these three papers, I can do no more than pose a series of questions. I cannot really interrelate them as they have no common theme.

Listening to Dr. Feldman, it is always difficult not to be carried away by his flood of oratory. When he takes cells that have been transformed *in vitro* with PHA and transfers them back into syngenic recipients, do they ever cause any enlargement of popliteal lymph nodes? Do allogenically sensitized cells have any syngenic cytotoxicity?

Dr. Hall reported interesting phenomena, based on experiments involving several different species of animals, which show some evidence that the injected cells were the same as those found at the lesions. In fact, the cells he showed us were heavily overlayed with grains in the film. How does he know that the radioactivity detected in the lesions initiated in the skin represents the migration of the labeled cells injected? I was not very impressed by the morphological evidence. Can he also say whether the immune state of the recipient, vis-à-vis the challenge, was of any importance? Did it make any difference if the animals were initially primed?

Dr. Hall showed a long and interesting series of substances which he had applied to the skin in addition to *C. parvum* and BCG—heat and radiation and all sorts of strange things. Did he have a similar kind of effect if he put in one of those glass skin windows?

Dr. Toujas described some of the effects of *C. parvum* injections. I was a little concerned in the first series of experiments about the injection of thymocytes, or bone-marrow or both; what is the histopathology of the enlarged spleens at which he looked? It was probably almost entirely red-pulp enlargement, as Dr. Milas told us.

When Dr. Toujas was talking about colony-forming units, I wondered whether he had done any studies on the suicidability of the CFU after injection of *C. parvum?* This would be a nice adjunct to the other work he has done.

FELDMAN: Dr. Davies always raises important questions. I cannot answer his first question—namely, whether lymphoid cells which are stimulated with lectins—say, PHA—re-inoculated *in vivo* will recruit—because such an experiment was not done. In fact, I would be extremely disappointed if they did recruit.

With regard to allosensitization, if A lymphocytes are sensitized *in vitro* against B allo-antigens and inoculated into an A recipient, there is recruitment. These recipient-recruited cells will kill B, but not A. They will retain their specificity against the sensitizing cells. However, if Dr. Davies meant whether sensitizing B lymphocytes and inoculating these into A has been tried, this was not done.

HALL: I can answer Dr. Davies's questions fairly directly. I agree that when radioactivity is being assessed, allegedly in the form of cells and tissues, it is important to check it by autoradiography and by some other means. In fact, the experiments with lesions in the rat were repeated using tritiated thymidine, and labeled cells were found to be present. Also, iododeoxyuridine cannot be reutilized, and we have shown that it is in the form of DNA in those lesions.

We have not done skin windows. They are difficult in rats. In sheep the cell population so recruited is dominated by polymorphs and it does not seem to be a very satisfactory technique. With regard to the immune status of the recipient rat, I am not clear what was meant by the question.

DAVIES: For example, was an attempt made to initially immunize an animal against *C. parvum,* so that an injection of *C. parvum* was followed, two or three weeks later, by another *C. parvum* injection as one of the lesion-initiating injections. Suppose the cells were then injected to see whether there was extravasion. That is the kind of immunity of which I was thinking.

HALL: We carried out one experiment in which the animal was sensitized systemically to DNCB, and then challenged with a challenging dose. In that case there was no entry.

We have not done any more experiments, although Johns Hopkins is, at present, doing some work in which animals are immunized against soluble antigens, followed by putting in the antigen-specific blast. However, I am inclined to the view that it will not make any difference.

DAVIES: I was intrigued by this, because one of the subjects about which we have heard little today is immunity against *C. parvum.* Does it indeed elicit an immune response? Can antibodies be titrated against *C. parvum?* Is it non-immunogenic? If so, this is a rather strange phenomenon.

HALL: It is extremely immunogenic, and it is very easy to titrate antibodies against it. In fact, it is used as a standard antigen because it is an antigen of convenience.

WHITE: May I tempt Dr. Hall to speculate a little more? Has he possibly done some experiments in which the cells were treated *in vitro* with, say, enzymes, to see whether they go through? Second, what about the effect of a heterologous delayed-type response at the periphery? Would that bring the labeled cells through?

HALL: I have not done experiments in which the cells were treated with enzymes for two reasons: first, in general terms, if lymphocytes of any sort are mishandled *in vitro*—which happens inevitably, even by labeling them—

the distribution tends to be impaired. Second, a fact which I ought to have stressed is that in these small skin lesions the percentage of the total dose of cells injected which reaches the lesion is, of course, 1% at the most, and is usually much less. Most of these cells go to the gut—but that is another story.

To detect a difference in behavior of this minority population is extremely difficult technically, which is why it is only with *C. parvum* and BCG, which were completely outside the range of the controls, that I am prepared to draw any conclusions. The approach suggested by Dr. White is a possible one, of course.

With regard to the second question, if the reaction to DNCB is accepted as a delayed-type hypersensitivity response, the immunoblasts do not seem to go in. Certainly, we have sensitized sheep to BCG and then raised a skin lesion with PPD, so that the inducing antigen is not present in the lesion; even there, we were unable to show any impressive entry vis-à-vis a satisfactory control. I cannot give an explanation of this.

BOMFORD: I have a comment which bears on the results presented by Dr. Hall about the accumulation of immunoblasts at the site of injection of *C. parvum*, and also on those of Dr. Milas about the prolongation of the life of skin homografts, which suggests a suppression of T-cell function by *C. parvum*.

I think these two phenomena may be connected. The first indication of this comes from the work of G. G. Allwood and G. L. Asherson [(1973). *Clin. Exp. Immunol.* 11:579], who showed that the delayed-type hypersensitivity response to picryl chloride could be suppressed by prior treatment with *C. parvum*. They also showed that the trapping of chromium-labeled lymphocytes in the draining lymph node from the site of picryl chloride application was reduced in mice pretreated with *C. parvum*.

The idea suggests itself that during these phenomena—in which there is apparent suppression of T-cell function—the antigenic stimulus provokes the T cells, but they get trapped on the way to the site of elicitation because of this phenomenon of more efficient extravascularization at the site of *C. parvum* injection.

Has Dr. Hall ever looked at the fate of labeled immunoblasts in mice, or other animals, which have been treated with *C. parvum* intravenously? Is it known where the immunoblasts go under those circumstances? It is the intravenous route which has been generally used to prolong skin homograft survival.

HALL: I cannot answer that satisfactorily. We have tried all sorts of ways to alter the basic distribution pattern of these cells when they are injected into rats: this includes distribution through the gut, the lungs, liver, spleen, and so on. It is extremely hard, even by the most draconian treatments, to alter this pattern. As I explained earlier, slight variations in minority sites, such as skin lesions, are extremely difficult to substantiate.

Asherson's experiments were dealing with lymph-node lymphocytes, which are a different population. Our experience has been that although there have been claims in the literature by C. Griscelli, P. Vassalli, and R. J. McCluskey, [(1969). *J. Exp. Med.* **130**:1423] that, for example, a lymph node draining the site of a *C. parvum* or BCG injection is specifically attractive to this form of blast, we have not been able to confirm that finding. In all these experiments, which appear to be rather similar at first sight, there is a very heterogeneous population of cells being used. We have to be careful in comparing their results.

McBRIDE: I should like to return to Dr. Davies's question with respect to immunity to *C. parvum*. It is now known that most species have naturally occurring antibodies against *C. parvum*. This is perhaps to be expected in view of the cross-reactions between the anaerobic *Corynebacteriaceae*.

With respect to the effects of *C. parvum* in B mice, is it possible that during lethal irradiation of the normal mice to make B mice that the primed T cells could exist against *C. parvum* and that these could be operative in a B mouse? That is, perhaps there could be a residual population of primed T cells in a B mouse.

DAVIES: The experiments relevant to your question were done some years ago. As far as could then be determined, the state of immunity engendered before thymectomy, irradiation, and injection of bone marrow was discernible 60 days after these various manipulations. It was not as good as that which would have resulted had the animal not been thymectomized and irradiated. But during that period of time, a switch had been made, and—by all criteria—the animal was a true radiation chimera in that, as far as could be determined, all its lymphoid cells—or nearly all of them—were donor type, rather than host type. It seems strange to have this persistence of immunity during such a traumatic event in the animal's life. I do not know the mechanism, or whether this persistence is due to a very small residue of radioresistant T cells, or transfer of information—perhaps along the lines which seem to be envisaged in Dr. Feldman's experiments.

WHISNANT: With regard to Dr. Feldman's beautiful and convincing presentation, I am interested in target cell/killer cell ratios which might come out of the model. If a normal population of cells is overlayed on, say, five sequential different H2 types, how many cells are lost? Is it possible to have an idea how many cells are required to kill a target cell? Second, I do not recall the specific antigen used to sensitize Dr. Hall's donor animal. Is it possible that a particular antigen is cross-reactive in a heterologous manner with BCG and *C. parvum?*

FELDMAN: In answer to the question of how many cells it takes to kill a target cell, the lytic kinetics of the reaction is first order kinetics, that is, one single hit by a lymphocyte is all that is needed to kill a target cell. Furthermore, there are no known cytotoxic substances released from killed cells which kill the neighboring cells. Alternatively, it may be said that fibroblasts live together in this situation, but die independently.

May I comment on a remark made by Dr. Bomford with regard to Asherson's experiments with picryl chloride? Could it be that in these experiments, as with the prolongation of the skin homografts, the *C. parvum* may have activated suppressor T cells which have prevented the development of effectors and, therefore, there is a decreased reaction to the picryl chloride?

WANEBO: First, did the timing of injection of *C. parvum* have an influence on the histopathology in the model studied? For example, during a study of the mouse at 14 days after injection versus one or two days after injection, is there a point at which there might be complete destruction of cortical lymphocytes at one point and a rebound phenomenon at another point? Second, could these extravasated lymphocytes be T cells or B cells? Has anybody investigated this possibility? Is *C. parvum* more of a B-cell "stimulator"?

TOUJAS: With respect to the effect of timing on the histology of the spleen, we have essentially studied the appearance of the giant cells. We were interested also in the T- and B-dependent area, and the histologist is studying this now.

HALL: There is no evidence that the immunological specificity of the blasts can play any role in guiding these cells to their destination. We have checked this thoroughly, although I will not go through all the evidence now. In many of these experiments *C. parvum* was used, but we first established using a whole range of antigens that it is immaterial which one is used.

From these experiments it is not possible to say whether the extravasated lymphocytes could be T or B cells. We know that both types of cells are likely to be present. I suspect that most of the cells which we were tracing were probably B cells. However, I would not like to give the impression that those cells which extravasate are necessarily implicated in, for example, tumor rejection, because we were using them only as an experimental model. Some of them may well have been T cells too, but I cannot give precise quantitations.

DIMITROV: An important piece of information given to us by Dr. Toujas was that, in addition to white cells, he found erythroblasts showing the greatest stimulation. This is important, because all patients with cancer have ineffective erythropoiesis. If this is due to poor stimulation of the stem cells, the attention of the clinicians must be drawn to it.

13

Inhibition of Thymidine Incorporation of Tumoral YC8 Cells Cultured *in Vitro* by Peritoneal Macrophages Activated with *Corynebacterium parvum*

BERNARD HALPERN, ANNE-MARIE LORINET, LOUCAS SPARROS, and ANTOINETTE FRAY

Abstract

Peritoneal cavity macrophages obtained from animals treated with *Corynebacterium parvum* inhibited the DNA synthesis of isogenic YC8 tumoral cells present in the culture to a considerable extent. Macrophages from control animals displayed a similar activity, but at a much lower level. Previous x-irradiation of the macrophages did not abolish their inhibitory activity.

BERNARD HALPERN, ANNE-MARIE LORINET, LOUCAS SPARROS, and ANTOINETTE FRAY, Department of Experimental Medicine, College of France, Paris, France.

Introduction

The inhibitory action of *Corynebacterium parvum,* a potent stimulant of the reticuloendothelial system (RES) (Halpern *et al.,* 1964), on tumor invasion raises the question of a possible implication of the macrophage population in this phenomenon (Halpern *et al.,* 1966; 1973; Fray *et al.,* 1975).

Materials and Methods

Five- to seven-week-old, male Balb/c mice were used throughout. Peritoneal cells were obtained from animals immediately after decapitation. Following laparotomy, the peritoneal cavity was rinsed with warm Hank's medium containing 10 units of calciparine.* The fluid was collected and centrifuged at 400*g* for 5 min in a cooled centrifuge. The cells were then resuspended in the same medium with 10% heat-inactivated fetal calf serum added. The cell concentration was adjusted to 2×10^6/ml. Then, 2 ml of this cell suspension was poured into sterile, falcon Petri dishes, 35 mm in diameter. The dishes were placed in an incubator at 37°C, and gassed with 10% CO_2 for 2 h. After removal of the supernatant, the adhering cells were washed twice with the culture medium.

Tumoral YC8 cells (Leclerc *et al.,* 1972; Halpern *et al.,* 1973) were obtained by puncturing the abdominal cavity of ascitic tumor-bearing mice with a glass pipette. The cells were then added to a Petri dish containing Hank's medium with heat-inactivated fetal calf serum. The final cell concentration was adjusted to 5×10^5 cells/ml; 10^5 cells (0.2 ml of suspension) were then added to the Petri dishes containing the layered peritoneal cavity cells obtained from control mice and mice treated with *C. parvum.* The relative cell concentrations of unseparated peritoneal cells were adjusted to have 40 effector cells for each target cell. When adherent cells were used, the relative cell concentrations were adjusted to 24:1. Other dishes containing only 10^5 YC8 cells (prepared under the same conditions) served as reference.

Tritiated thymidine† was appropriately diluted and added at a dose of 48 mCi/mmol to each dish, the final thymidine concentration being 4×10^6 M. The dishes were then incubated for 1 h at 37°C. Afterward, the cells were mechanically detached from the bottom of the Petri dish, contrifuged at 1000*g* for 10 min, and the supernatant was discarded; the cells were then treated with 10% trichloroacetic acid overnight. The precipitate was washed with trichloroacetic acid and then dissolved in 2 ml hyamine for scintillation counting. Counts were made for 10 min.

---

*Calciparine from Laboratoires Choay, Paris.
†Obtained from the Commissariat à l'Energie Atomique (CEA), Saclay, France.

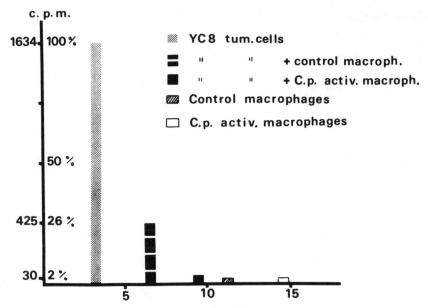

Fig. 1. [³H] thymidine incorporation rate. [³H] thymidine uptake by YC8 tumoral cells cultured alone or in the presence of control macrophages and macrophages activated by *C. parvum*. For comparison, [³H] thymidine uptake by the same numbers of control macrophages and macrophages activated by *C. parvum* culture alone is also shown.

Results

Effects of Macrophages from Control Animals and Animals Treated with *C. parvum* on Thymidine Incorporation by Tumoral YC8 Cells

In this group of experiments, *C. parvum*, as well as BCG,* was intravenously injected at a dose of 500 μg (dry weight), five days before the peritoneal cells were collected. The results are shown in Fig. 1.

It can be deduced from the results reported in Fig. 1 that peritoneal macrophages obtained from control animals consistently reduced the rate of thymidine incorporation by tumoral YC8 cells. The inhibition varied from one experiment to another, and ranged from 20–50%. However, the reduction was regularly greater when macrophages activated with *C. parvum* were used. In this case, 70–95% inhibition was observed. Preliminary experiments indicated that macrophages obtained from animals treated with live BCG, administered intravenously, were equally active.

*From the Pasteur Institute, Paris.

Table I. Normal and Irradiated Macrophages Inhibition of Thymidine Uptake by Tumoral YC8 Cell

Cells	Corynebacterium parvum (Mérieux)	Difference, %
YC8	1739	
YC8 + macrophage C. parvum	579	−67
YC8 + macrophage C. parvum, irradiated with 1500 R	719	−59
YC8 + macrophage C. parvum, irradiated with 5000 R	655	−63

Effects of Irradiation on Macrophages Inhibition of Thymidine Incorporation by YC8 Tumoral Cells

The inhibition by macrophages of the proliferation of isogenic tumor cells is, in itself, an intriguing phenomenon. As an approach to the study of the possible mechanism, a study was performed with x-irradiated cells. The macrophages were subjected to radiation doses of 1500 R and 5000 R, delivered by a cobalt source. The results, summarized in Table I, indicate that high doses of x-irradiation do not abolish the inhibitory effect of *C. parvum*-treated macrophages on the thymidine uptake of tumoral cells. Under our experimental conditions, neither the adherent nor the nonadherent cells showed uptake of tritiated thymidine in measurable amounts, regardless of whether the cells came from control animals or from animals treated with *C. parvum*.

Discussion

The results reported here deserve some comment. In our experimental model, peritoneal macrophages, especially macrophages stimulated by *C. parvum*, inhibited the multiplication of malignant cells by contact. It should be emphasized that YC8 cells are isogenic with the macrophage donor, and, consequently, this inhibition cannot be credited to histocompatibility factors. It should be stressed that the tumor cells which are inhibited in their proliferation are not killed by the contact with macrophages, as shown by the dye-exclusion technique. We are therefore dealing with a new phenomenon consisting of an arrest of DNA synthesis in the malignant cell. This phenomenon should be correctly called *cytostatic,* a term used to designate similar phenomena observed in bacteria. This property of the macrophages seems to be radioresistant. Prior irradiation with 5000 R did not abolish this activity. It is impossible to state, at present, whether the inhibition results from a cell-to-cell contact inhibition or whether it is mediated by some diffusible factors. This last problem is presently being investigated.

Inhibition of tumoral cell division is strongly displayed by activated macrophages. However, control macrophages also effect a significant reduction of thymidine uptake. This can be explained by the fact that under normal breeding conditions, the control animals are subjected to many bacterial aggressions which may nonspecifically activate a certain percentage of the macrophages. This hypothesis should, however, be checked by a comparative study using animals bred under germ-free conditions.

References

Fray, A., Sparros, L., Lorinet, A. M., and Halpern, B. (1975). Nonspecific cytotoxic activity of peritoneal exudate cells against tumoral cells in *Corynebacterium parvum*-treated animals, in this volume, pp. 181–186.

Halpern, B., Prévot, A., Biozzi, G., Stiffel, C., Mouton, D., Morard, J. C., Bouthillier, Y., and Decreusefond, C. (1964). Stimulation de l'activité phagocytaire du système réticuloendothélial provoquée par *Corynebacterium parvum. J. Reticuloendothel. Soc.* **1**:77.

Halpern, B., Biozzi, G., Stiffel, C., and Mouton, D. (1966). Inhibition of tumor growth by administration of killed *Corynebacterium parvum. Nature (Lond.)* **212**:853.

Halpern, B., Fray, A., Crepin, Y., Platica, O., Lorinet, A. M., Rabourdin, A., Sparros, L., and Isac, R. (1973). *Corynebacterium parvum*, a potent immunostimulant in experimental infections and in malignancies, in: *Immunopotentiation,* Ciba Foundation Symposium, 18 (new series), p. 217, Elsevier-Exerpta Medica-North Holland, Amsterdam.

Leclerc, J. C., Gomard, E., and Levy, J. P. (1972). Cell-mediated reaction against tumors induced by oncornaviruses. I. Kinetics and specificity of the immune response in murine sarcoma virus (MSV)-induced tumors and transplanted lymphomas. *Int. J. Cancer* **10**:589.

14

A Comparative, Scanning Electron Microscope Study of the Interaction between Stimulated or Unstimulated Mouse Peritoneal Macrophages and Tumor Cells

F. PUVION, A. FRAY, and B. HALPERN

Abstract

Both general morphology and cell interactions were investigated in adherent cell populations of peritoneal exudates incubated with YC8 cells. The capacity of stimulated macrophages to participate in the destruction of tumor cells was demonstrated by cytotoxic tests using ^{51}Cr (Fray et al., this volume, p. 181). In this study, possible associations between macrophages and tumor cells were observed with the scanning electron microscopy.

F. PUVION, A. FRAY, and B. HALPERN, Institut de Recherches sur le Cancer, Unité 124, INSERM, and Institut d'Immunobiologie, INSERM, CNRS, and EPHE, Hôpital Broussais, Paris 14e, France.

Materials and Methods

Macrophages

Peritoneal cells from both normal and stimulated, 3- or 4-month-old, female Balb/c mice were withdrawn from the peritoneal cavity.

Stimulation

Five days before harvesting, mice were intravenously injected with 500 μg of *Corynebacterium parvum.*

Tumor Cells

YC8 cells were withdrawn from the peritoneal cavities of female Balb/c mice which had been injected 6 days before with Moloney virus-induced lymphoma cells transplanted serially in the peritoneum of normal mice.

Macrophage Cultures

Peritoneal cells were suspended in 199 culture medium containing 5% fetal calf serum; their final concentration was 10^6 cells/ml. Aliquots containing 1 ml of this suspension were cultured in 35 $\times$ 10 mm falcon Petri dishes. The adherent nature of the macrophages was ascertained after 2 h of incubation at 37°C in a moist atmosphere containing 5% CO_2.

This first incubation was followed by intensive rinsing with culture medium. Such treatment eliminated nonadherent cells. The falcon dishes containing normal or stimulated adherent cells were reincubated for 18 h under the same conditions. Some of them were mixed with YC8 cells (in the proportion of 1 tumor cell to 40 adherent cells). This last incubation was followed by 3 washings.

Electron Microscopy

The falcon dishes containing peritoneal adherent cells were fixed for 15 min in 2.5% (v/v) glutaraldehyde in 0.1 M phosphate buffer, pH 7.4. The cells were rinsed with the same buffer, post-fixed for 1 h with OsO_4, according to the procedure of Parducz (1967), rinsed with distilled water, lyophilyzed, and coated with gold–palladium using an Edwards rotary-vacuum evaporator.

Control preparations of YC8 cells were processed in suspension, following the same schedule. After fixation and rinsing, one drop of the cell suspension was placed on the microscope-specimen holder, lyophilyzed, and coated with metal.

Specimens were observed with a scanning electron microscope (Cambridge Stereoscan S4) at 20 kV.

Results

Stimulated and unstimulated peritoneal adherent-cell specimens were constituted by three categories of cells, as established by their cellular morphology.

(1) Round cells, 4 or 5 μm in diameter, were present in stimulated preparations, but were rarely observed in normal, peritoneal, adherent cells. These round cells were small lymphocytes and had some fingerlike processess on their surfaces. (2) Round cells, 7 or 10 μm in diameter, were observed in both stimulated and normal specimens. Many microvilli were present on their surface (Fig. 1). (3) Elongated cells were also observed in both preparations. They were not as contrasted as round cells. Their surfaces were constituted by many juxtaposed leaves or by many short microvilli. Small lymphocytes were often at the periphery of flattened cells.

The attachment of YC8 cells to the surface of the plastic dish was never strong enough to resist successive washings. In normal adherent-cell preparations, no attachment of YC8 cells to the surface of adherent macrophages was observed, indicating that any link established between adherent and YC8 cells did not resist the washing procedure. In contrast, stimulated adherent-cell preparations contained YC8 cells which were close to round (Figs. 2, 3) or elongated adherent cells. They could be on top of the adherent cells or at their periphery. Sometimes, the flattened cell had emitted a narrow process binding it to the tumor cell. In other cases, contact was realized by the end of several short microvilli emitted by both adherent and tumor cells. Finally, in other cases, the

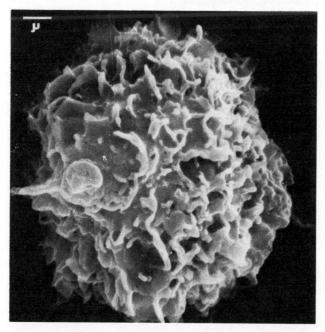

Fig. 1. A globular, adherent, *C. parvum*-stimulated cell showing a large number of microvilli. Microvilli are of fairly uniform diameter (0.1 μm), but of highly variable lengths. (8000 ✕)

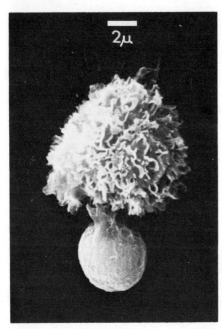

Fig. 2. This adherent *C. parvum*-stimulated cells is connected to a smooth **YC8** cell. Contact between these two cells is performed by an uropod emitted by the tumor cell. (4000 X)

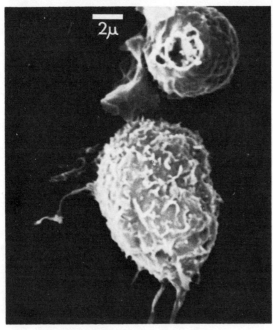

Fig. 3. The altered tumor cell is connected to the adherent, *C. parvum*-stimulated cell by an uropod. (4000 X)

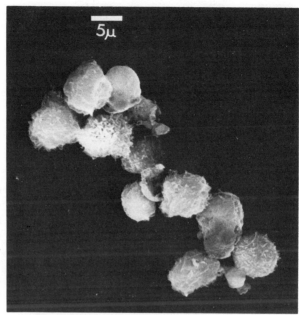

Fig. 4. YC8 cells of the control preperation display no uniformity in shape and size. Some cells have short microvilli, while others show a wrinkled or smooth surface. There are no cavities. (1600 ×)

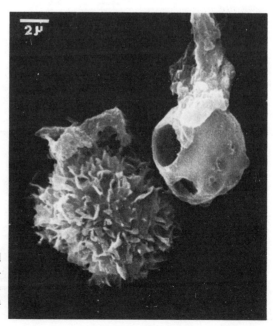

Fig. 5. The smooth tumor cell located near a globular, adherent, *C. parvum*-stimulated cell shows large cavities on its surface. (4000 ×)

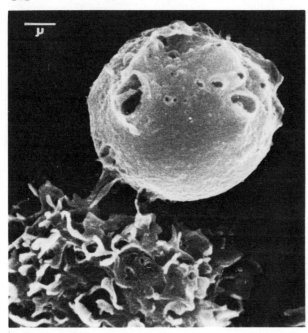

Fig. 6. An altered tumor cell is near a globular, *C. parvum*-stimulated, adherent cell. (8000 ×)

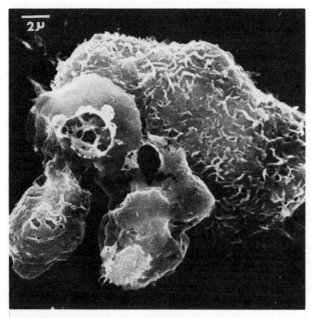

Fig. 7. An adherent cell derived from *C. parvum*-stimulated mice has fixed several altered tumor cells. (4000 ×)

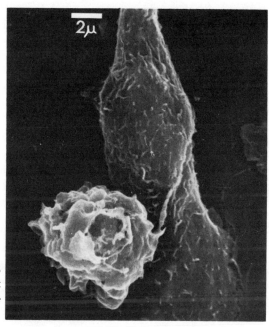

Fig. 8. Adhesion of a YC8 cell to a flattened adherent cell derived from *C. parvum*-treated mice. (4000 ✕)

tumor cell was attached to the adherent cell by an uropod. As in control preparations of YC8 cells incubated for 18 h in culture medium (Fig. 4), the surfaces of tumor cells were not uniform and ranged from cells with many microvilli to smooth cells. The smooth cells (Figs. 5–7) were in contact with round adherent cells and often had large cavities on their surfaces. On the other hand, tumor cells with microvilli or cytoplasmic veils were connected with flattened cells, the microvilli of which were rare (Fig. 8).

Discussion

The observations of control preparations of YC8 cells indicated that changes occurred on the outer membranes of tumor cells as a result of the biological activities of these cells. Indeed, their surfaces could be smooth, wrinkled, or bristling with fingerlike processes. These various aspects were also found when YC8 cells were incubated with stimulated adherent cells; moreover, smooth cells were often altered and presented large "holes." Smooth cells and cells with "holes" were near globular, adherent cells, while tumor cells with rough surfaces were connected with flattened, adherent cells.

These different aspects of tumor cells and adherent cells could correspond to various stages of biological cycles. For example, a stimulated adherent cell retaining a tumor cell could flatten and then curl when the tumor cell becomes altered. Another explanation could be that the tumor cell connected with a flattened, adherent cell might be released and then be captured by a globular, adherent cell.

In this study, it is not possible to know if one stimulated adherent cell is able to attract a tumor cell for a period long enough to lead to the death of the tumor cell or if this event requires the intervention of several stimulated adherent cells.

Our experiments lead us to affirm that contact between tumor cells and adherent peritoneal cells were found only when peritoneal cells were obtained from *C. parvum*-stimulated mice. Under these conditions, contacts were strong and were not broken by the washings which preceded aldehyde fixation.

Other investigators (Biberfeld *et al.*, 1973; Koren *et al.*, 1973) using electron microscopy have shown that a direct and close contact is a prerequisite for target-cell lysis. In these studies, the lymphocytes play an important role in the *in vitro* cytotoxic mechanism.

In our system, preliminary studies using ^{51}Cr release and [^{3}H]thymidine incorporation assays showed that the effect of the adherent *C. parvum*-stimulated peritoneal cells was stronger than the effect of nonadherent cells. These findings are in agreement with our observations.

Summary

Morphological observations on the contact-induced lysis of YC8 cells were carried out by means of scanning electron microscopy.

Unaltered target cells were located on the surface membranes of flattened, *Corynebacterium parvum*-stimulated adherent cells; altered target cells, on the other hand, established close contacts with globular, stimulated adherent cells. These contacts, leading to damage of the YC8-cell membrane, were not observed when YC8 cells were incubated with normal, unstimulated adherent cells.

Our findings provide direct evidence that *C. parvum*-stimulated adherent cells play an important role in the *in vitro* destruction of target cells and support the concept of contact-induced lysis.

Acknowledgments

The authors wish to thank Ms. A. Ponchel and Mrs. A. M. Lorinet for their skillful technical assistance.

References

Parducz, B. (1967). Ciliary movement and coordination in ciliates. *Int. Rev. Cytol.* 21:91–127.

Biberfeld, P., Biberfeld, G., Perlmann, P., and Holm, G. (1973). Cytological observations on the cytotoxic interaction between lymphocytes and antibody-coated monolayer cells. *Cell. Immunol.* 7:60–72.

Koren, H. S., Ax, W., and Freund-Moelbert, E. (1973). Morphological observations on the contact-induced lysis of target cells. *Eur. J. Immunol.* 3:32–36.

DISCUSSION

HALL: What is Dr. Halpern's reaction to the claim made by Evans, for example, about specific macrophage killing of tumor cells? Evans concedes to the occurrence of nonspecific killing—which is a nonlytic, cytotstatic event, but he also claims a specific killing by macrophages which he suggests is a lytic event.

Second, regarding the scanning electron micrographs showing the interaction between macrophages and tumor cell, some years ago B. Morris [(1968) Migration intratissulaire des lymphocytes du Mouton. *Nouv. Rev. Franç. d'Hématol.* 8:525–534.] published some data showing a similar, extremely close association between normal lymphocytes and macrophages from the same animal, with an extremely close junction of their cytoplasmic membranes as visualized in the electron microscope. In that situation, the lymphocytes were later allowed to escape by the macrophage. It seemed that one of the functions of a macrophage is to continually make intimate contacts with lymphocytes, just as though they were inspecting them, and then to let them go again. This event, which Dr. Halpern showed, could be a cytotoxic event, or is it merely the expression of a normal lymphocyte—macrophage interaction?

HALPERN: First, in our experiments we had two types of macrophages: those obtained from control animals and those obtained from *C. parvum*-stimulated animals. In other experiments, which I did not describe, we had macrophages from a tumor-bearing animal. The tumor had been implanted two weeks previously, so that the immunological reaction could have already occurred. We did not find any great difference in tumor-cell killing—or cytostasis—in the macrophages activated with *C. parvum,* whether they originated from tumor-bearing animals or not. We estimated this by the release of chromium-labeled cells.

The results were similar with irradiated macrophages. In some experiments, the cells received as much as 10,000 rads, yet the irradiated macrophages behaved exactly the same as the nonirradiated ones. Under both conditions, there was an inhibition of the incorporation of thymidine in the tumor cells when they were layered on a layer of macrophages.

The lack of effects of irradiation may be relevant to the well-known resistance of macrophages to x rays. Many years ago, we showed—with Georges Mathé [C. Stiffel *et al.* (1959). *Rev. Franç. Etud. Clin. Biol.* 6:164] measuring the phagocytic activity—that a total body irradiation with 1500 rads did not affect the phagocytic function. However, Feldman [R. Gallily and M. Feldman (1967). *Immunology* 12:197] has shown that x irradiation does impair the metabolic function of macrophages.

McBRIDE: Is it known whether it is the macrophages containing *C. parvum* that are cytotoxic, or another population of macrophages, activated in some other way? Could you also tell us how the *C. parvum*-activated macrophages were prepared?

HALPERN: We used macrophages obtained from peritoneal cavity exudate. It should be emphasized that *C. parvum* was injected intraperitoneally, and it can be presumed that the macrophages, or at least most of them, were in direct contact with the bacterial substrate. The so-called "activation" is reflected by several other properties. Thus, the activated macrophages spread much quicker than the nonactivated ones. It is likely that metabolic functions may be also modified. However, we have not investigated this problem thoroughly.

McBRIDE: Did they contain *C. parvum?*

HALPERN: No, we never saw *C. parvum* in the macrophages. In most of our experiments, in which *C. parvum* was given intraperitoneally, the macrophages were taken out several days after injection. However in other experiments, *C. parvum* was injected intravenously, and the macrophages were obtained by the i.p. route. The results did not differ in the two series of experiments.

BOMFORD: I should like to congratulate Dr. Halpern on his beautiful pictures. Has he seen a recent paper from Georges Klein's laboratory [F. Wiener, E. M. Fenyö, and G. Klein (1974). *Proc. Natl. Acad. Sci. USA* 71:148.] which made me wonder whether during the interaction between macrophages and tumor cells, cytoplasmic bridges can be established? These workers were looking at the formation of hybrid cells *in vivo* between injected tumor cells growing in the peritoneum and the host cells. They found quite a high frequency of hybrid cells, and presented evidence that the host component was probably a macrophage. I wonder whether a cytoplasmic bridge is established during the interaction, but, sometimes, instead of resulting in the death of the tumor cell, it enlarges and forms a hybrid between the macrophage and the tumor cell.

HALPERN: I do not want to make an incorrect statement; I showed pictures taken by Dr. Puvion and some of these show many macrophages strongly adhering to the cells. This was only seen frequently with macrophages obtained from *C. parvum*-treated animals. This event was not observed, or only rarely, with macrophages obtained from control animals. The adherence seems, therefore, to be dependent on activation with *C. parvum,* and probably relevant to the cytostatic or cytotoxic properties of activated macrophages.

FELDMAN: Remington and Hibbs have described some similar phenomena of the behavior of macrophages toward tumor cells. The macrophages were not from normal animals, nor from *C. parvum*-treated animals, but from toxo-plasma-treated animals. Remington and Hibbs indicated that such macrophages will either kill, or prevent the growth of tumor cells of a fibrosarcoma, but have no effect *in vitro* on normal fibroblast cells. That is, such cells can distinguish, if not recognize, between neoplastic and normal cells.

Has Dr. Halpern tested the behavior of his cells toward normal cells? If so, can he speculate about the properties of the tumor cells which enable the macrophages to recognize them?

HALPERN: This meeting started about a week too early. In several weeks I should be able to answer your question; this work is now in progress.

ATTIÉ: Dr. Halpern talked about three categories of macrophages: normal macrophages, stimulated ones, and those from tumor-bearing animals. There is a fourth category—macrophages from immunodepressed animals. Has this kind of macrophage been studied?

HALPERN: Not yet. I agree that there are many things still to be done in this domain.

15

The Macrophage-Stimulating Properties of a Variety of Anaerobic Coryneforms

ROBERT G. WHITE

Introduction

Over several years my colleagues and I investigated the adjuvant action of mycobacteria and related genera, such as the nocardias and corynebacteria. In 1965, on a visit to Professor Halpern in Paris, I learned of the remarkable microorganism which he was investigating called *Corynebacterium parvum*. Nothing stimulates like a paradox—and the paradox for me was that in my experience up to that time, true corynebacteria, in spite of their close taxonomical relationship with the mycobacteria and nocardias, did not show the same type of adjuvant properties. Thus, I propose to use the opportunity of this presentation to contrast the adjuvant properties of *C. parvum* and its relatives with those of mycobacteria and their relatives. This may be useful in clarifying our ideas on the way to search for the molecules involved in these two distinct types of biological activities.

Of course, we have to specify what we mean by the words "adjuvant activity." Mycobacterium and nocardia organisms facilitate the production of specific adaptive immunity by increasing both cell-mediated hypersensitivity and

ROBERT G. WHITE, Department of Bacteriology and Immunology, University of Glasgow, Scotland. Departmental Publication No. 7422.

humoral-antibody production. This means that when a protein antigen (usually a thymus-dependent one is chosen for this demonstration) in a water-in-oil emulsion is injected into an animal (typically, a guinea pig), there is a characteristic, severalfold increase in serum-antibody levels, involving γ_2 rather than γ_1 immunoglobulin (White *et al.*, 1963; White, 1963; 1967). Intense delayed-type hypersensitivity to the protein immunogen is also induced, and a large necrotic granuloma with complex histology, but involving a marked component of epithelioid and giant cells, develops at the site of the injection and within regional—and even remote—lymph nodes (Suter and White, 1954).

Most mycobacteria, whether pathogenic or nonpathogenic, atypical or saprophytic, and most true nocardias will produce the group of adjuvant effects of this type in the guinea pig. It is notoriously difficult to prove a negative, but the many corynebacteria which have been tested by us have failed to produce any of these effects. These include *Corynebacterium diphtheriae*, *Corynebacterium simplex*, *Corynebacterium xerosis*, *Corynebacterium ovis*, *Corynebacterium kutscheri (Corynebacterium murium)*, *Corynebacterium equi*, and *Corynebacterium hofmanni* (White *et al.*, to be published).

Taxonomy

Taxonomy is needed to understand the relationship between the organism designated *C. parvum* and the classical corynebacteria. An anaerobic coryneform organism referred to as *C. parvum* 936B was originally used by Halpern *et al.*, (1966) to increase the clearance of carbon from the blood of mice. In subsequent papers, the same and other anaerobic coryneform bacteria were used to inhibit tumor growth (Halpern *et al.*, 1966; Smith and Woodruff, 1968; Fisher *et al.*, 1970). It seems clear from the work of Johnson and Cummins (1972) that the term *Corynebacterium parvum* has no taxonomic definition, since bacteria with this designation appear in each of several serologically and biochemically defined, broad categories. Using investigations of cell-wall antigenic structure and DNA/DNA homology tests, these authors outlined a classification of anaerobic coryneform organisms based on three broad groups which are related to the type-strains *Propionibacterium acnes*, *Propionibacterium granulosum*, and *Propionibacterium avidum*. Specific antisera could be prepared against two groups of *P. acnes*, which can, therefore, be divided into the two groups: *P. acnes* I and II. Of 59 organisms which were collected under the designation "*C. parvum*," 29 were identified as *P. acnes* type I, 22 as *P. acnes* type II, 3 as *P. granulosum*, and 3 as *P. avidum* (Cummins and Johnson, 1974).

The lack of any taxonomic relationship with classical corynebacteria is clearly shown by the cell-wall sugar and amino-sugar compositions. In all but two of the 59 strains collected by Cummins and Johnson (1974), the diaminopimelic acid was present totally as the L isomer. Glycine regularly accompanied alanine, glutamic acid, and L-diaminopimelic acid (DAP); this association of glycine and L-DAP is also a feature of *Streptomyces* bacteria (Cummins and Harris, 1958). The cell-wall sugars also differ from those of mycobacteria, nocardias, and corynebacteria. For *P. acnes* type I, arabinose is uniformly absent and mannose uniformly present; for *P. acnes* type II, arabinose and galactose are uniformly absent and glucose and mannose uniformly present; for *P. granulosum* and *P. avidum,* arabinose is uniformly absent and mannose uniformly present.

In our work with mycobacteria, the extracted peptidoglycolipids were able to completely substitute for the biological (adjuvant) activities of whole bacilli in guinea pigs (White, 1965). These molecules appear in negatively-stained electron-micrograph preparations as filaments 133 Å (± 15 Å) in diameter. Mycobacterial cell walls carry on their surface a network of filaments of similar dimension. Nocardias and corynebacteria possess similar surface networks of filaments 87 Å (± 10 Å) in diameter and 59 Å (± 8 Å) in diameter, respectively (Gordon *et al.,* to be published). In contrast, negatively-stained preparations from representatives of each of the 4 groups of anaerobic coryneform organisms failed to show surface filamentous networks in culturally mature bacillary forms. A filamentous network appears to be present in the dividing bacilli from the early logarithmic phase of growth, but detaches from the surface at a later growth phase (Russell *et al.,* 1975).

Tests and Results

We tested a number of anaerobic coryneform organisms from each of the four categories [*P. acnes* I and II, *P. granulosum,* and *P. avidum,* according to the classification of Johnson and Cummins (1972)] for biological activity. In addition, we included several organisms of the "classical propionibacteria," as defined by van Niel (1928), and derived at their original cultural isolation from cheese, butter, and other dairy products. The first test chosen was the ability to clear a carbon suspension after intravenous injection (into mice by the method of Biozzi *et al.,* 1954). Of the 21 anaerobic coryneform strains tested, 15 were able to substantially increase (by at least 50%) the phagocytic index, K. The bacteria which were found effective in this way derived from each of the four serological groups of anaerobic coryneforms (O'Neill *et al.,* 1973). Organisms other than those designated *C. parvum* were active; thus, high activity could be found in *P. avidum* strains, e.g., *P. avidum* 4982 which increased K by 200%, and *P. granulosum* strains, e.g., *P. granulosum* 0507 which increased K by 210% (as compared with 160% for the Burroughs Wellcome *C. parvum* strain 6134, which serologically classifies as *C. acnes* type I). All members of the classical propionibacteria tested (*Propionibacterium freudenreichii, Propionibacterium arabinosum, Propionibacterium jensenii,* and *Propionibacterium rubrum*) failed to increase the phagocytic index significantly above that of controls.

All organisms found active in increasing the phagocytic index also caused an increase in the mass of the spleen. When this weight was plotted (as a ratio with the spleen weight of control animals injected intravenously with saline) against the proportional increase in phagocytic index, it was clear that there was a good correlation between the two.

We have also applied another method for detecting activation of the macrophage by anaerobic coryneform organisms. This method was developed in chickens and is an adaptation of the method of Myrvik *et al.* (1961) for obtaining alveolar macrophages for *in vitro* study. In our method (Cater and White, to be published), 6 mg of heat-killed bacteria were injected intravenously into a 6- to 10-week-old chicken. This resulted in a rapid increase, reaching a maximum on about day 7, in the enzyme content of macrophages, which were washed out of the lungs by tracheal perfusion post-mortem. We estimated acid phosphatase, β-D-glucuronidase, β-D-galactosidase, and phospholipase-A activity in the lysed macrophages. The increase in enzymes was partly accounted for by the increase in numbers and partly (up to twofold) by increase in enzyme content per cell.

In later experiments, it was found simpler to homogenize the whole lung and estimate enzyme levels on an aliquot. In such a test, 6 mg of heat-killed *Mycobacterium avium* uniformly produced, after intravenous injection, about a tenfold increase in acid phosphatase over that shown by saline-injected contemporaneous control birds (Table I). Other acid hydrolases, such as β-glucuronidase, β-galacturonidase, and phospholipase A increased in a similar ratio.

The test provides a rapid method for surveying the ability of anaerobic coryneforms and other bacteria to provoke the appearance of increased numbers of activated macrophages. Table I also includes the results of intravenously injecting a suspension of carbon particles. Assuming they are chemically inert, it was hoped that they might provide an indication of the metabolic activation which is merely a response to phagocytosis.

It can be seen that the responses to a variety of anaerobic coryneform organisms are scattered over a wide range, some—such as *P. avidum* 4982— providing responses which approach that of *M. avium* and others—such as *C. parvum* C—which are only just above the "carbon threshold." The degree of correlation between stimulation of enzyme increases (acid phosphatase) and phagocyte indices is shown in Fig. 1 (correlation coefficient $r = 0.74$; $P = 0.0006$).

This ability to activate the enzymes of macrophages or to realize an increase in the phagocytic index may, or may not, depend upon a direct interaction between the bacteria and the cells of the reticuloendothelial system. In the case of mycobacteria, which are outstanding in their ability to increase the phagocytic index, to cause macrophage proliferation, and to increase the cell content of hydrolases, it has been argued that the stimulation is mainly an indirect effect of the bacteria causing a stimulation of a population of T cells and increased cell-mediated hypersensitivity (White, 1971).

In the case of the anaerobic coryneforms, the same question was approached

Table I. Pulmonary Acid-Phosphatase Levels in Chickens, 6 Days after an Intravenous Injection of Different Heat-Killed Microorganisms

Genus	Organism or particle	Serological group	Acid-phosphatase K.A. units/ml	Mean
Mycobacteria	M. avium		220 235 260	238
Anaerobic coryneform	P. avidum 4982	4	186 195 209	196
	C. parvum 3085	1	160 165 174	166
	P. avidum 0589	4	156 161 170	162
	C. anaerobium 578	2	130 150 170	150
	C. parvum 0208	1	110 130 135	125
	C. liquefaciens 814	1	85 105 165	118
	C. parvum 1383	1	100 109 120	109
	C. parvum B	0	85 100 105	96
	C. parvum 6294	1	65 65 150	83

Table I continued

Genus	Organism or particle	Serological group	Acid-phosphatase K. A. units/ml	Mean
	P. granulosum 0507	3	68.7 74.3 65.3	69
	C. parvum 6292	2	52 59 72	61
	C. parvum C	3	20.2 33.4 36.1	30
	Carbon suspension		58.93 54.51 60.37	57.9
Classical propionibacteria	*P. freudenreichii* 10470		35 45 45	41.6
	P. jensenii 5960		30 24 32	28.6
	P. rubrum 8901		27 20 30	25.6
	P. arabinosum 5958		15 19 25	19.6
	Saline		20 16 22	19.6

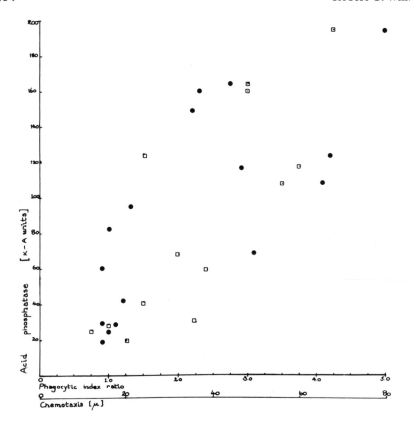

Fig. 1. Correlation between values obtained in measurements of chemotaxis and the increase in levels of acid phosphatase in the chicken lung, using different stains of anaerobic coryneforms. ● Solid dots: correlation phagocyte index and acid phosphatase. □ Open squares: correlation chemotaxis and acid phosphatase.

by an *in vitro* test for chemotactic activity (Wilkinson *et al.*, 1973). The test makes use of a type of double chamber separated by a millipore membrane, which Boyden developed for the measurement of chemotaxis by granulocytes (Boyden, 1962). However, instead of using a membrane with a 2-μm pore size, one designed to allow the transit of macrophages (8-μm pore size) was used.

Stimulation of chemotaxis occurred with organisms from each of the four groups of anaerobic coryneforms (Table II). The classical propionibacteria organisms (*P. freudenreichii, P. jensenii, P. rubrum,* and *P. arabinosum*) all failed to stimulate chemotaxis. As seen from the results at two levels of bacterial num-

Table II. Chemotactic Activity of Anaerobic Corynebacteria and Propionibacteria for Guinea Pig Peritoneal Macrophages[a]

Strain	Microns migrated toward bacterial suspension[b]	
	1500×10^6 organisms/ml	1500×10^4 organisms/ml
Group I: (*P. acnes* group)		
C. parvum 0208	20	40
C. parvum 3085	30	90
C. parvum 1383	20	120
C. liquefaciens 814	120	30
P. acnes 737 (VPI. No. 0389)	60	50
C. parvum A	30	50
Group II:		
C. diphtheroides 2764	100	10
C. anaerobium 578	90	40
C. parvum 10390[c]	30	30
C. parvum B	40	20
Group III: (*P. granulosum* group)		
C. parvum 10387	60	40
C. parvum C	30	60
P. granulosum 0507	40	40
Group IV: (*P. avidum* group)		
P. avidum 0575	70	50
P. avidum 4982	40	120
P. avidum 0589	30	90
Classical propionibacteria:		
P. freudenreichii	30	30
P. jensenii	20	N/T[d]
P. rubrum	20	10
P. arabinosum	30	20
Negative control, Gey's solution	20	
Positive control, casein 5 mg/ml	140	

[a]Data from Wilkinson *et al.* (1973). No plasma or serum were added to the tests shown in this table. The strain numbers of the bacteria in this table are numbers given by the Virginia Polytechnic Institute, by the Institut Pasteur, or by Burroughs Wellcome Co. The original sources can be learned from Table I in Johnson and Cummins (1972) and Table I in O'Neill *et al.* (1973).

[b]Chemotactic migration of macrophages; microns migrated through 8 μm filter in 130 min. Tests giving 10–30 microns migration are considered negative, 40–50 microns weakly positive, and 60 microns and above, unequivocally positive. Results are mean migration to the nearest 10 microns.

[c]A batch of *C. parvum* 10390 originally tested was strongly positive, but this result could not be repeated with subsequent batches.

[d]N/T = not tested.

bers, there was not a simple dose—response relationship. When the summed chemotactic effects at the two concentrations was plotted against the phagocytic index, a significant correlation was shown between the two functions ($P = 0.005$; correlation coefficient $r = 0.66$). Also, as seen in Fig. 1, a good correlation was apparent between the ability to increase acid phosphatase in the lung macrophages and the ability to increase chemotaxis ($P = 0.0004$; correlation coefficient $r = 0.79$).

It is noteworthy that the effect of the anaerobic coryneforms on chemotaxis *in vitro* represents a direct and a specific effect, i.e., direct in the sense that the effect occurred without the necessity for the presence of serum or plasma in the system, and specific in the sense that these organisms did not show chemotactic activity toward granulocytes. The chemical and physical characteristics of the chemotactic factor produced by anaerobic coryneforms and the conditions relating to its production in culture are discussed in a subsequent paper in this volume by Dr. P. C. Wilkinson.

Where we compared mycobacteria and the anaerobic coryneforms for their ability to exert chemotaxis, interesting differences were found. Until recently, mycobacteria failed to promote evidence of a chemotactic action on macrophages. Harris (1953) had found that macrophages responded to the same bacterial stimuli as granulocytes and that *Mycobacterium tuberculosis* strain H_{37} R_a attracted both types of cells equally. In contrast, Schär (1955) found that *M. tuberculosis* provided no direct chemotactic attraction for macrophages. She studied several constituents, including phosphatides, polysaccharides, and chloroform-soluble waxes. Phosphatide and wax fractions from a number of strains of *M. tuberculosis* showed weak leukotactic activity only at high concentrations. Meier and Schär (1957) later confirmed that polysaccharides from bovine strains of *M. tuberculosis* and from *Mycobacterium leprae* were not chemotactic for macrophages. More recently, Symon found that *M. tuberculosis* could exert a strong chemotactic effect for macrophages, providing that the test was set up in *plasma* (Symon *et al.*, 1972). Mycobacteria were found to attract macrophages more strongly than granulocytes. When tested in the absence of plasma, *M. tuberculosis* had virtually no ability to attract macrophages and, presumably, complement components are required for such plasma-dependent chemotaxis. The unique ability of the anaerobic coryneforms to activate macrophages for chemotaxis may provide a rapid biological test which could be immensely useful as a preliminary stage for defining the nature and source of a biological activity relating to the limitation of tumor growth.

All the foregoing tests stress the specific and positive stimulatory role of the anaerobic coryneforms for macrophages. To consider their biological effects, it may help to compare them with mycobacteria.

Like the mycobacteria, the anaerobic coryneforms have been reported to produce adjuvant effects on serum-antibody levels. We found these effects to be unimpressive when compared to mycobacteria. We tested the anaerobic coryneforms as adjuvants for the antibody response to sheep red cells in mice, for the response to human serum albumin in chickens, and for the response to ovalbumin in guinea pigs (O'Neill *et al.*, 1973). Only in guinea pigs did we find a convincing adjuvant effect on the serum-antibody levels. Three weeks after a single injection of antigen in water-in-oil emulsion with varying doses (200 μg, 1 mg, 2.5 mg dry weight) of anaerobic coryneforms, anti-ovalbumin levels were 2 and 3 times the control values for the two lower doses used (Table III). On immunoelectrophoresis of the guinea pig sera and after developing the precipitin arcs of the separated serum proteins against ovalbumin, almost all the antibody appeared as γ_1. Thus, there was little or no stimulation of the γ_2-precipitin arc, which is a characteristic feature of the adjuvant effect (at 3 weeks) of mycobacteria in complete Freund-type adjuvant (White *et al.*, 1963). This finding agrees with the fact that, after use of anaerobic coryneforms in the guinea pig, no elevation of antibody was detectable by complement fixation (Table III); it has been established that this test detects γ_2-immunoglobulin under these circumstances (Benacerraf *et al.*, 1963).

The guinea pig was also used for detecting the bacteria's ability to stimulate T cells and increase cell-mediated hypersensitivity. Thus, both intracorneal tests and skin tests (with 10 μg and 50 μg ovalbumin) were done 20 days after a single (footpad) injection of various coryneforms with ovalbumin in water-in-oil emulsion. Mycobacteria, in doses of 200 μg to 1 mg (dry weight), uniformly induced a strongly positive corneal test (cornea at 24 or 48 h was grossly thickened, grey, and opaque over whole extent) and strong delayed-type skin responses. In the case of the animals injected with anaerobic coryneforms (the strains used were those shown in Table III) from each of the four serological groups, the sizes of the intradermal skin responses read at 24 and 48 h did not differ from controls, and the corneal tests were uniformly negative to ovalbumin—after use of all the six strains in dosage of 200 μg, 1 mg, and 2.5 mg. Thus, in sharp contrast to mycobacteria, anaerobic coryneforms failed to stimulate cell-mediated hypersensitivity in the guinea pig. These results conflict with those obtained by Neveu *et al.* (1964), who claimed to produce a delayed-hypersensitivity effect equivalent to that of *Mycobacterium butyricum* by using picrylated HSA in the guinea pig. The comparative results of these and other tests using guinea pigs stimulated with mycobacteria and guinea pigs stimulated with anaerobic coryneforms are shown in Table IV.

The activity of mycobacteria when injected in water-in-oil emulsion characteristically results in the development of a slowly-evolving granuloma of complex histology and organization. The main cells are epithelioid cells which have developed from bone-marrow-derived monocytes and giant cells. In its latter stages (after 3–4 weeks), the granuloma includes large numbers of lymphocytes, which become organized into nodules, some of which include well-structured germinal centers (e.g., in the bird). Plasma cells can be present in large numbers, e.g., in the bird and rabbit, but not in the guinea pig. There is always a component of necrosis.

The lack of any stimulatory effect of anaerobic coryneforms in cell-mediated

Table III. Precipitins by Radial-Immunodiffusion in Arbitrary Units and by Complement Fixation as Titers (log$_2$ Dilution)

Serological group	Dose of organisms				
		200 µg		1 mg	2.5 mg
		Precipitation[a]	CFT[a]	Precipitation[a]	Precipitation[a]
C. parvum 0208	(I)	122	1.6	182	124
C. parvum 10390	(II)		2	192	137
C. anaerobium 578	(II)			220	
C. parvum 10387	(III)	223	2		80
P. granulosum 0507	(III)	163	2.6		93
P. avidum 4982	(IV)				85
Contemporaneous controls		75	2	73	110

[a] Average of group of three or four animals

Table IV. Comparison of the Immunobiological Actions of Mycobacteria and Anaerobic Coryneforms

Adjuvant effect	Mycobacteria	Anaerobic coryneforms
Antibody		
Precipitin	+++ (up to fivefold)	+ (two- and threefold)
Ig	γ_2	γ_1
CFT	+++ (over fivefold)	−
Cytophilic γ_2 at 3 wk	+	−
α-glob at 7 days	+	−
Cell-mediated hypersensitivity		
Skin, guinea pig	+++	−
Cornea, guinea pig	+++	−
Granuloma	large, with necrosis mixed macrophages, epithelioid and giant cells, lymphoid foci with germinal centers	inconspicuous, no necrosis, macrophages
Macrocytostimulant effects		
Chemotaxis	no direct effect, indirect on neutrophils and macrophages	direct effect, specific for macrophage
Phagocytic index	+	+
Increase of acid hydrolases	+++	++ to ±

hypersensitivity should lead to histological differences between their granulomatous reaction and the reaction following the injection of mycobacteria. As described by O'Neill *et al.* (1973), the local site of injection in the footpad of guinea pigs receiving various anaerobic coryneforms in suspension in mineral oil became occupied by a relatively simple proliferation of macrophages. Control animals receiving the mineral-oil vehicle showed an accumulation of some macrophages with foamy cytoplasm around oil vesicles. Animals receiving, in addition, anaerobic coryneforms had a larger, more compact, granuloma consisting of dense sheets of macrophages surrounding oil vesicles. Such macrophages, although densely packed in masses of cells with polygonal outline, did not show epithelioid morphology. Giant cells were not seen, and necrosis was absent.

In summary, the evidence I have surveyed suggests that the anaerobic coryneforms produce their main effects by directly and specifically activating macrophages. They do not activate the thymus-derived lymphocytes and in this, and many other ways, differ sharply in action from the mycobacteria and nocardias. We therefore propose that the active principles for the respective biological effects of mycobacteria and anaerobic coryneforms reside in totally different types of chemical entities.

References

Benacerraf, B., Ovary, Z., Bloch, K. J., and Franklin, E. C. (1963). Properties of guinea pig 7S antibodies. I. Electrophoretic separation of two types of guinea pig 7S antibodies. *J. Exp. Med.* **117**:937.

Biozzi, G., Benacerraf, B., Stiffel, C., and Halpern, B. N. (1954). *C. R. Soc. Biol.* **148**:431.

Boyden, S. V. (1962). The chemotactic effect of mixtures of antibody and antigen on polymorphonuclear leukocytes. *J. Exp. Med.* **115**:453.

Cummins, C. S. and Harris, H. (1958). Studies on the cell-wall composition and taxonomy of *Actinomycetales* and related groups. *J. Gen. Microbiol.* **18**:173.

Cummins, C. S. and Johnson, J. L. (1974). *C. parvum,* a synonym for *P. acnes. J. Gen. Microbiol.* **80**:433.

Fisher, J. C., Grace, W. R., and Mannick, J. A. (1970). Effect of nonspecific immune stimulation with *Corynebacterium parvum* on patterns of tumor growth. *Cancer* **26**: 1379.

Halpern, B. N., Biozzi, G., Stiffel, C., and Mouton, D. (1966). Inhibition of tumor growth by administration of killed *Corynebacterium parvum. Nature (Lond.)* **212**:853.

Harris, H. (1953). Chemotaxis of monocytes. *Br. J. Exp. Pathol.* **34**:276.

Johnson, J. L. and Cummins, C. S. (1972). Cell-wall composition and desoxyribonucleic acid similarities among the anaerobic coryneforms, classical propionibacteria and strains of *Arachnia propionica. J. Bacteriol.* **109**:1047.

Meier, R. and Schär, B. (1957). Vorkommen leukocytotaktischer polysaccharide in bakteriellem, pflanzlichem und tierischem Ausgangsmaterial. *Z. Physiol. Chem.* **307**:103.

Myrvik, Q. N., Leake, E. S., and Fariss, B. (1961). Studies on pulmonary macrophages from the normal rabbit: a technique to procure them in a high state of purity. *J. Immunol.* **86**:128.

Neveu, T., Branellec, A., and Biozzi, G. (1964). Propriétés adjuvantes de *Corynebacterium parvum* sur l'induction de hypersensitivité retardée envers les protéines conjuguées. *Ann. Inst. Pasteur, Paris* **106**:771.

O'Neill, G. J., Henderson, D. C., and White, R. G. (1973). Role of anaerobic coryneforms in specific and nonspecific immunological reactions. I. Effect on particle clearance and humoral and cell-mediated immune responses. *Immunology* **24**:977.

Russell, R. J., McInroy, R. J., Wilkinson, P. C., and White, R. G. (1975). Identification of a lipid chemo-attractant (chemotactic) factor for macrophages from anaerobic coryneform bacteria. *Behringwerke Mitt.* (in press).

Schär, B. (1955). Effects of constituents of tubercle bacilli on leukocyte migration. Cited by Kradolfer, F. in *Ciba Foundation Symposium on Experimental Tuberculosis,* p. 65, (Wolstenholme, G. E. W. and Cameron, M. P., eds.) Churchill, London.

Smith, L. H. and Woodruff, M. F. A. (1968). Comparative effect of two strains of *Corynebacterium parvum* on phagocytic activity and tumor growth. *Nature (Lond.)* **219**:197.

Suter, E. and White, R. G. (1954). The response of the reticuloendothelial system to the injection of the "purified wax" and the lipopolysaccharide of tubercle bacilli. A histologic and an immunologic study. *Am. Rev. Tuberc.* **70**:793.

Symon, D. N. K., McKay, I. C., and Wilkinson, P. C. (1972). Plasma-dependent chemotaxis of macrophages towards *Mycobacterium tuberculosis* and other organisms. *Immunology* **22**:267.

Van Niel, C. B. (1928). *The Propionic Acid Bacteria.* Baissevain, Haarlem.

White, R. G. (1963). Factors affecting the antibody response. *Br. Med. Bull.* **19**:207.

White, R. G. (1965). The role of peptidoglycolipids of *M. tuberculosis* and related organisms in immunological adjuvance. In *Molecular and Cellular Basis of Antibody Formalin,* p. 71 (Šterzl, J., ed.), Czechoslovak Academy of Sciences, Prague.

White, R. G. (1967). Role of adjuvants in the production of delayed hypersensitivity. *Br. Med. Bull.* **23**:39.

White, R. G. (1971). Factors controlling the adjuvant of immunosuppressive actions of antigens in complete Freund-type mixtures. *Ann. Sclavo* **13**:821.

White, R. G., Jenkins, G. C., and Wilkinson, P. C. (1963). The production of skin-sensitizing antibody in the guinea pig. *Int. Arch. Allergy Appl. Immunol.* **22**:156.

Wilkinson, P. C., O'Neill, G. J., and Wapshaw, K. G. (1973). Role of anaerobic coryneforms in specific and nonspecific immunological reactions. II. Production of a chemotactic factor specific for macrophages. *Immunology* **24**:997.

16

Macrophage-Stimulating Effects of Anaerobic Coryneform Bacteria *in Vitro*

P. C. WILKINSON

Introduction

Studies of the potentially therapeutically useful biological effects of the anaerobic coryneform bacteria have centered on the ability of these organisms to protect the whole animal against tumors or infections and on their ability to act as immunological adjuvants. It has become apparent that these properties of anaerobic coryneform bacteria depend largely on their ability to stimulate the functions of cells of the mononuclear phagocyte system. However, whole animal models can only give limited information about the steps involved. Therefore, in this paper I wish to describe studies of the direct and immediate effects of these bacteria on mononuclear phagocytes *in vitro*.

Macrophage-Stimulating Substances

Macrophage-stimulating substances can be divided into two categories according to the nature and duration of their action. First, there are those

P. C. WILKINSON, Department of Bacteriology and Immunology, University of Glasgow, Glasgow G11 6 NT, Scotland, Departmental Publication No. 7414.

substances—such as glycogen—which, in the presence of complement, stimulate macrophages within a period of minutes or hours, as judged by lysosomal hydrolase release or chemotaxis *in vitro* or by mobilization of cells *in vivo*. The effects of such substances are not sustained, so that macrophage activity reverts to prestimulation levels within a few days. In the second category, into which the anaerobic coryneform bacteria fall, are those agents which likewise cause an immediate activation of mononuclear phagocytes, but whose action is sustained so that, after injection of the bacteria *in vivo,* increased numbers of "activated" macrophages may be observed at the site of injection for weeks afterward. Since, for biological activity *in vivo,* a sustained activation of macrophages is needed, only agents in this second category are likely to show immunological adjuvant or antitumor effects. Immediate activation may result from a cell-membrane mediated stimulation of intracytoplasmic events in mononuclear phagocytes following direct physical contact with the stimulating agent. With certain agents, the process seems to stop there, whereas with other agents, the membrane-mediated events are followed both by new protein synthesis and by cell division and differentiation. The molecular and cellular biology of this sequence of events is not the least bit clear.

Effects of Anaerobic Coryneforms

Before proceeding further, it is necessary to emphasize that in this paper we are not discussing the biological effects of a single organism named *Corynebacterium parvum.* Johnson and Cummins (1972) demonstrated that the term *C. parvum* was taxonomically imprecise. Bacteria bearing this name appear in each of several serologically distinct groups. Moreover, within the same serological group, organisms designated *C. parvum* appear side by side with organisms bearing other designations. Previous investigations in this laboratory have shown that many organisms from each of Johnson's and Cummins's groups I to IV activate macrophages, as judged by carbon clearance *in vivo* and chemotaxis *in vitro,* whereas the "classical" propionibacteria—derived from dairy products and often regarded as closely related to the anaerobic coryneforms—do not (O'Neill *et al.,* 1973; Wilkinson *et al.,* 1973b). The activities to be considered are common to the organisms named collectively the "anaerobic coryneform bacteria" by Johnson and Cummins (1972), but not to the aerobic corynebacteria, the propionibacteria, or the nocardias. Details of the individual strains of anaerobic coryneform bacteria which show these effects, and their sources, are given in an earlier publication from this laboratory (O'Neill *et al.,* 1973).

Starting with the observation of Halpern *et al.* (1964) that the injection of *C. parvum* into animals enables the reticuloendothelial system to clear subsequently injected carbon from the circulation much more rapidly than is possible in normal control animals, O'Neill *et al.* (1973) showed that enhancement of carbon clearance was a property of the majority of strains of the anaerobic coryneform group. The enhanced clearance was associated with the development of hepatosplenomegaly and with a great increase in the population of Kupffer cells in the liver. Furthermore, as described below, this measure of mononuclear phagocyte function *in vivo* could be correlated very well with other indices of macrophage stimulation measured *in vitro*.

In an investigation contemporaneous with that of O'Neill *et al.* (1973) and using the same bacteria, we were able to demonstrate a chemotactic factor in cultures and culture filtrates of many strains of the anaerobic coryneforms (Wilkinson *et al.*, 1973b). This factor was unusual among the numerous chemotactic factors described to date (Wilkinson, 1974a) inasmuch as, in a serum-free medium, it strongly attracted mononuclear phagocytes from all sources tested, i.e., human blood monocytes, mouse peritoneal and alveolar macrophages, and guinea pig peritoneal macrophages. However, it had almost no chemotactic effect on neutrophils or eosinophils. The correlation between chemotactic activity and the ability to enhance carbon clearance was very striking when different strains were tested (Fig. 1). Almost all of the anaerobic coryneform bacteria which had originally been derived from human skin or from other human sources and which were active in one test were also active in the other. This raises the possibility that, at the molecular level, the recognition mechanism for macrophage chemotaxis and for particle clearance might be very similar. The classical propionibacteria showed no activity in either test (Wilkinson *et al.*, 1973b). In the presence of plasma, the anaerobic coryneforms could be shown to generate some chemotactic activity for neutrophils, probably because they can activate complement through the alternative pathway (McBride *et al.*, 1975).

A third property of the anaerobic coryneform bacteria which has been investigated in our laboratory is the effect of these organisms on the lysosomal hydrolases of macrophages. The first type of experiment was designed to show how incubation of macrophages with the anaerobic coryneform bacteria for a short period *in vitro* would affect the levels of these enzymes in macrophages. Monocytes were taken from human peripheral blood, or peritoneal or alveolar macrophages from the guinea pig or mouse, and the cells were incubated for 1 h with a suspension or culture filtrate of the test organism. At the end of the incubation, the cells were lysed, and the amount of acid phosphatase, β-glucuronidase, and β-galactosidase present in the lysate was assayed, using appropriate controls, in terms of the quantity of substrate digested (Wilkinson *et al.*, 1973a). Compared with a control batch of cells incubated in the absence of bacteria, the anaerobic coryneforms caused an increase in the total content of available enzyme in mononuclear phagocytes during the short period of incubation. However, these bacteria had little effect on acid hydrolase levels in granulocytes (Wilkinson *et al.*, 1973a). A high proportion of the enzymes released from blood monocytes appears to be secreted into the extracellular medium. This was determined by incubating the monocytes with the bacterial factor, then removing the cells and assaying the quantity of free enzyme in the supernatant

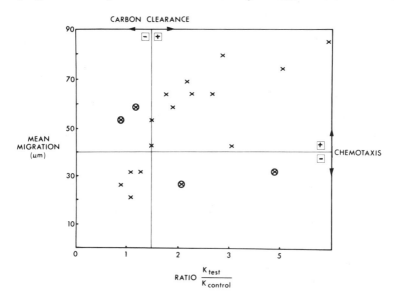

Fig. 1. Correlation of clearance-enhancing capacity of individual strains of anaerobic coryneforms with the chemotactic activity of the same strain. Each cross represents a single strain. Those organisms to the right of the vertical line are active in enhancing carbon clearance (K_{test} = 1.5 $\times$ $K_{control}$ or greater). Those above the horizontal line are active in macrophage chemotaxis (macrophage migration $>$40 μm in 130 min). Clearance tests were done in mice; chemotaxis tests were done using guinea pig macrophages. Fifteen out of 19 organisms fell either into the upper right-hand block (positive for both functions) or the lower left-hand block (negative for both functions: all of these 4 were classical propionibacteria, not anaerobic coryneforms). From Wilkinson *et al.* (1973b) and originally published in *Immunology*.

fluid. Since these procedures caused almost no increase in trypan-blue uptake by the monocytes, it was concluded that living monocytes were able to release lysosomal enzymes into the medium.

The second method of examining lysosomal hydrolase activity in macrophages was designed to explore long-term activation of these enzymes. The anaerobic coryneform bacteria were injected *in vivo*, either intravenously into chickens (White *et al.*, 1973) or intraperitoneally into mice or guinea pigs (Penney, McInroy, Cater, and Wilkinson, unpublished observations), and the levels of acid hydrolases were estimated in tissue macrophages (alveolar in chickens; peritoneal in mice and guinea pigs) at time intervals up to 3–4 weeks thereafter. These experiments showed that the enzyme content per cell increased gradually during this time period, so that the stimulated animal finished with a population of macrophages far more heavily armed with hydrolases several weeks after the injection of anaerobic coryneforms (and even more so after injection of myco-bacteria) than unstimulated animals. It is likely that this increase in acid hydrolase levels reflects a different process from that described above. Immedi-ate release of lysosomal enzymes from phagocytes is not inhibited by inhibitors of protein synthesis such as actinomycin and puromycin (Wilkinson, McKay, and Cater, in prep.) and probably results from mobilization of a preformed enzyme. The enzyme may exist in the normal cell in a lysosomal membrane-bound form which is not accessible to substrate, whereas activation causes the enzyme to be released in soluble form and to become immediately available to the substrate. However, over a period of several weeks *in vivo*, an increase in lysosomal hydrolase content in cells is likely to result not from release of preformed enzyme, but from synthesis of new enzyme. Compared with resting macro-phages, the macrophages taken three weeks after stimulation with coryneform bacteria or mycobacteria show an increased content of endoplasmic reticulum, as judged by electron microscopy (Cater and White, unpublished observations).

In defining the immediate effects of anaerobic coryneforms on macrophages *in vitro*, it is very advantageous to have a reliable, quick, and reproducible assay which measures macrophage stimulation. The measurement of chemotaxis has proved ideal for this purpose. It allows a reproducible determination of the activity of up to ten different organisms, or of fractions derived from them, using the same batch of cells on the same day. We now use human blood monocytes in all these experiments, since the blood monocyte is the cell whose function it is to respond to stimulation by emigration into the tissues, rather than using exudate macrophages—which have already performed this function and may be engaged in digestive activities which render them less capable of responding by locomotion to a renewed stimulus. Furthermore, the behavior of the human blood monocyte should be of more direct relevance than that of macrophages from other mammals when the properties of a group of organisms which are being used to treat human diseases are being considered.

The assay system used is a modification of the micropore-filter technique of Boyden (1962). Monocytes placed on top of a micropore filter (8-μm pore size) are allowed to migrate into the filter in response to factors derived from the anaerobic coryneforms which are placed in the lower chamber and allowed to diffuse through the filter toward the cells. The distance traveled by the leading front of macrophages in a gradient of the chemotactic substance during a fixed time is determined (Zigmond and Hirsch, 1973).

Using this assay, it has been possible to commence the task of determining the conditions under which anaerobic coryneforms produce macrophage-stimu-lating factors. The chemotactic factor is produced by the organisms during growth and begins to be released into the culture filtrate during the logarithmic growth phase (Wilkinson *et al.*, 1973b). This substance is soluble and diffusible. Only soluble factors are capable of exerting an effect in Boyden-type assays, where the monocytes and bacteria are physically separated from one another by a filter. Nevertheless, the close correlation between chemotactic-factor release and clearance enhancement by these organisms suggests that the same molecule which (when released from bacteria) activates migration of free macrophages, may (possibly when attached to the bacterial surface) interact with the membranes of fixed macrophages, e.g., Kupffer cells to enhance their clearance functions. Release of the chemotactic factor can be demonstrated from dead, as well as living, bacteria. Release does not depend on an energy-requiring secretion from the bacterial cell. If heat-killed lyophilized bacteria are suspended in a physiological medium and immediately tested for chemotactic activity, only weak activity is seen. However, if the organisms are left in suspension for a day or two at 4°C, the supernatant fluid becomes strongly active, indicating that the factor is being slowly released from the bacteria on storage. The chemotactic factor may, therefore, be superficially placed in the bacterial cell and loosely attached, so that it can be released easily without disruption of the architecture of the cell. It may be shown to diffuse through a dialysis membrane—but slowly—so that a proportion of the activity can be recovered from the dialysate after 2 days, which suggests that its molecular weight is not more than a few thousand. However, in attempting to define the size of the factor more accurately by permeation chromatography on Sephadex gels in physiological salt solutions, it was found that it behaved as a polydisperse substance. Chemotactic activity could be recovered from a whole range of fractions, with calculated molecular weights between 100,000 and 5000 or less daltons. This suggests that individual molecules of the factor readily form complexes, either with each other or with other molecules released from the bacteria. The chemotactic activity of culture filtrates of anaerobic coryneforms can be reduced by incubation with proteolytic enzymes, such as trypsin or chymotrypsin (Table I). This suggests that the active fraction contains a peptide moiety, although it is quite possible that the peptide may be linked to nonpeptide molecules—such as lipid or polysaccharide.* This factor is released by the anaerobic coryneforms, but not by other organisms—such as the aerobic corynebacteria, mycobacteria, or the nocardias. Those organisms may activate chemotaxis, but only indirectly by their action on serum complement (Symon *et al.*, 1972), and their action is not macrophage specific since they also attract neutrophils. We feel that the release of this factor, which possesses unique macrophage-stimulating actions *in vitro*, is likely to be relevant to—and possibly a prerequisite for—long-term macrophage activation and the enhanced ability of macrophages to kill target cells *in vivo*.

These experiments, therefore, suggest that the anaerobic coryneform bacteria stimulate macrophages on direct contact by virtue of possession of a molecule, or molecules, with unusual physicochemical properties, which may be released under physiological conditions from the bacterial cell. It is likely that this molecule possesses an affinity for macrophage membranes. A study of the

*See *Note Added in Proof,* p. 170.

Table I. Effects of Treating a Culture Filtrate of *Corynebacterium anaerobium* with Enzymes on Its Chemotactic Activity for Guinea Pig Peritoneal Macrophages

Treatment of culture filtrate (all enzymes tested at 500 μg/ml)	Macrophage migration (μm in 130 min in 8-μm pore size filter)
No treatment	95
Trypsin (30 min)	66
Trypsin (4 h)	58
α-Chymotrypsin (30 min)	88
α-Chymotrypsin (4 h)	73
Ribonuclease	96

molecular nature of chemotactic proteins and their interactions with cell membranes has beeen made in this laboratory (Wilkinson and McKay, 1971, 1972; Wilkinson, 1973, 1974b). These molecules were shown to contain solvent-exposed hydrophobic sites which have an affinity for and are available to interact with the hydrophobic interior of the phospholipid bilayer of the phagocytic cell membrane. Such molecules are usually more surface-active at water–air interfaces than typical, folded, native proteins. It is possible that by interacting with the membrane bilayer, such proteins can activate actin–myosin interactions in microfilaments. These interactions are certainly important in cell locomotion and in the release of secretory granules from many types of cells (Huxley, 1973). However, the macrophage-activating factor from the anaerobic coryneforms has not yet been purified sufficiently to determine directly whether it acts by the mechanism suggested above.

To perform effectively, the mononuclear phagocyte must be able to respond immediately to stimulation by migration, by phagocytosis, and by release of digestive enzymes. These events probably all involve the activation of microfilaments or microtubules, or similar intracytoplasmic contractile structures and may all, therefore, be initiated by interactions of appropriate stimulants with the cell membrane. However, having achieved these immediate functions, the macrophage may become temporarily depleted of hydrolases and other substances essential for further effective responses. The cells may then go into a quiescent phase while they rebuild their digestive machinery. Following a period of increased protein synthesis, differentiation, and cell division, a population of macrophages may emerge which is more effective functionally than the population from which the macrophages originated. It is probable that macrophage activation by the anaerobic coryneforms requires such a sequence of events. It is probably also necessary that new macrophages be continuously recruited, so that conditions resembling those described in "high-turnover granulomata" (Spector and Ryan, 1970) are created. It is not yet possible to explain these events in molecular terms. When well-defined macrophage-activating factors from the anaerobic coryneform bacteria become available in a pure state, they will serve as useful tools for exploring long-term macrophage activation under better defined conditions than are presently available.

Summary

The anaerobic coryneform bacteria produce and release a factor, or factors, which stimulate the activity of mononuclear phagocytes *in vitro*. Among the functions stimulated by this factor are chemotaxis and release of lysosomal acid hydrolases. Stimulation of these functions can be correlated with enhancement of particle clearance *in vivo*. Human blood monocytes and peritoneal and alveolar macrophages from mice or guinea pigs are all stimulated on contact with the anaerobic coryneforms. It is suggested that a factor—at present poorly characterized, but possibly partly peptide in nature—released from this group of bacteria, has an affinity for the mononuclear phagocyte-cell membrane and can thus activate contractile events in the cell which are necessary for locomotion and exocytosis or endocytosis. Following this short-term activation, the macrophages show enhanced protein synthesis and differentiation in the long term. The mode of action of the anaerobic coryneforms in activating these long-term changes is not understood.

Acknowledgments

This work was supported by Grant No. 972/200/B from the Medical Research Council.

References

Boyden, S. V. (1962). The chemotactic effect of mixtures of antibody and antigen on polymorphonuclear leukocytes. *J. Exp. Med.* **115**:453.

Halpern, B. N., Prévot, A. R., Biozzi, G., Stiffel, C., Mouton, D., Morard, J. C., Bouthillier, Y., and Decreusefond, C. (1964). Stimulation de l'activité phagocytaire du système réticuloendothéliale provoquée par *Corynebacterium parvum. J. Reticuloendothel. Soc.* **1**:77.

Huxley, H. E. (1973). Muscular contraction and cell motility. *Nature (Lond.)* **243**:445.

Johnson, J. L. and Cummins, C. W. (1972). Cell-wall compositions and deoxyribonucleic acid similarities among the anaerobic coryneforms, classical propionibacteria and strains of *Arachnia propionica. J. Bacteriol.* **109**:1047.

McBride, W. H., Weir, D. M., Kay, A. B., Pearce, D., and Caldwell, J. R. (1975). Activation of the classical and alternate pathways of complement by *Corynebacterium parvum*. *Clin. Exp. Immunol.* **19**:143.

O'Neill, G. J., Henderson, D. C., and White, R. G. (1973). Role of anaerobic coryneforms in specific and nonspecific immunological reactions. I. Effect on particle clearance and humoral and cell-mediated immune responses. *Immunology* **24**:977.

Spector, W. G. and Ryan, G. B. (1970). The mononuclear phagocyte in inflammation. In: *Mononuclear Phagocytes*, p. 219, (R. van Furth, ed.), Blackwell, Oxford and Edinburgh.

Symon, D. N. K., McKay, I. C., and Wilkinson, P. C. (1972). Plasma-dependent chemotaxis of macrophages towards *Mycobacterium tuberculosis* and other organisms. *Immunology* **22**:267.

White, R. G., O'Neill, G. J., Henderson, D. C., Cater, J., and Wilkinson, P. C. (1973). The adjuvant activity of "*Corynebacterium parvum*" in specific and nonspecific immunity. In: *Nonspecific Factors Influencing Host Resistance*, p. 285 (W. Braun and J. Ungar, eds.), Karger, Basel.

Wilkinson, P. C. (1973). Recognition of protein structure in leukocyte chemotaxis. *Nature (Lond.)* **244**:512.

Wilkinson, P. C. (1974a). *Chemotaxis and Inflammation*, Churchill-Livingstone, Edinburgh.

Wilkinson, P. C. (1974b). Surface and cell-membrane activities of leukocyte chemotactic factors. *Nature (Lond.)* **251**:58.

Wilkinson, P. C. and McKay, I. C. (1971). The chemotactic activity of native and denatured serum albumin. *Int. Arch. Allergy Appl. Immunol.* **41**:237.

Wilkinson, P. C. and McKay, I. C. (1972). The molecular requirements for chemotactic attraction of leukocytes by proteins. Studies of proteins with synthetic side groups. *Eur. J. Immunol.* **2**:570.

Wilkinson, P. C., O'Neill, G. J., McInroy, R. J., Cater, J. C., and Roberts, J. A. (1973a). Chemotaxis of macrophages: the role of a macrophage-specific cytotaxin from anaerobic corynebacteria and its relation to immunopotentiation *in vivo*. In: *Immunopotentiation*, p. 121 (G. E. Wolstenholme and J. Knight, eds.), Associated Scientific Publishers, Amsterdam.

Wilkinson, P. C., O'Neill, G. J., and Wapshaw, K. G. (1973b). Role of anaerobic coryneforms in specific and nonspecific immunological reactions. II. Production of a chemotactic factor specific for macrophages. *Immunology* **24**:997.

Zigmond, S. H. and Hirsch, J. G. (1973). Leukocyte locomotion and chemotaxis. New methods for evaluation and demonstration of cell-derived chemotactic factor. *J. Exp. Med.* **137**:387.

Note Added in Proof. Chemotactic activity has recently been isolated in a lipid fraction released from anaerobic coryneforms, which does not contain peptide [Russell, R. J., McInroy, R. J., Wilkinson, P. C., and White, R. G. (1975). *Behringwerke Mitt.*, in press].

DISCUSSION

BOMFORD: Dr. Halpern found that macrophages from mice treated with *Corynebacterium parvum* exhibit cytostatic activity against tumor cells *in vitro*. Together with Massimo Olivotto at Beckenham, I obtained similar results using an almost identical system in which the macrophages were grown as a monolayer on the bottom of a Petri dish, and the target tumor cells—syngenic lymphoma cells—were grown in suspension [Olivotto M. and Bomford R. (1974). *Int. J. Cancer* **13**:478].

Recently, together with George Christie, we have been approaching the problem of the mechanism of macrophage activation by *C. parvum* (Christie and Bomford, manuscript submitted for publication). This afternoon's presentations made mention of two materials in *C. parvum* which may be capable of activating macrophages in some way by direct contact—the phospholipid discussed by Dr. Fauve and the chemotactic material discussed by Dr. Wilkinson.

We wished, to discover whether macrophages could be induced to show antitumor activity by simple contact with *C. parvum*. We suspected this not to be the case because it had already been mentioned by Alexander and Evans at the Ciba Symposium on Immunopotentiation that this could not be done. This was also our experience. We could discover no conditions under which exposing normal macrophages to *C. parvum* activated them to show a cytostatic action against tumor cells. However, we were able to bring about activation by exposing macrophages to *C. parvum* and immune lymphocytes from the spleens of mice sensitized to *C. parvum*.

I think this is an expected result. Other workers have published data showing macrophage activation by products of sensitized lymphocytes [Evans and Alexander (1970). *Nature (Lond.)* **228**:620; Godal *et al.* (1971). *Clin. Exp. Immunol.* **8**:625]. Clearly, we are not seeing a phenomenon which is unique to

C. parvum. However, we have evidence that macrophage activation also by *C. parvum in vivo* proceeds by an immunological pathway.

Summarizing this evidence, in mice previously sensitized to *C. parvum* and are then resensitized, there was a recall effect in macrophage activation—it occurred more rapidly. Also, the spleen cells of these mice were able to mediate macrophage activation earlier *in vitro*. The converse experiment was to use T-cell-depleted mice. In this situation, the time course of macrophage activation appeared normal, but there was a delay in the ability of spleen cells to mediate activation *in vitro*. We are not certain why T-cell depletion failed to affect macrophage activation. Either there were sufficient residual T cells to mediate activation, or there was a direct nonimmunological mechanism of macrophage activation by *C. parvum* operating *in vivo* which we could detect *in vitro*.

17

Comparative Studies on the Effect of *Corynebacterium parvum* on Bone-Marrow Cell Colony Formation *in Vitro*

NIKOLAI V. DIMITROV, SIMONNE ANDRE,
GEORGE ELIOPOULOS, and BERNARD HALPERN

Introduction

Bone-marrow cells are able to proliferate in agar cultures and form distinct colonies of granulocytes or macrophages if stimulated by the colony-stimulating factor (Bradley and Metcalf, 1966; Metcalf, 1970; Pike and Robinson, 1970; Paran and Sachs, 1968). This factor is necessary for the initiation and maintenance of colonies *in vitro* and probably as a regulator of granulopoiesis and monocyte formation *in vivo*. Colony-stimulating factor (CSF) is detectable in the serum and urine of normal mice and humans and appears to be unique for

NIKOLAI V. DIMITROV, Hahnemann Medical College, Philadelphia, Pa. SIMONNE ANDRE, GEORGES ELIOPOULOS, and BERNARD HALPERN, Institute of Immunobiology, Hospital Broussais, Paris, France.

This work was undertaken during the tenure (N.V.D.) of an American Cancer Society–Eleanor Roosevelt–International Cancer Fellowship, awarded by the International Union against Cancer.

the granulopoiesis and monocyte formation (Paran and Sachs, 1968; Price *et al.*, 1973; Paran *et al.*, 1968; Craddock *et al.*, 1973; Landau and Sachs, 1971). It has been extensively studied, and its activity, biochemical property, and inhibition have been determined (Robinson *et al.*, 1967; Ichikawa *et al.*, 1967; Stanley *et al.*, 1968; Stanley and Metcalf, 1969; Chan *et al.*, 1971).

Our study was undertaken to investigate the effect of *Corynebacterium parvum* on formation of colonies *in vitro* under different experimental conditions.

Materials and Methods

For all experiments, adult $C_{57}Bl$ mice (10–12 weeks old) were used. The agar bone-marrow culture (technique of Mintz and Sachs, 1973) was the most suitable technique for our experimental conditions. *C. parvum* was given i.p. (500 μg), and the bone-marrow cells and serum were collected after 4 h (one injection) and after 48 h (two injections with an interval of 24 h). For comparison, injections of endotoxin (30 μg, i.p.) were used, following the same schedule (Table I).

Procedure

Under nembutal anesthesia, the animals were bled through the angle of the eye followed by intracardiac aspiration. The bone marrow was obtained using the perfusion technique of the femur. The specimen was kept in Eagle's medium in the form of a well-dispersed suspension. Dialyzed, pooled mouse serum was used as the source of CSF. The condition of the bone-marrow culture has been previously described (Quesenberry *et al.*, 1972).

Table I. Experimental Groups of Adult $C_{57}Bl$ Mice

Group	Treatment
I	Control animals for serum and bone marrow
II	Vaccination (one injection *C. parvum* or endotoxin) Collection of serum or bone marrow 4 h later
III	Vaccination (two injections of *C. parvum* or endotoxin) at a 24-h interval Collection of serum or bone marrow 48 h after the first injection

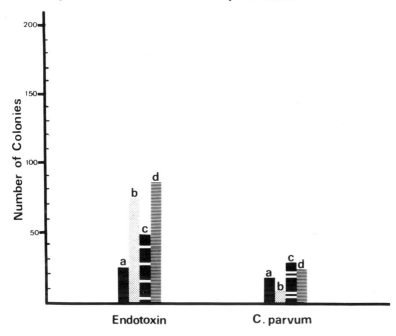

Fig. 1. Mean values of three experiments for controls and mice injected with a single 500-μg i.p. dose of *Corynebacterium parvum* or 5-μl i.p. dose of endotoxin. (a) Bone marrow and serum from nontreated animals; (b) bone marrow from nontreated animals and serum from treated animals; (c) bone marrow from treated animals and serum from nontreated animals; and (d) bone marrow and serum from treated animals.

Each experiment consisted of four combinations: (1) bone marrow and serum from nontreated animals (control); (2) bone marrow from nontreated animals and serum from animals treated with *C. parvum* or endotoxin; (3) bone marrow from animals treated with *C. parvum* or endotoxin and serum from nontreated animals; and (4) bone marrow and serum from animals treated with *C. parvum* or endotoxin.

Colonies were counted after 7 days and included only clusters with 50 or more cells. In order to obtain time curves in the same experiments, the counting of the colonies was done daily thereafter.

Results

The optimal experimental conditions for this study had been determined previously (Dimitrov *et al.*, 1975). The results from the first group showed that the numbers of colonies in all the experiments were similar to the control (Fig. 1). There was no significant effect of *C. parvum*, either on the colony-forming cells or on the CSF when the specimens were taken 4 h after a single injection with the vaccine. On the other hand, specimens taken 4 h after a single injection with endotoxin showed a significant increase in the number of colonies when the serum of these animals was used as a source of CSF (Fig. 1). No significant changes were noted when the bone marrow of the same animal was cultured in the presence of normal serum. Increased numbers of colonies were formed when the bone-marrow culture was done with bone-marrow cells and serum from animals injected with a single dose of endotoxin.

The results from the second group showed that serum from mice with two injections of *C. parvum* exhibited a certain inhibitory effect on colony formation in cultures using normal mouse bone marrow (Fig. 2). Identical experiments performed with serum from mice receiving endotoxin showed slight increases in the number of colonies. In another combination, serum from normal mice and bone marrow from mice injected with *C. parvum*, the number of the colonies was significantly increased (Fig. 2). Such stimulation was not observed in the corresponding group of mice injected with endotoxin. An increase in colony formation to a lesser degree was present in cultures with bone marrow and serum obtained from mice treated with *C. parvum*. The count of colonies was significantly higher than with serum and bone marrow from animals injected with two doses of endotoxin. The relationship between time and the appearance of colonies was observed by daily counting of the colonies (Table II).

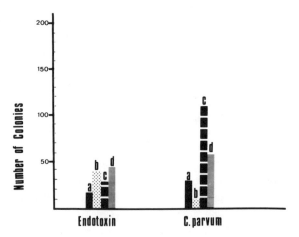

Fig. 2. Mean values of three experiments for controls and mice injected with two 500-μg i.p. doses of *Corynebacterium parvum* or two 30-μl i.p. doses of endotoxin at an interval of 24 h. (a) Bone marrow and serum from nontreated animals; (b) bone marrow from nontreated animals and serum from treated animals; (c) bone marrow from treated animals and serum from nontreated animals; and (d) bone marrow and serum from treated animals.

Table II. The Relationship between Time and the Appearance of Colonies

	Day 1	Day 2	Day 3	Day 4	Day 5	Day 6	Day 7	Day 8
Normal control (number of colonies)	—	4	2	21	33	42	43	43
Bone marrow from animals injected with *C. parvum* (number of colonies)	—	1	1	5	27	71	152	163

Bone-marrow cultures using normal bone-marrow cells and normal serum as a source of CSF were compared to cultures containing bone-marrow cells obtained from animals previously injected with *C. parvum* (two injections) and normal serum as a source of CSF. The colony-forming capacity during the first two days was minimal and similar in both groups. A slight increase was noted on the third day and was found to be more pronounced on days 4 and 5. During this period of time, the number of colonies in cultures with normal bone marrow was significantly higher than in the cultures with bone marrow obtained from mice injected with *C. parvum*. After the fifth day, the number of colonies in the normal bone-marrow cultures did not change and remained level until the termination of the culture. The number of colonies in cultures with bone marrow from mice injected with *C. parvum* continued to increase, and on the seventh day, the colony count showed more than a threefold increase. The counting of the colonies was discontinued after day 8 because many colonies aggregate and the count becomes inaccurate.

Discussion

The results of this study show that the colony-forming cells undergo a rapid expansion in bone-marrow cultures when the donor animal is pretreated with *C. parvum*. The enhancement effect of *C. parvum* on bone-marrow cultures appears to be rather unique. A single intraperitoneal injection of *C. parvum* has no effect on CSF or on bone-marrow cells. On the other hand, a single intraperitoneal injection of endotoxin is capable of stimulating the activity of CSF. The latter finding has been described by other investigators, and endotoxin has been used for stimulation of CSF before the serum is used in culture (Craddock *et al.*, 1973; Metcalf, 1971; Quesenberry *et al.*, 1972).

It appears that the mechanism of the effect of endotoxin differs substantially from that of *C. parvum*. This difference was more pronounced in the experiments in which two injections were used and the marrow collected 24 h after the second injection (Fig. 2). Use of serum from animals treated with *C. parvum* as a source of CSF resulted in inhibition of colony formation, an effect which was not seen in experiments with serum obtained from animals pretreated with endotoxin. The mechanism of the inhibitory effect of *C. parvum* on the activity of CSF is not clear. It is possible that *C. parvum* binds to the CSF and forms a protein complex which is not capable of exercising a stimulating activity in bone-marrow cultures. It has been shown that the active fraction of the CSF is a glycoprotein which may be altered, losing its biological properties when the vaccine is present in the serum of the experimental animals. We have performed experiments with dialyzed serum, both from controls and from animals treated with *C. parvum,* and found no difference in the activity when compared to experiments with nondialyzed serum. The inhibitory effect of *C. parvum* in the treated groups remained unchanged.

The significant increase in the number of colonies when bone-marrow cells from pretreated animals were cultured in the presence of no normal serum indicated that *C. parvum* had a direct effect on the colony-forming cells of the bone marrow. This effect appears to be delayed and is probably dose-dependent (after two injections). The cells present in the colonies are monocytes and granulocytes, with a preponderance of monocytes. In some preliminary experiments we replaced serum as a source of CSF with supernatant of macrophage homogenate obtained after peritoneal washing. The stimulating effect of *C. parvum* was also present in these experiments. One may speculate that the direct effect of *C. parvum* could be on the monocyte and its precursors. More information is needed if we are to draw further conclusions concerning the mechanism of action and the elective effect of this vaccine.

The stimulation of colony formation is a time-related process and occurred after the fifth day after initiation of the cultures. This indicates that the colony-forming cells require a certain time for adaptation to *in vitro* conditions.

The results of these experiments opened many questions regarding the maximum activity of the CSF and the precursor cells capable of forming colonies. The fundamental questions to be answered are whether the stimulating activity is stable and when the optimal effect of *C. parvum* occurs. This will require additional experiments with cells collected several days after the last injection.

The enhancement effect of some other antigens on precursors of bone-marrow cells capable of forming colonies *in vitro* mediated through CSF has been reported by Metcalf (1971) and McNeill (1970). Bacterial endotoxin, heterologous erythrocytes, and bacterial flagellum preparations are capable of stimulating colony formation in normal mouse bone-marrow cultures (McNeill, 1970). The effect of these antigens is mostly on the CSF and shows a rise in colony-stimulating activity very soon after a single intravenous injection (Metcalf, 1971; McNeill, 1970). Our results differ substantially from the results of Metcalf and McNeill, probably because of the involvement of different mechanisms and, to a certain degree, because of differences in experimental conditions. We injected *C. parvum* intraperitoneally, whereas they used intravenous injections of various antigens. Similar results were reported by Wolmark and Fisher (1974), using subcutaneous injections of *C. parvum* in tumor-bearing mice.

Whatever the mechanism of action, the most important information obtained from this study is that *C. parvum* can stimulate bone-marrow cells capable of proliferation. This finding suggests that the vaccine may be used as a valuable adjuvant during radiation or chemotherapy, which may result in a well-known side effect—myelodepression. This suggestion deserves further experimentation with *C. parvum* for more conclusive information and practical application.

References

Bradley, T. R. and Metcalf, D. (1966). The growth of mouse bone-marrow cells *in vitro*. *Aust. J. Exp. Biol. Med. Sci.* **44**:287–299.

Chan, S. H., Metalf, D., and Stanley, E. R. (1971). Stimulation and inhibition by normal human serum of colony formation *in vitro* by bone-marrow cells. *Br. J. Haematol.* **20**:329.

Craddock, C. G., Hays, E. F., Forsen, N. R., and Rodensky, D. (1973). Granulocyte–monocyte colony forming capacity of human marrow: a clinical study. *Blood* **42**:711–720.

Dimitrov, N. V., Andre, S., Eliopoulus, G., and Halpern, B. (1975). Effect of *Corynebacterium parvum* on bone-marrow cultures. *Proc. Soc. Exp. Biol. Med.* **148**:440–442.

Ichikawa, Y., Pluznik, D. H., and Sachs, L. (1967). Feedback inhibition of the development of macrophages and granulocytes colonies. Inhibition by macrophages and granulocyte colonies. Inhibition by macrophages. *Proc. Natl. Acad. Sci. USA* **58**:1480.

Landau, T. and Sachs, L. (1971). Characterization of the inducer required for the development of macrophage and granulocyte colonies. *Proc. Natl. Acad. Sci. USA* **68**:2540–2544.

McNeill, T. A. (1970). Antigenic stimulation of bone-marrow colony forming cells *in vitro*. *Immunology* **18**:39–48.

Metcalf, D. (1970). Studies on colony formation *in vitro* by mouse bone-marrow cells. II. Action of colony stimulating factor. *J. Cell. Comp. Physiol.* **76**:89–100.

Metcalf, D. (1971). Antigen-induced proliferation *in vitro* of bone-marrow precursors of granulocytes and macrophages. *Immunology* **20**:727–738.

Mintz, U. and Sachs, L. (1973). Difference in inducing activity of human bone-marrow colonies in normal serum and serum from patients with leukemia. *Blood* **42**:331–339.

Paran, M. and Sachs, L. (1968). The continued requirement for inducer for the development of granulocyte and macrophages colonies. *J. Cell. Comp. Physiol.* **72**:247.

Paran, M., Ichikawa, Y., and Sachs, L. (1968). Production of the inducer for macrophage and granulocyte colonies by leukemic cells. *J. Cell. Comp. Physiol.* **72**:251.

Pike, B. L. and Robinson, W. A. (1970). Human bone-marrow colony growth *in vitro*. *J. Cell. Comp. Physiol.* **76**:77.

Price, G. B., McCullogh, E. A., and Till, J. E. (1973). A new human low molecular-weight granulocyte colony-stimulating activity. *Blood* **42**:341–348.

Quesenberry, P., Morley, A., Stohlman, F. S., Richard, K., Howard, D., and Smith, M. (1972). Effect of endotoxin on granulopoiesis and CSF. *N. Engl. J. Med.* **286**:227–231.

Robinson, W., Bradley, T. R., and Metcalf, D. (1967). Effect of whole-body irradiation on colony production by bone-marrow cells *in vitro*. *Proc. Soc. Exp. Biol. Med.* **125**:388.

Stanley, E. R. and Metcalf, D. (1969). Partial purification and some properties of the factor in normal and leukemic human urine stimulating mouse bone-marrow colony growth *in vitro*. *Aust. J. Exp. Biol. Med. Sci.* **47**:467–483.

Stanley, E. R., Robinson, W. A., and Ada, G. L. (1968). Properties of the colony-stimulating factor in leukemic and normal mouse serum. *Aust. J. Exp. Biol. Med. Sci.* **46**:715–726.

Wolmark, N. and Fisher, B. (1974). The effect of single and repeated administration of *Corynebacterium parvum* on bone-marrow macrophage colony production in sygenic tumor-bearing mice. *Cancer Res.* **34**:2869–2872.

18

Nonspecific Cytotoxic Activity of Peritoneal Exudate Cells against Isogenic Tumoral Cells in Animals Treated with *Corynebacterium parvum*

A. FRAY, L. SPARROS, A. M. LORINET,
and B. HALPERN

Abstract

Peritoneal exudate cells obtained from animals treated with *Corynebacterium parvum* displayed a cytotoxic action on YC8 isogenic tumoral cells as evidenced by the ^{51}Cr-release method. It was found that the cytotoxic effect was shared by nonadherent and adherent cells. In this respect, the adherent cells were more active (by a factor of about two) than the nonadherent cells. The induction of the cytotoxic effects of the peritoneal exudate lymphocytes appears to be due to the proper action of *C. parvum* and independent of the presence of the tumor, since no difference in the cytotoxic potency was observed between control and tumor-bearing animals.

A. FRAY, L. SPARROS, and A. M. LORINET, Institute of Immunobiology, Hôpital Broussais, Paris, France and B. HALPERN, Collège de France, Paris, France.

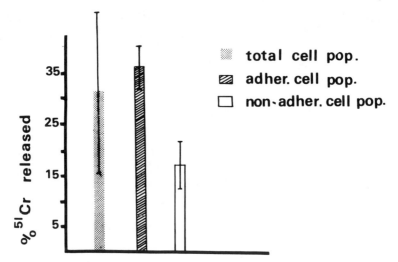

Fig. 1. Cytotoxic effects of peritoneal exudate cells obtained from animals treated with *Corynebacterium parvum* on YC8 tumor cells. The cytotoxicity was measured by the ⁵¹Cr release. The effector cells were, respectively, the whole cell population and the adhering and nonadhering cells. The nonadherent effector cells display a protective effect.

Introduction

Earlier investigations from this laboratory provided evidence that treatment of tumor-bearing animals with *Corynebacterium parvum* increased the cytotoxic effects of nonadherent peritoneal exudate cells when incubated *in vitro* with tumoral isogenic cells (Halpern *et al.*, 1973a,b).

Experiments were performed in order to establish whether the cytotoxic activities displayed by the peritoneal cells were due to an eventual immune reaction against the tumor antigens or whether they were due to a nonspecific stimulation produced by *C. parvum*. In addition, it was of interest to investigate whether the adherent cells were also involved in this phenomenon.

Materials and Methods

In all experiments, 6- to 8-week old, male, Balb/c mice from the breeding center of the CNRS (Orléans-la-Source, France) were used. The animals used in these experiments were either control Balb/c mice or animals to which *C. parvum* "Mérieux" had been administered at a uniform dose of 500 μg (dry-weight) intraperitoneally in a volume of 0.25 ml, seven to eight days before the cells were taken. A certain number of these animals also received a subcutaneous inoculum of 3×10^6 YC8 tumoral cells obtained from an ascitic tumor (Halpern *et al.,* 1974). The peritoneal exudate cells were obtained following a peritoneal injection of 5 ml of medium 199 containing 10% heat-inactivated fetal calf serum and calciparine (10 U/ml).

The collected exudate was centrifuged, and after three washings with the medium, the cells were resuspended and finally adjusted to a concentration of 2×10^7 cells/ml; 0.5 ml of the cell suspension (10^7 cells) was distributed in sterile falcon Petri dishes, 35 mm in diameter, containing 2.5 ml medium 199 to which 10% heat-inactivated fetal calf serum had been added. After incubation for 30–45 min at 37°C in a moist atmosphere containing 5% CO_2, the supernatant was withdrawn, and the nonadherent cells were counted and adjusted to a concentration of 2×10^7 cells/ml.

The number of the adherent cells is calculated by the difference: Total cell population − nonadherent cells = adherent cells. In order to maintain the initial concentrations in the two cell populations, after separation 0.50 ml medium was poured on the adherent cell layer, resulting in a final cell concentration of 8×10^6/ml.

For the nonadherent cells, 0.15 ml of the 2×10^7 cell suspension was added to 0.35 ml of medium, resulting in a final concentration of 3×10^6 cells. In these conditions, three groups of cell suspension were obtained: (1) the mixed peritoneal exudate cells; (2) the nonadherent cells; and (3) the adherent cells.

In all cases, 0.50 ml [^{51}Cr]-YC8 cell suspension at a concentration of 1×10^5 cells/ml was added in the following proportions: (1) 200/1 for the non-separated peritoneal exudate cells; (2) 60/1 for the nonadherent cells; (3) 140/1 for the adherent cells.

The Petri dishes were then incubated at 37°C in a moist CO_2-enriched atmosphere for 16 h, and chromium release was measured in a scintillation counter, as reported previously (Halpern *et al.,* 1973a,b).

Results

The Relative Percentage of Adherent and Nonadherent Cells in the Peritoneal Cavity Exudates in Control Animals and Animals Treated with *C. parvum*

In this experiment, *C. parvum* was administered seven days before collecting peritoneal exudate cells. The Petri dishes containing the cells were incubated at 37°C for 45 min. The figures representing a mean of 9–11 individual experiments are summarized in Table I. They suggest that there is an increase in the number of adherent cells in the peritoneal exudate population in animals receiving *C. parvum*.

Table I. Percentage of Adherent and Nonadherent Cells in the Peritoneal Exudate of Controls and Balb/c Mice Treated with *C. parvum*

Treatment	% Nonadherent cells	% Adherent cells
None (controls)	36 (mean of 11 experiments)	64
C. parvum i.p. 500 µg 7 days before	24 (mean of 9 experiments)	76

Table II. Percentage of ^{51}Cr Release from YC8 Cells Incubated with Peritoneal Exudate Cells from Controls and Animals Treated with *C. parvum*

		Groups treated with *C. parvum*		
		Percentage of YC8 tumoral cells killed as calculated from the ^{51}Cr release		
Control group (mean of experiment)	Days after *C. parvum* treatment	Unseparated cells	Nonadherent cells	Adherent cells
	8	36	12.3	43
	7	28.7	8	27
±10%	7	12.6	24.7	36
	7	54.6	21.6	44.4
	7	29.6	17	31.6
	Mean	32 ± 15	17 ± 7	36 ± 4

Cytotoxic Effects of Peritoneal Exudate Adherent and Nonadherent Cells from Control Animals and Animals Treated with *C. parvum* on YC8 Tumoral Cells

YC8 tumoral cells tagged with ^{51}Cr were incubated at 37°C for 18 h, during which time peritoneal exudate cells were either unseparated or separated into adherent and nonadherent cells, and the ^{51}Cr release in the supernatant was calculated according to the formula

$$\% \,^{51}Cr = \frac{R - S}{T - S} \times 100$$

where R is the release of ^{51}Cr from YC8 cells in the presence of effector cells, T the total release from tagged cells, and S the spontaneous ^{51}Cr release in the presence of an equal concentration of control cells.

The results are reported in Table II. The figures indicate that peritoneal exudate cells activated with *C. parvum* were able to lyse YC8 tumoral cells *in vitro*. The percentage of the lysed cells is approximately 32 ± 15% with unseparated cells, about 17 ± 7% with the nonadherent cells, and about 36 ± 4% with the adherent cells. It can therefore be assumed that the cytotoxic activity of the peritoneal exudate cell population is attributable to both the adherent and the nonadherent cell populations, the adherent cell population being roughly twice as active as the nonadherent cell population.

It should be noted that the cytotoxic action displayed toward YC8 tumoral cells by the peritoneal exudate cells was of the same magnitude whether obtained from tumor-bearing animals or from control animals treated with *C. parvum*.

Discussion

The method described here for obtaining nonadherent and adherent cells from the peritoneal exudate presents a number of advantages: the two cell populations can be obtained and counted without damaging the cells; it suffices to subtract the nonadherent cell population from the total cell population. This technique is economical and avoids time-consuming manipulations. It also avoids traumatization of the adherent cells.

The results obtained show that peritoneal exudate cells activated by *C. parvum* display cytotoxic activity toward YC8 syngenic tumoral cells. As this activity has been observed in tumor-bearing as well as in nontumor-bearing animals, the cytotoxic activity so observed cannot be attributed to specific immune factors and represents another example of tumor-cell aggression by cells activated by *C. parvum*. In this respect, the study of the nonadherent and adherent cell populations revealed that the cytotoxic activity was displayed by both, although the efficiency of the adherent cell population was twice as high as that of the nonadherent cell fraction.

Peritoneal cells obtained from the peritoneal exudate of control animals were never found to display cytotoxic action on YC8 tumor cells. They were found to exert a rather protective action on spontaneous chromium release by the tumoral cells, in accordance with similar findings reported by other authors (Brunner *et al.*, 1968).

It appears from the figures reported in Table I that the sum of the cytotoxic activities of the two cell populations is significantly greater than that observed in the nonseparated cell population. Moreover, when the mixed population of adherent and nonadherent cells was reconstituted after previous separation, the total cytotoxicity rate returned to that observed with the unseparated cells. It seems, therefore, that in this model, the two cell populations exert a mutual inhibitory effect. This last observation can be interpreted in the light of the observations of Scott (1972a,b), who has shown a depressive influence of macrophages activated by *C. parvum* on the thymidine-incorporation rate by lymphocytes stimulated *in vitro* with phytohemagglutinin.

References

Brunner, K. T., Mauel, J., Cerottini, J. C., and Chapuis, B. (1968). Quantitative assay of the lytic action of immune lymphoid cells on ^{51}Cr-labeled allogenic target cells *in vitro*. Inhibition of isoantibody and by drugs. *Immunology* **14**:181.

Halpern, B., Fray, A., Crepin, Y., Platica, O., Sparros, L., Lorinet, A. M., and Rabourdin, A. (1973a). Action inhibitrice du *Corynebacterium parvum* sur le développement des tumeurs malignes syngéniques et son mécanisme. *C. R. Acad. Sci. (Paris)* **276**:1911.

Halpern, B., Fray, A., Crepin, Y., Platica, O., Lorinet, A. M., Rabourdin, A., Sparros, L., and Isac, R. (1973b). *Corynebacterium parvum:* a potent immunostimulant in experiment infections and in malignancies. In: *Immunopotentiation,* Ciba Foundation Symposium **18**:217, Elsevier-Exerpta Medica-North Holland, Amsterdam.

Halpern, B., Lorinet, A. M., Sparros, L., and Fray, A. (1974). Inhibition of thymidine incorporation by tumor YC8 cells cultured *in vitro* by peritoneal macrophages activated with *Corynebacterium parvum*. In this volume, p. 132–136.

Scott, M. T. (1972a). Biological effects of the adjuvant *C. parvum* I. Inhibition of PHA, mixed lymphocyte and GVH reactivity, *Cell. Immunol.* **5**:459.

Scott, M. T. (1972b). Biological effects of the adjuvant *C. parvum* II. Evidence for macrophage T-cell interaction. *Cell. Immunol.* **5**:469.

DISCUSSION

HALPERN: Dr. Sachs, we would like to hear some comments from you as a new member of the *Corynebacterium parvum* Club.

SACHS: I am extremely grateful to Dr. Halpern for showing us, in a typically French manner, that a scientific meeting should combine science and art. Clearly, the beautiful pictures which have been shown are to impress on us the ancient and obvious nature of French civilization.

Since, I unfortunately do not work with this magnificent organism, perhaps I might say a little about the kind of things we have heard here, and what we might perhaps think about.

Clearly, there is a variety of cell types. For those concerned about cells which might be involved, we have heard about lymphocyte, macrophage, and granulocyte involvement. Macrophages have two types of effects: the obvious, quick, cytostatic effect and a cytotoxic effect which takes much longer. We have also learned that this material can be used for stimulating bone-marrow cell division.

There are a number of matters about which we need to know: what makes them divide, what makes them differentiate, and what makes them kill?

Furthermore, *C. parvum* can stimulate certain activities directly and rapidly—certain enzymatic changes. This might be interesting but, as we have heard, these changes do not kill the tumor cells. What causes these delayed effects?

From Dr. Dimitrov's results, perhaps we can make the following simple hypothesis: in order to get these activities to differentiate, certain additives are required. The direct effect of the *C. parvum* does not appear to be the stimulation of any of these activities to differentiate. It is known that, with colony-forming cells, there are certain compounds produced by the body which will make the precursor cells differentiate. In fact, there are two substances which are involved. The first is the activity enabling the precursor to divide—otherwise there would not be a colony—and the other is the activity which enables *these* two to differentiate.

One can suggest that *C. parvum* is therapeutic for cancer treatment for a number of reasons: it can stimulate certain processes directly, but this does not seem to be particularly important from the point of view of being deleterious to cancer. It stimulates the release of a variety of substances in the body which stimulate the differentiation of the growth-inhibitory cells. This would explain why the addition of *C. parvum* to the cells does not by itself do what is required.

Therefore, to look for a direct effect of *C. parvum* on these cells may be incorrect. We should look to see what happens to the capacity of *C. parvum*-treated animals' sera to induce stimulation, and then determine to what extent this may be useful in therapy.

Another point is that the material which induces differentiation of the normal cells also has an effect on malignant cells. For example, in the case of granulocytic leukemia, granulocytic cells from man and mouse can be placed in tissue culture and a material inducing the differentiation of normal cells can be added. In certain types of leukemia, this material can induce a normal differentiation of the leukemic cell, so that it becomes like a normal cell and may stop dividing. Thus, if there is an effect on myeloid leukemia, and perhaps on other leukemic cells—as may happen—this could be built into the following scheme: When an excess of greater production of the particular chemical substance(s) (yet unidentified) is added (which will not only induce differentiation of normal cells but also help to overcome the effect of chemotherapy), it may be a material not directly produced by the action of *C. parvum* on these cells, but by the animal, which has induced differentiation.

Therefore, it is not at all unlikely that by means of this material—and *C. parvum* may help here—there may be an indirect action in that it produces a release of substances which are essential for the differentiation of these cell types—either differentiation of the normal cells or the normal differentiation of leukemic cells. The so-called adjuvant effect of *C. parvum* may be no more than that.

Part V
Corynebacterium parvum in Experimental Tumors and Metastasis

19

An Analysis of the Increase in Host Resistance to Isogenic Tumor Invasion in Mice by Treatment with *Corynebacterium parvum*

BERNARD HALPERN, YVONNE CREPIN,
and ANNE RABOURDIN

Abstract

This study deals with the effects of *Corynebacterium parvum* on the resistance of the host to transplantable isogenic tumors. Differences have been observed depending on the nature of the tumor, the size of the inoculum, the mode of introduction, and the time interval between the tumor inoculum and the treatment with *C. parvum.*

In the case of the YC8 Balb/c isogenic lymphoma, remarkable results were obtained when both malignant inoculum and *C. parvum* were applied intraperitoneally. The results were still consistent, although less favorable, when the malignant challenge and the immunostimulator were administered intravenously. In this experimental model, visceral metastases affecting the lung, liver, kidney,

BERNARD HALPERN, Collège de France, Paris, France, and YVONNE CREPIN and ANNE RABOURDIN, Institute of Immunobiology, Hôpital Broussais, Paris, France.

and spleen were frequently observed in the control animals. Treatment with *C. parvum* produced a remarkable inhibition of the metastasic dissemination.

The resistance of F_1 (Balb/c $\times$ $C_{57}B1$) hybrid hosts to the invasion of YC8 lymphoma was not consistently different from the resistance of the parental Balb/c strain. Treatment with *C. parvum* did not significantly increase the resistance of the F_1 hybrids against tumor dissemination, a finding at variance with that previously reported for **AKR** leukemia.

The effects of *C. parvum* on the evolution of the isogenic Graffi tumor were less favorable than the effect on YC8 lymphoma. It follows from the results reported here that the enhancement of resistance of the host against isogenic tumors by *C. parvum* is conditioned by a variety of factors, such as the nature of the tumor, the route of inoculation, and the time interval between the treatment and the tumor challenge. There is clearly a need for further experimentation to find optimal conditions of administration of *C. parvum* for the extension of these data to human applications.

Introduction

The enhancement of host resistance against tumor invasion following treatment with killed *Corynebacterium parvum* has been reported by many investigators (Halpern *et al.*, 1966; Woodruff and Boak, 1966; Lamensans *et al.*, 1968; Currie and Bagshawe, 1970; Smith and Scott, 1972; Woodruff *et al.*, 1972; Israel and Halpern, 1972; Halpern *et al.*, 1973a,b; Woodruff and Dunbar, 1973; Likhite and Halpern, 1973). Emphasis has been placed on the fact that this phenomenon seems to depend on a variety of ill-defined factors, such as the genotype of the host, the nature of the tumor, and the route of administration of the tumor cells.

The time interval between the administration of the immunopotentiator and the tumor graft also seems to be critical (Woodruff and Dunbar, 1973). It is therefore not surprising that the results reported from various laboratories are not always concordant.

The aim of these studies was to analyze and define some of these factors in a well-established model.

Material and Methods

Most of our experiments were performed with the isogenic YC8 tumor, a murine lymphoma induced primarily in Balb/c strain mice by the Moloney virus and maintained by serial passages in ascitic form. *C. parvum* was obtained from the Mérieux Institute (Lyon) in the form of a heat-killed suspension, containing 2 mg/ml (dry weight) bacteria to which $8^\circ/_{oo}$ formalin had been added. Six- to eight-week-old Balb/c male mice were mainly used. They were obtained from the C.N.R.S. breeding center, Orléans-la-Source.

Tumor grafts were transplanted in the form of ascitic cells taken from donors which had received an intraperitoneal inoculum of 150,000 YC8 cells or 500,000 Graffi tumor cells 8 days previously. The cells were obtained from ether-asphyxiated animals by sterile puncture of the peritoneal cavity, usually after a previous intraperitoneal injection of 2 ml of warm sterile Hank's solution (Pasteur Institute); then 0.5 ml of ascitic liquid was diluted in 50 ml of Hank's solution, and the tumor cells were counted. The percentage of their viability was controlled using a trypan-blue dye-exclusion technique (0.2 ml of cell suspension + 0.05 ml of a 2% trypan-blue solution). The tumor cell concentration was adjusted to have an inoculum dose contained in 0.2 ml. The cell suspensions containing less than 90% viable cells or contaminated with blood were discarded. The inocula generally represented a pool of cells obtained from three donors.

The *C. parvum* vaccine was administered at a uniform dose of 500 μg dry weight, either intraperitoneally or intravenously, in a volume of 0.25 ml. The time intervals between the tumor inoculation and the injection of *C. parvum* varied in different groups of experiments, as indicated hereafter.

The animals were inspected daily during the course of the experiments, and the mortality rate recorded. All deceased animals were autopsied, and the macroscopic pathological features reported.

Results

The results will be reported in three parts with regard to the genotype of the strain and the nature of the tumor inoculated. In each of the three sections, the results will be analyzed in different series depending on the parameters adopted.

Division I. YC8 Tumor in Balb/c Mice

Series I

The intraperitoneal route of administration was used. The animals included in this series were divided into two groups.

Group A: Group A included animals receiving uniform tumor inoculum of 500,000 live cells by intraperitoneal administration and *C. parvum* in the same manner at a dose of 500 μg. The animals were divided into four subgroups of 15–20 animals each. One group served as control, the three others received *C. parvum* at various time intervals with respect to the tumor inoculum. The results of experiment A are reported in Fig. 1. In the control group, the mortality reached 100% by the 21st day following tumor implantation. In all treated groups, the survival time was consistently increased. The most favorable results were obtained when *C. parvum* was administered on day −2; in this group, more than 50% of survivors were observed on day 42, and there were more than 30% of definitive survivors.

The results were somewhat similar in the group of animals receiving *C.*

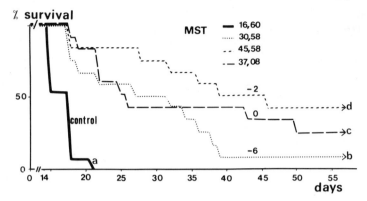

Fig. 1. Group A: In this series the Balb/c mice received intra-peritoneally a uniform inoculum of 500,000 live YC8 cells on day 0. The animals were divided into four groups (15–20 each): (a) Control group; (b) Group 0, animals injected i.p. with *Coryne-bacterium parvum* on day −6; (c) group of animals injected i.p. with *C. parvum* on day 0; (d) group of animals injected i.p. with *C. parvum* on day −2.

parvum on day 0. However, on the whole, the survival rates were lower, although still higher than for the control groups or for the animals receiving *C. parvum* on day −6.

   Group B: The animals in this group were divided into three subgroups, each receiving a different dose of YC8 cells by peritoneal inoculation: (a) 10^5 cells, (b) 10^4 cells, and (c) 10^3 cells. Each of these subgroups received a uniform dose of *C. parvum* by intraperitoneal injection on day −2. The results are summarized in Fig. 2.

   In the control group, the mortality was nearly 100% within 60 days for the subgroups receiving 10^5 and 10^4 cells, and 70% for the subgroup receiving 10^3 cells. In the treated groups, no mortality was noted within 150 days of observations of the subgroup receiving 10^3 cells; the mortality was, respectively, 20% and 30% in the groups receiving 10^4 and 10^5 malignant cells.

   The results observed in this series clearly indicate a remarkable increase in host resistance to tumor invasion following the administration of *C. parvum* into the peritoneal cavity two days prior to inoculation. These results are much more remarkable if one considers the severity of the malignant challenge which, in the control groups, led to 100% mortality.

Series II

   In this series of experiments, the neoplastic inoculum of YC8 cells, as well as the *C. parvum*, were administered intravenously.

   As in the preceding series, one group of experiments was performed by

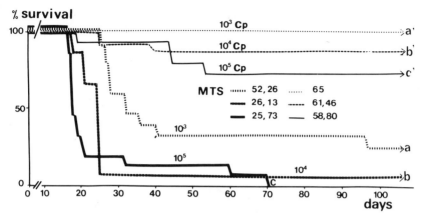

Fig. 2. Group B: In the control experiment, three groups of 20 Balb/c mice received, respectively, an intraperitoneal inoculum of (a) 10^3, (b) 10^4, and (c) 10^5 YC8 cells on day 0. In the treated series, three similar groups of animals received identical intraperitoneal inoculations two days after intraperitoneal injection of 500 μg of *Corynebacterium parvum:* (a') 10^3, (b') 10^4, and (c') 10^5.

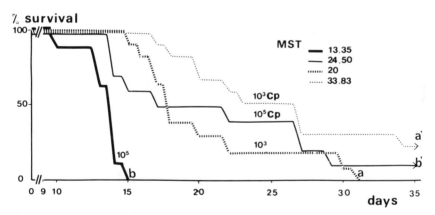

Fig. 3. Patterns of the inhibition of tumor growth in the isogenic host by *Corynebacterium parvum* when both the tumor inoculum and the immunostimulant were administered intravenously. In this experiment the doses of the tumor inoculum varied, while the time interval between the injection of *C. parvum* and the tumor inoculum was kept constant. The recipient Balb/c mice were divided into four groups of 20 animals each. Two of the four groups served as controls and received (a) 10^3 or (b) 10^5 YC8 tumor cells, respectively, on day 0. The animals of the treated groups received an intravenous injection of 500 μg of *C. parvum* on day −4 and on day 0, respectively, (a') 10^3 or (b') 10^5 YC8 tumor cells.

varying the dose of the malignant cells and keeping the time interval constant, while in the second group, the malignant inoculum was kept constant and the time intervals were varied.

The data reported in Fig. 3. shows the results. The groups of animals received malignant inocula of 10^5, 10^4, 10^3, and 2×10^2 cells, respectively, by intravenous injection, while *C. parvum* was similarly administered by the intravenous route on day −4.

The mortality in the control subgroups was 100% with all doses of malignant cells inoculated. The differences consisted only in the length of survival time, which ranged from 15 days for the greatest to 32 days for the smallest tumor-cell doses.

In the treated groups, consistent prolongation of the survival time was observed in all subgroups. With the smaller inocula, definitive survivors reaching 20–30% were observed.

The results of the assays in which the time factor was studied are summarized in Fig. 4. In the subgroups receiving the highest malignant challenge (10^5 and 10^4 cells), leading to 100% mortality in less than 3 weeks in the control groups, pretreatment of the animals on day −4 with a single injection of *C. parvum* resulted only in a prolongation of the survival time. The results were similar when *C. parvum* was given on day +6. Moreover, when the immunostimulant was given on both day −4 and day +6, the survival time was greatly increased, the first death in the treated group occurring when all animals in the control group had already succumbed. In addition, as many as 40% of the treated animals survived indefinitely.

Metastases

In animals receiving high challenges of 10^3 or more YC8 cells intravenously, metastases were regularly observed in various organs—the lung, liver, spleen, and kidney. Treatment with *C. parvum* regularly reduced and often suppressed the incidence of metastases in animals sacrificed ten days after the tumor challenge.

Division II. YC8 Tumor Development in Hybrids (Balb/c × $C_{57}Bl/c)F_1$ and the Action of *C. parvum*.

The resistance exhibited by F_1 hybrids to the growth or dissemination of a grafted tumor syngenic with one of the parental strains has been found to vary, depending on genotype as well as on the nature of the tumor. The sarcoma J of Betz, a spontaneous tumor syngenic with the $C_{57}Bl/c$ mouse, was found to be more virulent when inoculated into F_1 (C_{57} Bl × C_3H) hybrids (Halpern *et al.*, 1963). On the other hand, more recent research reported from this laboratory (Lamensans *et al.*, 1968) showed that when AKR leukemia was transferred from leukemic parents to young recipients, either from the AKR strain or F_1 (AKR × CBA) hybrids, the degree of resistance was not consistently different in the

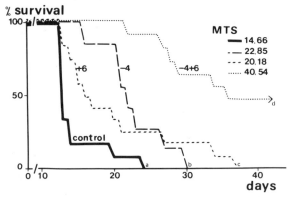

Fig. 4. Patterns of inhibition of the tumor invasion in the isogenic host by *Corynebacterium parvum*. In this experiment, the doses of the tumor cells remained constant, while the time interval between the injection of *C. parvum* and the tumor inoculum varied. The recipient Balb/c mice were divided into four groups: Group (a) served as control and received an intravenous injection of 10^5 YC8 cells on day 0. Similar inocula were given i.v. to the three other groups of animals pretreated with an intravenous injection of 500 μg of *C. parvum* on the following dates: Group (b) on day −4; Group (c) on day +6; and Group (d) on days −4 and +6.

untreated animals. However, treatment with *C. parvum* has been found to be much more efficient in the hybrids than in the syngenic strain animals.

The effect of *C. parvum* was consequently investigated in F_1 (Balb/c X C_{57} Bl) hybrids using the YC8 tumor, which is syngenic with the Balb/c strain and to which the C_{57} Bl/6 mice are fully resistant.

The results suggest that, on the whole, the susceptibility of the hybrids to the YC8 tumor was not greatly different from that of the parental Balb/c strain. As to the action of *C. parvum,* no evidence of increase in the resistance of the F_1-hybrid recipient against the invasion of this tumor could be obtained.

Division III: Graffi Tumors in C_{57} Bl Mice

The Graffi tumor is another virus-induced tumor transplantable in C_{57} Bl mice in the form of an ascitic tumor. Figure 5 summarizes the effect of *C. parvum* when both the tumor cells and *C. parvum* (500 μg per animal) were given intraperitoneally on day 0. In a range of tumor-cell doses, varying from $10^6 - 10^2$ cells, treatment against the tumor invasion was not effective. When *C. parvum* was administered intravenously on day −4 and the tumoral inoculum given by the same route, a regular and consistent protection reaching 70% of definitive survivors was obtained with tumoral inocula which were still 100% lethal in the controls.

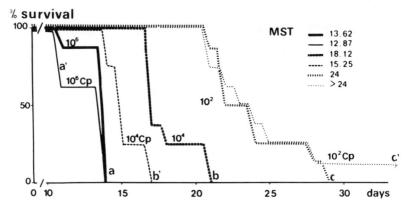

Fig. 5. Patterns of inhibition of tumor growth in the isogenic host by *Corynebacterium parvum*. In this experiment, different doses of Graffi tumor cells were injected intraperitoneally into groups of C_{57} B1 mice on day 0. The animals were divided into six groups: three control groups (a, b, and c) received, respectively, 10^6, 10^4, or 10^2 Graffi tumor cells. The animals of the three treated groups (a', b', c') received, on the same day, an intraperitoneal injection of a uniform dose of 500 μg *C. parvum* and 10^6, 10^4, or 10^2 tumor cells, respectively.

Discussion

The general impression that emerges from an analysis of the experimental data reported here is that treatment with *C. parvum* leads to a consistent increase in the resistance of the host against tumor challenges. However, the magnitude of this resistance depends on a great number of factors, of which only a limited number have been investigated so far. The prominent feature is an increase in the survival times observed in all groups of mice treated with *C. parvum*. Optimal protection depends on the mode of administration and the time interval between the tumor inoculation and the *C. parvum* treatment.

Augmentation of host resistance associated with *C. parvum* treatment was best evidenced in the experiments employing the YC8 lymphoma when tumor cells and *C. parvum* were injected into the peritoneal cavity. However, treatment by the intravenous route yielded consistently favorable results with a large percentage of definitive survivors under conditions in which 100% mortality was observed in the control group. Highly significant survival rates were obtained in groups of animals receiving *C. parvum* inoculations. However, when *C. parvum* was given on day −2 and repeated on day +4, the results were much more favorable in comparison with those obtained in comparable experiments using only a single treatment of *C. parvum*.

It was surprising to note that in the experiments dealing with YC8 lymphoma cells inoculated into F_1 hybrids, the so-called "hybrid phenomenon," usually expressed by increased resistance, was not observed. This is in contrast to what had been reported for AKR leukemia (Lamensans *et al.*, 1968).

References

Currie, G. A. and Bagshawe, K. P. (1970). Active immunotherapy with *Corynebacterium parvum* and chemotherapy in murine fibrosarcomas. *Br. Med. J.* 1:541.

Geran, R. I., Greenberg, N. H., MacDonald, M. N., Schumacher, A. M., and Abbott, B. J. (1972). Protocols for screening chemical agents and natural products against animal tumors and other biological systems (Third Edition). *Cancer Chemother. Rep. 3.*

Halpern, B., Biozzi, G., and Stiffel, C. (1963). Action de l'extrait microbien Wxb 3148 sur l'évolution des tumeurs expérimentales. In *Rôle du système réticulo-endothélial dans l'immunité antibactérienne et antitumorale, Colloque International du CNRS* 115:221.

Halpern, B., Biozzi, G., Stiffel, C., and Mouton, D. (1966). Inhibition of tumor growth by administration of killed *Corynebacterium parvum. Nature (Lond.)* 212:853.

Halpern, B., Fray, A., Crepin, Y., Platica, O., Sparros, L., Lorinet, A. M., and Rabourdin, A. (1973a). Action inhibitrice du *Corynebacterium parvum* sur le développement des tumeurs malignes syngéniques et son mécanisme. *C. R. Acad. Sci. (Paris)* 276:1911.

Halpern, B., Fray, A., Crepin, Y., Platica, O., Lorinet, A. M., Rabourdin, A., Sparros, L., and Isac, R. (1973b). *Corynebacterium parvum,* a potent immunostimulant in experimental infections and in malignancies. In: *Immunopotentiation* (Ciba Foundation Symposium 18), p. 217, Elsevier-Excerpta Medica-North Holland, Amsterdam.

Israel, L. and Halpern, B. (1972). Le *Corynebacterium parvum* dans les cancers avancés. *Nouv. Presse Med.* 1:1.

Lamensans, A., Stiffel, C., Mollier, F., Laurent, M., Mouton, D., and Biozzi, G. (1968). Effet protecteur de *Corynebacterium parvum* contre la leucémie greffée AKR. Relations avec l'activité catalasique hépatique et la fonction phagocytaire de système réticuloendothelial. *Rev. Fr. Etud. Clin. Biol.* 13:773.

Likhite, V. V. and Halpern, B. (1973). The delayed rejection of tumors from the administration of tumor cells mixed with killed *Corynebacterium parvum. Int. J. Cancer* 12:699.

Smith, S. E. and Scott, J. (1972). Biological effects of *Corynebacterium parvum.* III. Amplification of resistance and impairment of active immunity to murine sarcoma. *Br. J. Cancer.* 26:361.

Woodruff, M. F. A. and Boak, J. L. (1966). Inhibitory effect of injection of *Corynebacterium parvum* on the growth of tumor transplants in isogenic hosts. *Br. J. Cancer* 20:343.

Woodruff, M. F. A. and Dunbar, N. (1973). The effect of *Corynebacterium parvum* and other reticuloendothelial stimulants on transplanted tumors in mice. In: *Immunopotentiation* (Ciba Foundation Symposium 18), p. 287, Elsevier-Excerpta Medica-North Holland, Amsterdam.

Woodruff, M. F. A., Inchley, M. P., and Dunbar, N. (1972). Further observations on the effect of *Corynebacterium parvum* and antitumor globulin on syngenically transplanted mouse tumors. *Br. J. Cancer* 26:67.

DISCUSSION

FELDMAN: Have any experiments been done in which the tumor and the *Corynebacterium parvum* were given in two different sites, namely say, the tumor intraperitoneally and the *C. parvum* intravenously?

HALPERN: Yes, we have such data, but I did not elaborate on these results because of lack of time. I thought that these aspects of the problems would be brought up during the discussion.

If the *C. parvum* was injected intravenously and the tumor was inoculated intraperitoneally, the results were consistently good. But, in the reverse situation, when *C. parvum* was injected intraperitoneally and the tumor intravenously, the results were not so good.

FELDMAN: You have shown that the YC8 is extremely susceptible to the effect produced by the *C. parvum,* whereas the Graffi tumor is dramatically less susceptible. At the end of the conference, it would be interesting if Dr. Halpern would tell us how many tumors out of those investigated were found to be susceptible and how many not susceptible. This would give us an important indication regarding the state of our knowledge on the subject.

HALPERN: My intention in presenting these results was to be provocative, and to show that it is not possible to extrapolate or to generalize. This was my main reason for showing so much data. One of the problems which I want to emphasize is that, in spite of the nonspecificity of immunostimulation, the results depend on the nature of the tumor, or rather on the host–tumor relationship.

MILAS: Have you done any studies in which animals were immunized and then challenged with the viable tumor cells?

HALPERN: Yes, to a certain extent and with certain tests. But these data were published in the CIBA Foundation Symposium on Immunopotentiation which came out of print a few months ago [(1973). *Immunopotentiation* (Ciba

200

Foundation Symposium), Elsevier, North Holland]. We have shown that peritoneal cavity and spleen lymphocytes of these animals were cytotoxic *in vitro* for these tumor cells.

MILAS: What is the immunogenicity of the YC8 tumor?

HALPERN: We did not succeed immunizing the Balb/c mice against this tumor by administering sublethal doses of tumor cells. This tumor is extremely virulent, and the 100% lethal dose is situated between 10^1 and 10^2 cells. There is no evidence that an immune condition can be obtained which will enable animals to reject a tumor. The only evidence available is that lymphocytes of tumor-bearing animals become cytotoxic *in vitro* for the tumor cells. More-over, the cytotoxic effects become manifest about 7–9 days after the tumor implantation and persist 18–20 days. At any time, the proportion of lympho-cytes/target cells was 200/1.

WRBA: Returning to Dr. Feldman's comments, everybody is looking for a working system and also showing positive results. In my talk I will be mentioning a lot of negative results with a variety of tumors. From the cytostatic screening we know this, but it is a different mechanism in this case. We hope to discover why it works in some systems and not in others. This is a very important point; everybody is looking for a beautifully functioning system, and people who do not work in this field receive the impression that *C. parvum* is effective in all tumors, but this is not true.

COHEN; Since there are these great differences in the two tumors studied, have any comparable studies been made with BCG in these two tumors to see whether it would act differently than *C. parvum?*

HALPERN: No systematic comparative study has been done by us.

BIOZZI: I think Dr. Feldman's suggestion is very good. It would be helpful to make a list of tumors which are susceptible or resistant to the protective effect of *C. parvum.* However, in practice this is difficult to do because the protec-tion depends greatly on the experimental conditions used. Dr. Mazurek is working with us on this problem. The two tumors used, a mammary carcinoma and a lymphosarcoma, are rather resistant to *C. parvum,* since intravenous injection of *C. parvum* does not protect against a subcutaneous graft of these tumors. However, when *C. parvum* and tumor cells are given by the same route, either intravenously or intraperitoneally, there is a protective effect. In the same way, when the tumors are grafted subcutaneously, *C. parvum* is effective if injected in the same site, while no protection occurs when the injection site is far from the graft area. The protective effect in that case seems to be due to a local effect of *C. parvum.*

Thus, it is extremely difficult to make a general statement of whether a given tumor is resistant; all the possible combinations of treatment must be tried.

20

Effect of Inactivated *Corynebacterium* on Different Experimental Tumors in Mice

M. ROUMIANTZEFF, M. MUSETESCU, G. AYME, and M.C. MYNARD

Introduction

The immunostimulant activities of inactivated *Corynebacterium parvum* suspension are well described in the work of Halpern *et al.* (1963). We investigated this nonspecific immunostimulation by measuring the effect of *C. parvum* on RES-organs stimulation, humoral-adjuvant activity, carbon-clearance stimulation, interferon induction, and protection versus bacterial and viral challenges. All these tests are quantitative and accurate enough to check experimental production precisely, judge different parameters, and control the batches used for animal or clinical trials.

The potential of *C. parvum* as an agent in tumor immunotherapy is dependent on reliable evidence of its antitumor activity. The antitumor activity of *C. parvum* has been well-documented since the pioneering work of Halpern *et al.* (1966). However, consistent quantitative measurements are difficult to obtain with experimental tumor systems. This report presents our experience with 3 experimental tumors in mice; the principal purpose of our study was to develop

M. ROUMIANTZEFF, M. MUSETESCU, G. AYME, and M. C. MYNARD, Institut Français d'Immunologie, Fondation Mérieux, Marcy l'Etoile, 69260 Charbonnières-les-Bains, France.

standardized tests to compare different batches and measure the production quality of antitumor immunostimulants.

In this paper, *C. parvum* antitumor activity is estimated for some well-defined experimental conditions and compared to the activity of other immunostimulants.

Materials and Methods

Immunostimulant

All *C. parvum* preparations were made from strain Prévot 3607. The bacterial suspensions were totally inactivated (1 h at 65°C and formaldehyde addition) and standardized to 2 mg/ml (dry weight after dialysis) suspensions. Table I shows the different lots used: experimental lots, pilot lots, and lots for clinical use.

Other immunostimulants were engaged in a comparative study with *C. parvum*: *Corynebacterium granulosum*, a reticulostimulin from the Institut Pasteur (2 mg/ml); BCG from the Institut Mérieux (2 mg/ml); *Brucella* extracts from Prof. Pilet's laboratory and our own laboratory (2 mg/ml); mycobacteria

Table I. Immunostimulant Material: *Corynebacterium parvum* Lots All Issued From Strain IM 1585, and Other Immunostimulants

Immunostimulant : *Corynebacterium parvum* IM

Strain	$\begin{cases} \text{Prévot 3607} \\ \text{IM 1585} \end{cases}$	Classified	$\begin{cases} \textit{Corynebacterium parvum} \\ \text{(Prévot 1954)} \\ \textit{Propionibacterium avidum} \\ \text{(Cummins and Johnson, 1974)} \end{cases}$

Bacterial suspension, 65°C, 1 h inactivation and formaldehyde
2 mg/ml (dry weight)

Experimental lots : 1 − 2 − 5 − 6 − 7 − 8bd − 11a.g − 14a.g −16b − 17− 18b − 19 − 21 − 22
Pilot lots : 4 − 7 − 8 − 10 − 12 − 15 − 16 − 18 − 20 − 22
Experimental lots for clinical use (SO) : SO195 − 225 − 260 − 274 − 282 − 301

Other immunostimulants (for comparative study)

Reticulostimulin *Corynebacterium granulosum* (Institut Pasteur)
BCG
Mycobacteria extracts, *Brucella* extracts (Prof. Pilet), *Trypanosa* extracts, . . .
Levamisole, tetramisole, . . .

Table II. Methods: Three Tumor Systems and General Methodology for Stimulation and Challenge

		Tumor systems			
Tumor	Mouse strain	Relationship	Tumor cells	Clinical expression	Total mortality control
Ehrlich's ascitic tumor	Swiss (inbred) 18–20 g	Nonisogenic	10^3	Profuse ascite	20–30 days
AKR leukemia	AKR 16–18 g	Isogenic	10^3	RES tumors: spleen, nodes, thymus, liver	18–26 days
YC8 ascitic tumor[a]	Balb/c 16–18 g	Isogenic	10^3	Ascite	18–32 days
		General methodology			

Stimulation, i.p. (or other) route(s), 0.5 ml
Challenge, i.p. route, 0.2 ml
Control challenge, always 100% tumor mortality

[a]YC8 ascitic tumor (Leclerc *et al.*, 1972).

extracts from our laboratories (4 mg/ml); *Trypanosa* extracts from the Institut
Mérieux (75–350 μg total nitrogen/ml); Levamisole and Tetramisole.*

Tumor Systems

We routinely used three tumor systems, which we attempted to standardize
on mice. Table II gives the main characteristics of these three tumors: (1)
Ehrlich's ascitic tumor cells were used on 18- to 20-g nonisogenic, inbred Swiss
mice from our own colony. (2) AKR leukemia cells were used on 16- to 18-g
AKR mice obtained from IFFA-CREDO, Saint-Germain sur l'Arbresle.* (3) YC8
ascitic tumor cells,† described by Leclerc *et al.* (1972), were used on 16- to 18-g
isogenic Balb/c mice from our colony. The three tumor lines were maintained
and processed in our laboratory.

*Levamisole sulfate and Tetramisole chlorhydrate were gifts from Dr. G. H. Werner,
  SUCRP, Vitry sur Seine, France.
†YC8 ascitic cells and mice were kindly provided by Prof. B. Halpern.

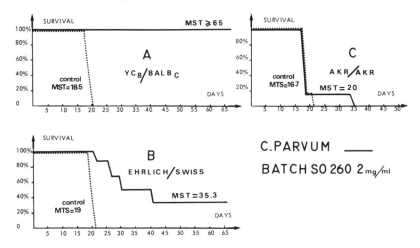

Fig. 1. Stimulation by *Corynebacterium parvum* and protective effect against challenges by three tumor systems. Effect of a single, 0.5-ml, intraperitoneal injection of *C. parvum*, 1000 µg per mouse, 4 h before challenges: (A) YC8 on Balb/c mice stimulated — and control ·····. (B) Ehrlich's tumor on Swiss mice stimulated — and control ·····. (C) AKR on AKR mice stimulated — and control ·····. Percentage survival curves and calculation of mean survival times for 65 days of observations were done. Challenge for stimulated groups and controls (10^3 cells; 0.2 ml, i.p. route) lead to 100% mortality in control mice for the three systems.

Table II also summarizes the general protocol: Generally one injection by the intraperitoneal (i.p.) route was administered (details or variations are given in table or figure legends). Challenge was by the i.p. route (0.2 ml): The challenge was always separated from stimulation by a minimal 4-h delay to avoid an eventual direct action of stimulating agent on tumor cells. The challenge, judged on control group, must always be sufficient to give a 100% tumor mortality.

All the results are expressed as median survival time and chiefly as mean survival time (MST), following the NCI 11 protocol for tumor-test evaluation described by Geran *et al.* (1972).

Results

Corynebacterium Activity on the Three Tumor Systems

Routinely, different *C. parvum* batches were tested in parallel on the three systems: YC8, Ehrlich's, and AKR tumors. Figure 1 illustrates a typical experiment: the same preparation, *C. parvum* SO 260, was used to stimulate (i.p. route, 0.5 ml, 4 h before challenge) the three groups of mice. Challenges were similarly administered (i.p. route, 0.2 ml, 10^3 viable cells) and had (in control

Table III. YC8 Tumor Challenge Titration and Stimulation of Protective Activity for Three Different Challenge Levels[a]

C. parvum		SO 260	500 μg
Stimulation	i.p.	0.5 ml	−4 h
Challenge	i.p.	0.2 ml	

Mean survival time (65 days of observation)		
Challenge	Control	Stimulation
10^3 cells/mouse	19.7	> 65
10^4 cells/mouse	17.7	19.2
10^5 cells/mouse	16	15.3

[a]Challenge activity and protective activity expressed as mean survival time after 65 days of observation.

groups) similar effects on the three groups: 100% mortality and mean survival times were in the same range (16.7 for AKR, 18.5 for YC8, and 19 for Erlich's tumor).

The survival curves and the calculated mean survival times (at 65 days) showed a dramatic difference in *C. parvum* effect on the three systems: Absolutely no effect on AKR leukemia (Fig. 1C). A very significant protective effect on Ehrlich's ascite: delay of ascite and mortality, and some complete recovery (MST = 35.3) (Fig. 1B). A complete protective effect on YC8 tumor (MST at 65 days was maximal: $\geqslant 65$) (Fig. 1A).

Challenge Levels and Protective Activity

The protection by *C. parvum* stimulation is dependent on the challenge level. We regularly observed protection in Ehrlich and YC8 systems, even with severe challenges which always lead to 100% mortality on controls in a very short period of time (see Table V for MST averages). However, the protective effect was reduced or completely abolished if the challenges were increased. Table III illustrates an assay where this challenge dependence was especially marked: for YC8 system, 500 μg *C. parvum* gave total protection (MST > 65) for a normal challenge level of 10^3 cells, which—in a short period of time (MST = 19.7)—killed 100% of the control mice. But the same stimulation was not able to protect mice against challenges of 10^4 and 10^5 cells.

Comparison of *C. parvum* and Other Immunostimulants

Working on several immunostimulants, we often set up parallel experiments with different *C. parvum* preparations and other immunostimulants, using the same standardized tumor tests.

Table IV. Results of Stimulation by *Corynebacterium parvum* and Other Immunostimulants in Different Standardized Assays for Two Tumor Systems: Ehrlich's on Swiss Mice and YC8 on Balb/c Mice[a]

	Dose	No.	Ehrlich's ascite	No.	YC8/Balb/c
C. parvum	1000 µg/mouse	11 assays	$\overline{44.6}$ (25.1–54.3)	5 assays	$\overline{>65}$
C. parvum	500 µg			9 assays	$\overline{62.6}$ (57–>65)
C. parvum	200 µg	5 assays	$\overline{29.1}$ (27–33.5)		54–65–>65
C. parvum	40 µg				25–43–59
C. granulosum	1000 µg		38.3–34.7		>65 >65
BCG	1000 µg		23.3		46
Brucella ext.	1000 µg		52		50.5
Mycobacteria ext.	2000 µg		34.4–31.1–24.7		>65–64–53.5
Trypanosa	75 and 350 µg NT		18.8 and 23.7		18.3–18.3–27.5
Levamisole and tetramisole	30 µg		21 and 26		
Control challenge			$\overline{21.9}$ (19–25.7)		$\overline{21}$ (18–26)

[a]Effect of a single, 0.5-ml, intraperitoneal injection of the different immunostimulants: dose per mouse is indicated for each case. The unique stimulating injection was always given 4 h before challenge.

Challenge for stimulated groups and controls (0.2 ml, i.p. route) always lead to 100% mortality in control mice; averages for control mean survival times were calculated: 21.9 for Ehrlich's and 21 for YC8, and the limits observed are given in brackets.

Protective activities for the different cases are expressed as mean survival time after 65 days of observation. If more than four different assays were run, an average value was calculated, and the limits observed are given in brackets.

Table IV summarizes some of the results observed in comparative studies with the i.p. route of stimulation, 4 h before i.p. challenge, for both Ehrlich and YC8 systems. *C. parvum* assays were numerous, allowing us to establish averages, and *C. parvum* was often engaged at different doses.

The figures (averages or separated values), expressed as mean survival times after 65 days of observation, show that *C. parvum* (and *C. granulosum*) preparations had the best protective effect in standardized assays for both nonsyngenic Ehrlich's and syngenic YC8 tumors. At equivalent or superior doses, only some mycobacteria extracts and perhaps *Brucella* extracts had a similar protective effect; BCG, under our conditions, was less active.

Dose—Response Effects

Figures 2 and 3 show the sharp dose—response effects observed for Ehrlich's and YC8 tumor assays. Fivefold dilutions (50 mg/kg, 10 mg/kg, and 2 mg/kg) of *C. parvum* preparation lead to different protection levels clearly illustrated by the survival curves, median survival times, and mean survival times.

Standardized Assays as Control Tools for Production

Table V gives results obtained with the two standardized assays by the i.p. route (YC8 and Ehrlich's tumor assays) in the study of different production factors: all the figures are mean survival time (at 65 days of observation).

C. parvum—without complete inactivation, accidentally or voluntarily ob-

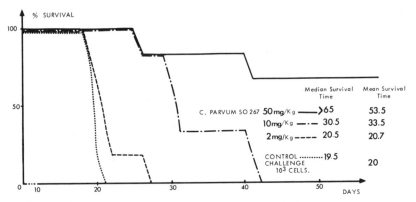

Fig. 2. Dose—response effect of single, 0.50-ml intraperitoneal injection of *Corynebacterium parvum* at 3 fivefold dilutions (50 mg/kg ———; 10 mg/kg —·—·—; 2 mg/kg – – –) against Ehrlich's ascite challenge. Stimulations were done 4 h before challenge on 18- to 20-g inbred Swiss mice. Challenge for stimulated groups and control group (10^3 cells, 0.2 ml, i.p. route) lead to 100% mortality in control mice ·····. Percentage survival curves, median survival time, and mean survival time (65 days of observation) were established for the three stimulating doses and control.

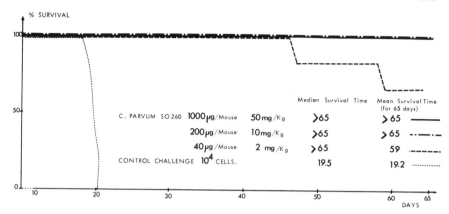

Fig. 3. Dose–response effect of a single, 0.50-ml intraperitoneal injection of *Corynebacterium parvum* at 3 fivefold dilutions (50 mg/kg ——; 10 mg/kg — · —; 2 mg/kg - - - - -) against YC8 tumor. Stimulations were done 4 h before challenge on 16- to 18-g Balb/c mice. Challenge for stimulated groups and control group (10^3 cells, 0.2 ml, i.p. route) lead to 100% mortality in control mice · · · · ·. Percentage survival curves, median survival time, and mean survival time (65 days of observation) were established for the three stimulating doses and control.

tained—did not lead to better stimulation. Formaldehyde concentration variation did not give significant differences for protective activity. Other inactivating agent—such as phenol—may allow a satisfactory inactivation without significantly changing the protective activity. Other conditions for growing *C. parvum* i.m. 1585 do not seem to change the activity of the final preparation.

Table VI summarizes the results obtained in similar YC8 tumor assays, expressed as mean survival times, at different levels of our development of *C. parvum* production. For experimental lots, in small volume and with intentional variations of some parameters, MST showed some variations, which are generally not statistically significant. For pilot lots—at semi-industrial scale, and especially for clinical use batches—MST variations were reduced.

Long-Range Observation

Our different tumor assays were daily observed and recorded for a period of 65–90 days. For logistic reasons, this observation time seemed reasonable, and our official mean survival times were established after 65 days. However, some experiments were kept for a longer period: between 5–6 months. Figure 4 illustrates one of these long-term observations, revealing interesting facts. Three different pilot lots were compared in the same trial; as usual, we gave only one stimulation at day 0, and the YC8 challenge was severe, but normal (control MST = 18).

Table V. Comparison for Different Production Factors[a]

	Mean survival time (65 days of observation)	
	Balb/c YC8	Ehrlich's ascite
C. parvum without inact.	59–60	54.3
C. parvum formaldehyde inact. (concentration)		
< 100 µg/ml	59–60	40–42.7
100 µg/ml	57–>65–>65	26.2–32.5–34.3
200 µg/ml	64.5–>65–>65–>65	28.7–35.3–36–42.3–43.5
800 µg/ml	57–59–>65–>65	25.1–33.7–33.7–34.7–38.3
C. parvum phenol inact. (concentration)		
0.1%	> 65	54.3
0.5%	60	49
Liquid medium	60–>65	33–37
Challenge control (average)	$\overline{21}$ (18–26)	$\overline{21.9}$ (19–25.7)

[a]Results of stimulation by different experimental *C. parvum* preparations in different standardized assays for two tumor systems: Ehrlich's tumor on Swiss mice and YC8 on Balb/c mice.

Effect of a single, 0.5-ml, intraperitoneal injection of the different preparations. The unique stimulating injection was always given 4 h before challenge. Challenge for stimulated groups and controls (0.2 ml, i.p. route) always lead to 100% mortality in control mice; averages for control mean survival times were calculated: $\overline{21}$ for YC8 and $\overline{21.9}$ for Ehrlich's. The limits observed are given in brackets.

Protective activities for the different cases are expressed as mean survival time after 65 days of observation.

Table VI. Comparison for Different Productions[a]

	Mean survival time (65 days of observation)
Experimental lots	57–59–59–60–60–>65–>65
Pilot lots	57–64.5–>65–>65–>65–>65
Batches for clinical use	>65–>65–>65–>65–>65
Control challenge	$\overline{21}$ (18–26)

[a]Results of stimulation by different *C. parvum* preparations–experimental lots, pilot lots, and lots for clinical use–in different standardized assays for YC8 tumor on Balb/c mice.

Effect of a single 0.5-ml, intraperitoneal injection of the different productions given 4 h before challenge. Challenge for stimulated groups and controls (0.2-ml, i.p. route) always leads to 100% mortality in control mice; average for control mean survival time was calculated: $\overline{21}$. The limits observed are given in brackets.

Protective activities for the different cases are expressed as mean survival time after 65 days of observation.

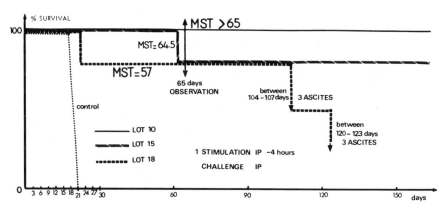

Fig. 4. Long-term observation (5 months) in YC8-standardized assay after a single 0.5 ml, intraperitoneal injection of three different pilot lots of *Corynebacterium parvum*. The same stimulation, 500 μg/mouse, 4 h before challenge was used for the three lots. The same challenge was used for the three stimulated groups and control group. After 65 days of observation establishment of the mean survival times for the three different products were established, but observation was extended up to 150 days (about 5 months). Percentage survival curves show the difference observed during this long-term assay, especially the 6 specific (ascite) deaths observed for pilot lot 18.

When the assays were estimated after 65 days, the three lots did not appear to differ, varying only by one specific (ascite) mortality; so the three mean survival times were not the same ($\geqslant$ 65, 64.5, and 57), but the differences were not statistically significant. However, if the observation period was extended to 150 days, dramatic differences appeared: (a) For lot 10, MST > 65 (65 days of observation) showed no change; there was complete protection for 5 months, following a single injection. (b) For lot 15, MST = 64.5 (65 days of observation), again, there was no change. (c) For lot 18, MST = 57 (65 days of observation), the situation was completely new. Three mice died with specific ascite between 104–107 days; three more died around 120 days.

These facts reveal that after a unique stimulation, a protective effect could be definitive or only temporary, and conditions of the test must be well discussed, i.e., number of animals, observation delay, etc., to get enough accurate separation between comparison products and to get statistically different MST values.

Variations of the Test Parameters

Immunostimulation Routes

The standardized system used in this study was the intraperitoneal route. Some preliminary studies indicated that this stimulation was most efficient for Ehrlich's and YC8 tumor challenge.

A systematic comparison demonstrated that a very poor protective effect, just at the limit of significance, occurred with a single intravenous (i.v.) or subcutaneous (s.c.) *C. parvum* stimulation administered just 4 h before intraperitoneal Ehrlich's tumor challenge, which rapidly killed 100% of controls. No protective effect for single i.v. *C. parvum* stimulation and no limit effect for single s.c. stimulation were observed when stimulation was done 4 h before the intraperitoneal YC8 tumor challenge, which killed 100% of controls.

Number of Stimulations

Experiments were performed with both Ehrlich's and YC8 tumor systems to compare the effects of one, two, or three stimulations. To explore these types of stimulation, it was obligatory to separate the multiple stimulations clearly. So the i.p. injections were distributed before or after challenge, from −14 days to +14 days. No real differences were observed among one, two, or three stimulations; each dose being 500 μg/mouse with a 3-day interval. This kind of experiment clearly shows that if the number of stimulations has very little importance, the timing of the stimulations is crucial.

Time of Immunostimulations and Challenge

With systematic studies, for both tumor systems, it was possible to observe a protective effect from day −21 to day +10. Table VII illustrates the effect observed against Ehrlich's tumor challenge with three stimulations at 3-day

Table VII. Comparison for Different Three-Stimulation Protocols: Immunoprevention and Immunotherapy Protocols[a] (Ehrlich's Tumor Challenge)

Time of the 3 stimulations (days)			Mean survival time (65 days of observation)
−14	−10	−7	48
−10	−7	−3	52.5
−7	−3	0	42
−3	0	+3	54
0	+3	+7	57
+3	+7	+10	37.5
Control			27

[a]Results for different stimulation protocols, all with 3 stimulations, each with *C. parvum* SO 260, 500 μg in 0.50 ml, intraperitoneal injection. Stimulations were at 3-day intervals from day −14 to day +10. Stimulation at day 0 means, as usual, stimulation given 4 h before challenge.

Challenge for stimulated groups and control (0.2 ml, i.p. route) were done all together at day 0, and lead to 100% mortality in control mice.

Protective activities are expressed as mean survival time after 65 days of observation.

intervals, before, at the time of challenge, and after the challenge. Normal protection was observed for the different schedules.

For immunoprevention protocols with Ehrlich's tumor challenge—even with only a single stimulation, a regular protection was observed from day −14 to day 0, but not at day −21.

For immunoprevention protocols with YC8 tumor challenge—even with only a single stimulation, a strong protection was observed from day −21 to day 0.

For immunotherapy protocols, with both Ehrlich's and YC8 tumor challenges, good protection was observed from day 0 to day +7 or +14. The best protective effect was regularly obtained by stimulation at day +7.

On the other hand, when the first stimulation was given too late—at day +14—no significant effect was observed for the steep challenges used in these experiments.

Discussion

The practical intention of this work was to get standardized, reliable tests for measuring tumor activity in order to control immunostimulants, especially *C. parvum* batches.

From the first report by Halpern *et al.* (1966), several publications showed evidence for *C. parvum* activity against different rodent tumor systems (Woodruff and Boak, 1966; Lamensans *et al.*, 1968; Mathé *et al.*, 1969; Amiel *et al.*, 1969; Fisher *et al.*, 1970; Halpern *et al.*, 1973a). However, these works are difficult to compare because of the great variety of nonisogenic and isogenic tumors and the greater diversity of *Corynebacterium* preparations and, especially, of experiment conditions.

Some works used nonisogenic systems: Betz's sarcoma and Ehrlich's ascite. (Halpern *et al.*, 1966, 1973a), L 1210 leukemia (Mathé *et al.*, 1969; Mathé, 1973), and Lewis solid tumor (Mathé, 1973). Other works used isogenic systems: either chemically-induced sarcomas or fibrosarcomas (Woodruff and Boak, 1966; Fisher *et al.*, 1970; Currie and Bagshaw, 1970; Milas and Mujagic, 1972; Woodruff and Dunbar, 1973), spontaneous A mammary carcinoma (Woodruff and Boak, 1966), E ♂ G2 leukemia (Amiel *et al.*, 1969), AKR leukemia (Lamensans *et al.*, 1968; Biozzi *et al.*, 1972), Graffi leukemia (Chirigos *et al.*, 1973), or YC8 lymphoma (Halpern, 1973; Halpern *et al.*, 1973b).

The nature of *Corynebacterium* preparations also varied: generally, a classical *C. parvum* killed by heat and formaldehyde was used. Only three works compared two (Smith and Woodruff, 1968) or three preparations (Halpern *et al.*, 1963; Woodruff and Dunbar, 1973). Always, the *C. parvum* concentrations actually used were very difficult to define. The routes of injection were often different, but few publications compare two (Halpern *et al.*, 1966; Lamensans *et al.*, 1968) or more routes (Halpern *et al.*, 1973a).

The variable timing used for stimulation and challenge in these experiments makes it even more difficult to compare their results, especially with regard to immunoprevention and immunotherapy protocols. However, these previous works provide the basis for tests controlling antitumor activity of *C. parvum* preparations.

Our work confirms that the activity of *C. parvum* is very variable from one tumor system to another: no effect on AKR, a potent effect on Ehrlich, and a very potent effect against YC8. However within one tumor system, it seems possible to standardize the stimulation procedure and the challenge conditions to get a reproducible test. Of course, this test is designed to be carried out under favorable conditions: to observe an average protective effect, doses, routes, timing, and titration were regularly performed.

A crucial parameter, as previously published by Amiel *et al.* (1968), Woodruff and Boak (1966), and Halpern *et al.* (1973b), is the challenge dose. Excessively high levels of tumor cells erase the potential protective activity, a reasonable challenge, just sufficient to give a 100% tumor mortality in the control group, must be established.

In our assays, these equilibrated conditions, *C. parvum* (as compared to other products) appeared to be a potent immunostimulant for both nonsyngenic Ehrlich's ascite and syngenic YC8 tumor. These results are in agreement with those previously published by Halpern *et al.* (1966) and Woodruff and Dunbar (1973) who compared two or several immunostimulants, but are not in complete agreement with the results of Mathé (1973).

Standardized assays for Ehrlich's and YC8 tumor systems offer accurate tools to compare different productions or production parameters quantitatively. A careful comparison, especially of the mean survival time calculations, allows the selection of better conditions for potent *C. parvum* immunostimulation and the control of different batches intended for experimental or clinical trials.

It is clear that the animal models we possess demonstrate evidence that some factors are essential for stopping a malignant process. The route of administration for each model must be clearly established. The number of repeated stimulations seems nonessential, but the schedule of treatment is crucial. Our results confirm that a therapy starting after challenge can stop the tumor, as several times demonstrated by Woodruff and Boak (1966).

These results suggest that it is possible to measure, under defined conditions, an antitumor activity in *C. parvum* preparations. These quantitative values could be useful to determine the best preparations, but only the most sophisticated studies combining immunotherapy and chemotherapy in different animal models and clinical investigations will provide evidence of adjuvant action for antitumor defense in patients (Israël, 1973; Israël and Halpern, 1972).

Summary

Our experience with 3 experimental tumors in mice is presented. The principal aim was to get standardized tests for antitumor activity to compare different immunostimulants—especially *Corynebacterium parvum* batches—and to measure their potential antitumor activity.

The three tumor systems—nonsyngenic Ehrlich's ascite, syngenic AKR leukemia, and syngenic YC8 tumor—with standardized conditions of assays, are presented. Challenge levels necessary and sufficient to get 100% tumor mortality in controls are discussed.

C. parvum activity on the 3 systems under the defined conditions is presented: there was no effect on AKR, a significant protective effect on Ehrlich's tumor, and a strong protective effect on YC8 tumor.

Comparison, in parallel standardized assays, between *C. parvum* and other stimulants, provides evidence of the special potent activity of *C. parvum* under the conditions specified.

The remarkable dose—response effects are analyzed. These intraperitoneal-route, standardized tests on Ehrlich's and YC8 tumors, appear to be accurate tools for comparing different productions or production parameters and for checking the different batches, especially with mean survival time calculations. Long-range observations after a single stimulation permit us to discuss the conditions necessary to get statistically valid values. Studies about stimulation parameters show that the route of stimulation is a fundamental factor; the number of stimulations does not seem to be essential, but the schedule of immunostimulations is a crucial factor which, however, allows both immuno-prevention and immunotherapy experimental assays.

Acknowledgments

The authors would like to thank Mr. C. Stellman and G. Béranger for statistical work. The expert assistance of Mrs. D. Vorel and Miss O. Barge for technical work, and Mrs. C. Cambet and Miss M. Saubin for secretarial work is gratefully acknowledged.

References

Amiel, J. L., Litwin, J., and Bérardet, M. (1969). Essais d'immunothérapie active non spécifique par *Corynebacterium parvum* formolé. *Rev. Fr. Etud. Clin. Biol.* **14**:909.

Biozzi, G., Stiffel, C., Mouton, D., Bouthillier, Y., and Decreusefond, C. (1972). Importance de l'immunité spécifique et non spécifique dans la défense antitumorale. *Ann. Inst. Pasteur, Paris* **122**:685.

Chirigos, M. A., Pearson, J., Woods, W., and Spahn, G. (1973). Immunotherapy and chemotherapy in murine leukemia. *Virus Tumorogenesis and Immunogenesis.* p. 335, (W. S. Ceglowski and H. Friedman, eds.), New York, Academic Press.

Currie, G. A. and Bagshawe, K. D. (1970). Active immunotherapy with *Corynebacterium parvum* and chemotherapy in murine fibrosarcomas. *Br. Med. J.* **1**:541.

Fisher, J. C., Grace, W. R., and Mannick, J. A. (1970). The effect of nonspecific immune stimulation with *Corynebacterium parvum* on patterns of tumor growth. *Cancer* **26**:1379.

Geran, R. I., Greenberg, N. H., MacDonald, M. M., Schumacher, A. M., and Abbott, B. J. (1972). Protocols for screening chemical agents and natural products against animal tumors and other biological systems (third edition). *Cancer Chemother. Rep.* **3**.

Halpern, B. (1973). Inhibition of malignant tumor growth by *Corynebacterium parvum* and its mechanism. I.R.C.S. Intern. Res. Commun. System (April 1973).

Halpern, B. N., Prévot, A. R., Biozzi, G., Stiffel, C., Mouton, D., Morard, J. C., Bouthillier, Y., and Decreusefond, C. (1963). Stimulation de l'activité phagocytaire du systéme réticuloendothélial provoquée par *Corynebacterium parvum. J. Reticuloendothel. Soc.* **1**:77.

Halpern, B. N., Biozzi, G., Stiffel, C., and Mouton, D. (1966). Inhibition of tumor growth by administration of killed *Corynebacterium parvum. Nature (Lond.)* **212**:853.

Halpern, B., Fray, A., Crépin, Y., Platica, O., Lorinet, A. M., Rabourdin, A., Sparros, L., and Isac, R. (1973a). *Corynebacterium parvum,* a potent immunostimulant in experimental infections and in malignancies. *Immunopotentiation,* p. 217 (Ciba Foundation, New Series), Elsevier-Excerpta Medica, North-Holland, Amsterdam.

Halpern, B., Fray, A., Crepin, Y., Platica, O., Sparros, L., Lorinet, A. M., and Rabourdin, A. (1973b) Action inhibitrice du *Corynebacterium parvum* sur le développement des tumeurs malignes syngéniques et son mécanisme. *C. R. Acad. Sci.* **276**:1911.

Israël, L. (1973). Preliminary results of nonspecific immunotherapy for lung cancer. *Cancer Chemother. Rep.* **4**:283.

Israël, L. and Halpern, B. (1972). Le *Corynebacterium parvum* dans les cancers avancés. Première évaluation de l'activité thérapeutique de cette immunostimuline. *Nouv. Presse Med.* **1**:19.

Lamensans, A., Stiffel, C., Mollier, M. F., Laurent, M., Mouton, D., and Biozzi, G. (1968). Effet protecteur de *Corynebacterium parvum* contre la leucémie greffée AKR. Relation avec l'activité catalasique hépatique et la fonction phagocytaire du système réticulo-endothélial. *Rev. Fr. Etud. Clin. Biol.* **23**:773.

Leclerc, J. C., Gomard, E., and Lévy, J. P. (1972). Cell-mediated reaction against tumors induced by oncornaviruses. I. Kinetics and specificity of the immune response in murine sarcoma virus (MSV) induced tumors and transplanted lymphomas. *Int. J. Cancer* **10**:589.

Mathé, G. (1973). Attempt at using systemic immunity adjuvants in experimental and human cancer therapy. *Immunopotentiation*, p. 305 (Ciba Foundation, New Series), Elsevier-Excerpta Medica, North-Holland, Amsterdam.

Mathé, J. L., Pouillart, P., and Lapeyraque, F. (1969). Active immunotherapy of L1210 leukemia applied after the graft of tumor cells. *Br. J. Cancer* **23**:814.

Milas, L. and Mujagic, H. (1972). Protection by *Corynebacterium parvum* against tumor cells injected intravenously. *Rev. Eur. Etud. Clin. Biol.* **17**:498.

Smith, L. H. and Woodruff, M. F. A. (1968). Comparative effect of two strains of *Corynebacterium parvum* on phagocytic activity and tumor growth. *Nature (Lond.)* **219**:197.

Woodruff, M. F. A. and Boak, J. L. (1966). Inhibitory effect of injection of *Corynebacterium parvum* on the growth of tumor transplants in isogenic hosts. *Br. J. Cancer* **20**:345.

Woodruff, M. F. A. and Dunbar, N. (1973). The effect of *Corynebacterium parvum* and other reticuloendothelial stimulants on transplanted tumors in mice. *Immunopotentiation*, p. 287 (Ciba Foundation, New Series), Elsevier-Excerpta Medica, North-Holland, Amsterdam.

21

Results of Investigations with *Corynebacterium parvum* in an Experimental Animal System

BERNARD FISHER, NORMAN WOLMARK,
and E. R. FISHER

Introduction

Increasing evidence is accumulating from animal model systems (J. C. Fisher *et al.*, 1970; Halpern *et al.*, 1966; Smith and Scott, 1972; Woodruff and Boak, 1966) and from studies in patients (Israel, 1973; Israel and Halpern, 1972; Israel and Edelstein, 1973), to suggest that various strains of anaerobic coryneforms are capable of tumor-growth inhibition. Mice harboring an array of experimental tumors have received *Corynebacterium parvum* as the only form of therapy by various routes and at a multiplicity of times. Although the experimental models varied greatly, there were certain conditions in which *C. parvum* afforded a degree of host protection. All investigators have reported that growth of tumors was more readily inhibited when *C. parvum* was administered to mice prior to,

BERNARD FISHER and NORMAN WOLMARK, Department of Surgery, University of Pittsburgh Medical School, Pittsburgh, Pennsylvania 15261 and E. R. FISHER, Institute of Pathology, Shadyside Hospital, Pittsburgh, Pennsylvania 15232.

Supported by USPHS Grants CA 05949, CA 12102, and CA 14972.

at, or shortly after tumor-cell inoculation. Practically no evidence has been presented to demonstrate its effectiveness when given to mice with established, visible, palpable, or measurable tumors.

Since immunopotentiators are presumed to be effective in hosts harboring a minimal tumor burden, there exists a rationale for their use against overt tumors in combination with tumor-cell destructive agents, providing the latter do not interfere with mechanisms responsible for effectiveness of the former. Only a few reports have provided information regarding the effects of administration of *C. parvum* in combination with chemotherapy to experimental animals with solid tumors (Currie and Bagshawe, 1970; Woodruff and Dunbar, 1973), and to date, only one group of investigators has recorded its experience employing such a combination against solid tumor in humans (Israel, 1973; Israel and Halpern, 1972; Israel and Edelstein, 1973).

As yet, no unifying concept is available to account for the observed inhibition of tumor growth. While numerous investigations have been directed toward elucidating the mechanisms involved, it remains to be conclusively demonstrated that there is participation of the immune system. Attempts to identify a particular cell type participating in *C. parvum*-mediated tumor-growth repression have resulted in a number of divergent observations. Findings have demonstrated that restraint of tumor growth as a consequence of *C. parvum* administration can proceed in animals whose T cells have been severely depleted (Woodruff *et al.*, 1973) or who have been treated with antilymphocyte serum (Castro, 1973), tending to minimize the effector functions of that cell type in the adjuvant suppression of tumor growth. The demonstration that such a phenomenon is independent of host capacity to produce humoral antibody lessens the likelihood of B-cell participation (Biozzi *et al.*, 1972). Moreover, presently reported findings demonstrating that *C. parvum*-mediated tumor-growth inhibition can be improved by B-cell depressant cytostatic agents, such as cyclophosphamide, further support that contention. While such observations tend to diminish the importance of the lymphocyte in *C. parvum*-mediated tumor repression, others have recently reported that lymph-node and peritoneal lymphocytes taken from normal animals pretreated with *C. parvum* displayed *in vitro* destruction of syngenic tumor cells (Halpern *et al.*, 1973). Such findings have been characterized as "nonimmune cytotoxicity."

Increasing attention has been focused on the cytotoxic role of the macrophage (Evans and Alexander, 1972). While a tumor cytostatic effect has been attributed to *C. parvum*-activated macrophages (Halpern, this volume), little or no evidence is available to indicate that such cells are cytotoxic. While their role in *C. parvum*-mediated cytotoxicity may be questionable, a host of evidence does implicate the importance of such cells in *C. parvum*-elicited immunopotentiation (Frost and Lance, 1973; Howard *et al.*, 1973a,b; Scott, 1972a,b).

A series of investigations are being carried out in our laboratory (a) to obtain further information as to whether a specific cellular immune mechanism participates in *C. parvum*-induced tumor-growth inhibition and, if so, (b) to elucidate the types of cell(s) involved, as well as (c) to gain information which might aid in formulating a rational regimen for the administration of *C. parvum* in patients with cancer.

This communication presents findings relative to (1) the effect of *C. parvum* in single and repeated inoculations on bone-marrow-macrophage precursors of both normal and tumor-bearing animals; (2) the effect of *C. parvum* on *in vitro* cytotoxicity of regional and nonregional lymph-node cells from animals either having a tumor present or from those in which a tumor had been previously removed; and (3) the effect of utilizing prolonged administration of *C. parvum* alone and in combination with cyclophosphamide for the treatment of established, measurable, C_3H mammary tumors.

Effect of *C. parvum* on Bone-Marrow Macrophage-Colony Production

Method

Adult male and female C_3HeB/FeJ mice (Jackson Memorial Laboratories, Bar Harbor, Maine) were utilized when 8–12 weeks old. *C. parvum*—American Culture Collection Number 6134 (batch PX289 and PX365A)—was obtained from Burroughs-Wellcome Company, North Carolina.* Preparations consisted of 7 mg dry weight per ml of formalin-killed organisms suspended in saline (containing 0.01% Thiomersol). The dose of a single administration consisted of 1.4 mg. *Mycobacterium bovis* (strain BCG) was obtained from the Research Foundation, Chicago, Illinois. The dose of a single injection consisted of 1.0 mg.

The tumor used was a spontaneous, syngenic, mammary adenocarcinoma which originated in a C_3H female and was maintained by transfer into female mice. Tumor implantation consisted of the subcutaneous trocar transfer of a 1- to 2-mm fragment of tumor into the left hind leg distal to the popliteal node.

All injections were administered subcutaneously into the left hind leg of all animals, except in one experiment in which the effectiveness of i.p. and i.v. inoculations was compared. In tumor-bearing mice, the injection was between the tumor and regional (popliteal and inguinal) lymph nodes. A modification of the method of Bradley and Metcalf (1966), described in detail elsewhere (Baum and Fisher, 1972), was employed to assay bone-marrow macrophages.

Results

Normal Mice

In Experiment I, a single injection of *C. parvum* or BCG produced an essentially similar pattern of bone-marrow macrophage-colony production (Fig. 1). Stimulation commenced very early and achieved levels considerably greater than controls by two days. At seven days, stimulation was rapidly subsiding, and

*Provided by Dr. John K. Whisnant.

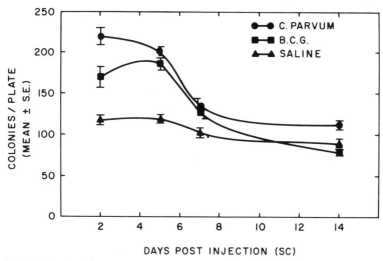

Fig. 1. Single injection of *Corynebacterium parvum* or BCG in normal mice, macrophage-colony production.

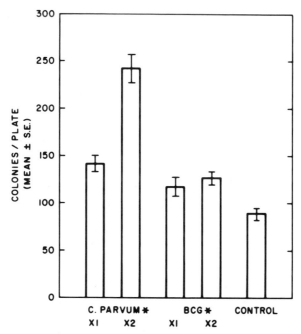

Fig. 2. Repeated injection of *Corynebacterium parvum* or BCG in normal mice, macrophage-colony production.

only a minimal effect was detectable at 14 days. Although *C. parvum* produced a statistically significant greater response than BCG at 2 and 14 days, the differences are not reflected in a changed pattern of stimulation.

Results of Experiment II (Fig. 2), demonstrated a marked difference in colony production between mice receiving two doses of *C. parvum* and those receiving two doses of BCG. When macrophage assay was performed 7 days after the last injection, a second inoculation of *C. parvum,* given 14 days after the first—at a time when stimulation from the initial injection was terminating, resulted in a synergistically greater stimulation than that achieved by a single injection. In fact, the number of colonies obtained seven days after the second injection (Fig. 2) approximated the maximum number obtained two days after a single injection (Fig. 1). In contrast to results with *C. parvum,* a second inoculation of BCG failed to stimulate the production of macrophage colonies more than a single inoculation, and the number produced was markedly less than that observed after two inoculations of *C. parvum.*

Experiment III was undertaken to compare routes of *C. parvum* administration on macrophage-colony production. It was observed (Fig. 3) that i.v. and i.p. administration was more effective than s.c. inoculation in stimulating and prolonging macrophage-colony production.

Tumor-Bearing Mice

Results of Experiment IV (Fig. 4) demonstrated that the presence of an established, growing tumor had no stimulatory effect on bone-marrow macro-

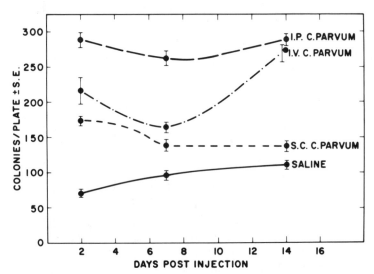

Fig. 3. Effect of route of administration on *Corynebacterium parvum* bone-marrow macrophage production in normal mice.

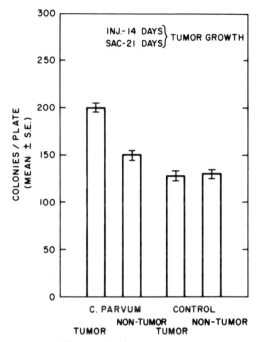

Fig. 4. Effect of *Corynebacterium parvum* on macrophage-colony production in tumor-bearing mice.

phage-colony production at 21 days of tumor growth, the levels observed being no greater than non-tumor-bearing controls. If, however, *C. parvum* was administered to an animal with a tumor at 14 days of growth, significantly greater bone-marrow macrophage-colony production was achieved at 21 days than when a similar inoculation was administered to a non-tumor-bearing animal.

Results of Experiment V (Fig. 5) indicated that a single administration of either *C. parvum* or BCG at 24 days of tumor growth increased bone-marrow macrophage-colony production to a similar degree. As in Experiment IV, the presence of a growing tumor no longer had any bone-marrow macrophage-stimulating properties at 31 days, with levels obtained being no different from non-tumor-bearing controls. Two inoculations of *C. parvum* administered on days 10 and 24 of tumor growth achieved a much greater bone-marrow macrophage-colony production than did two similarly administered doses of BCG. Two inoculations of *C. parvum* had a considerably greater bone-marrow macrophage stimulation than did a single inoculation given at 24 days of tumor growth. In contrast, two administrations of BCG were no better than a single administration of either BCG or *C. parvum* given on day 24 of tumor growth.

When the effectiveness of treatment was assessed, only animals receiving two

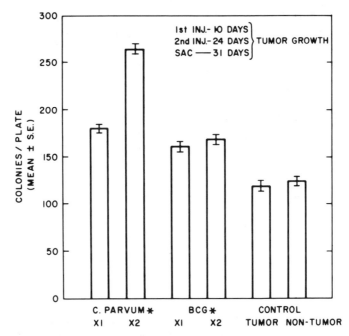

Fig. 5. Repeated injection of *Corynebacterium parvum* or BCG in tumor-bearing mice, macrophage-colony production.

inoculations of *C. parvum* demonstrated any significant inhibition of tumor growth at 31 days when compared to untreated mice.

Comment

Previous investigations conducted in this laboratory have demonstrated that the presence of an established, growing, syngenic tumor is capable of augmenting the production of bone-marrow macrophage colonies (Baum and Fisher, 1972). This stimulus was, however, transient and at 14 days of tumor growth was no longer effective, in spite of the continuing presence of progressively increasing levels of tumor antigen. The present results confirm those findings in that no stimulatory effect was noted at 21 days of tumor growth. When *C. parvum* was administered after 14 days of tumor growth, i.e., at a time when stimulation of marrow-macrophage precursors would have been expected to have ceased, a synergistic augmentation in macrophage-colony production was noted. Although available tumor antigen was not in itself still acting as a stimulus to marrow-macrophage production, it probably had a sensitizing effect on macrophage precursors, permitting levels of stimulation by *C. parvum* greater than that occurring when *C. parvum* was administered to normal animals. If, as previously speculated by us (Baum and Fisher, 1972), the transient duration of bone-marrow macrophage-colony production by tumor antigen is due to a negative-feedback inhibition, it might be postulated that *C. parvum* functions by interrupting such an inhibitory mechanism, as well as independently stimulating available marrow-macrophage precursors, thus effecting a synergistic augmentation.

The present observations confirm and, more importantly, extend findings utilizing BCG (B. Fisher *et al.,* 1975), and they compare findings resulting from use of BCG with those following *C. parvum* administration. The stimulatory effect of *C. parvum* or BCG on bone-marrow macrophage-colony production occurs very soon after administration. At a time (after 48 h) when the peak stimulation resulting from s.c. *C. parvum* injection has passed, the phagocytic index and weight of peripheral lymphoid organs (Halpern, 1974) are beginning to increase. Such observations suggest that bone-marrow macrophage precursors may be the initial target for adjuvant stimulation and that there is a subsequent migration and population of peripheral lymphoid tissues, as well as the entire reticuloendothelial system (RES) by those cells. An explanation for the increased RES activity observed as a result of this growth and following administration of immunopotentiating agents is thus available. The observation that i.v. or i.p. inoculation was more effective than s.c. injection is in keeping with our findings, discussed in depth later, that i.v. or i.p. *C. parvum* more effectively inhibits tumor growth.

The demonstration that a repeated inoculation of s.c. *C. parvum* given at the termination of the activation phase of the first injection is able to produce a synergistic augmentation, whereas BCG is completely refractory, suggests that these agents could stimulate macrophages differently in both tumor and non-tumor-bearing animals. Such findings are in keeping with those of others (Biozzi *et al.,* 1965), who observed that mice reinjected with BCG toward the end of the reticuloendothelial stimulation phase produced by the first injection showed no further hyperphagocytic activity, whereas *C. parvum* was able to successfully "restimulate" mice under the same conditions.

Determination of patterns of bone-marrow macrophage stimulation may provide a useful method for elucidating an optimum therapeutic regimen for the administration of various immunological adjuvants. If a correlation between bone-marrow macrophage stimulation and inhibition of tumor growth can be substantiated, then utilization of the presently employed technique for the screening and monitoring of prospective immunotherapeutic agents would have merit. Moreover, it would provide a method for determining the dose and schedule of administration so that a sustained, elevated, level of bone-marrow macrophage stimulation could be maintained. This would be of particular pertinence when immunostimulants are utilized together with myelosuppressive chemotherapeutic agents (Israel, 1973; Israel and Edelstein, 1973; Israel and Halpern, 1972). Under such circumstances, an optimum bone-marrow protective effect could be achieved as a result of maximum marrow stimulation. From the present findings, it is likely that repeated administrations of *C. parvum* is apt to be more effective than BCG.

Effect of *C. parvum* on Cytotoxicity of Regional and Nonregional Lymph-Node Cells from Animals with Tumors Present or Removed

Method

The mice, tumors, and *C. parvum* employed, as well as BCG, were all similar to those described previously.

Popliteal and regional nodes of tumor-bearing legs are designated as regional lymph nodes (RLNs), and cells from those nodes as RLNCs. Nodes from the right foreleg and axilla of mice with tumor are referred to as distant or nonregional lymph nodes (NRLNs), and their cells as NRLNCs. The corresponding nodes from non-tumor-bearing animals served as controls. The technique employed in this laboratory for cytotoxicity testing of RLNCs and NRLNCs has been described (B. Fisher *et al.*, 1974). Wells were scored using a scale of 0–5, according to the amount of well free of tumor cells, 0 indicating complete coverage by tumor cells and 5 complete absence of cells. The data are presented as the percent of tumor-cell destruction. This represents the amount of tumor remaining in treated wells compared to tumor in nontreated control wells.

Results

Normal Mice

The injection of a single or two weekly inoculations of *C. parvum* failed to produce cytotoxicity by LNCs from nodes adjacent to the inoculation, which was significantly different from its effect on LNCs from saline-injected controls (Fig. 6).

Tumor-Bearing Mice

The single inoculation of *C. parvum*, either into a tumor or between a tumor, and its RLNs (paratumor) resulted in a significant increase in cytotoxicity by varying numbers of RLNCs removed 14 days, but not 7 days, after injection (Fig. 7). In one of the experiments using 3.7×10^4 RLNCs, one injection of *C. parvum* did not significantly enhance tumor destruction by such LNCs (42%) as compared to results from untreated tumor-bearing animals (37%). Intratumor inoculations of two doses of *C. parvum* a week apart did, however, markedly enhance *in vitro* tumor-cell destruction (80% versus 37%). In a single instance where i.p. *C. parvum* was employed, cytotoxicity of LNCs was not enhanced.

NRLNCs from mice bearing tumors (21–28 days) displayed significant cytotoxicity, but less than that displayed by such cells from RLNs. A single injection of *C. parvum*, either intra- or paratumor, had only a slight effect in altering

	SALINE	C.PARVUM	
		DAYS -14	DAYS -7,-14
RLNCs	4*	6	7
NRLNCs	3	4	3

Fig. 6. Effect of *Corynebacterium parvum* on cytotoxicity of RLNC, and NRLNCs, non-tumor-bearing mice. Percent tumor-cell destruction (*). LNCs = 1 X 10^5.

tumor destruction by NRLNCs (Fig. 8). When two intratumor injections (days −7 and −14) were given, NRLNC cytotoxicity (39%) was significantly greater than was achieved by a single injection given on day −14 (25%).

An experiment was repeated three times to evaluate the effect of BCG injected into tumors on cytotoxicity of RLNCs (Fig. 9). Neither 7 nor 14 days following such treatment was a significant effect noted.

*RLNCs	SALINE		CORYNEBACTERIUM PARVUM					
			INTRA-TUMOR			PARA-TUMOR		IP
			DAY-7	DAY-14	-14 & -7	DAY-7	DAY-14	DAY-14
1X10⁵	5*	61	61	77	−	−	−	−
1X10⁵	3	66	64	−	−	61	−	−
5X10⁴	4	60	−	80	−	−	78	−
5X10⁴	8	38	−	59	−	−	43	37
3.7X10⁴	9	52	−	84	−	−	73	−
3.7X10⁴	1	37	−	42	80	−	−	−

Fig. 7. *Corynebacterium parvum* and RLNC cytotoxicity, tumor-bearing mice. Percent tumor-cell destruction (*).

#RLNCs	SALINE		CORYNEBACTERIUM PARVUM			
			INTRA TUMOR		PARA TUMOR	IP
			DAY-14	DAYS-14&-7	DAY-14	DAY-14
7.5×10^5	6*	27	30	—	24	—
1×10^5	2	25	30	39	—	—
1×10^5	6	26	37	—	30	29

Fig. 8. *Corynebacterium parvum* and NRLNC cytotoxicity, tumor-bearing mice. Percent tumor-cell destruction (*).

Following Tumor Removal

Following removal of a tumor which had been present for 14 days, cytotoxicity of RLNCs was lost (Fig. 10). By 3 weeks post-tumor removal the cytotoxicity was not significantly different from cytotoxicity produced by LNCs from normal, non-tumor-bearing mice. In a series of experiments where treatment was carried out 14 days after removal of a primary tumor, a comparison was made between the ability of a second tumor, a single injection of *C. parvum* or BCG, or a second tumor plus *C. parvum,* to restore cytotoxicity when injected in proximity to nodes regional to the first tumor. Neither *C. parvum* nor BCG was effective. A second tumor growing for 7 or 14 days did restore

	SALINE		BCG	
			DAY-7	DAY-14
I	12*	52	46	41
II	5	74	73	70
III	4	74	60	71

Fig. 9. Effect of BCG on RLNC cytotoxicity in tumor-bearing mice. Percent tumor-cell destruction (*). LNCs = 1×10^5.

# RLNCs	DAYS POST TREATMENT	TUMOR REMOVAL	SALINE		2nd TUMOR	C. PARVUM	BCG	2nd TUMOR + C. PARVUM
1×10^5	7	21	9*	4	73	13	9	91
1×10^5	7	21	7	8	61	11	9	82
3.7×10^4	14	28	9	7	39	8	4	92
3.7×10^4	14	28	2	1	32	4	3	96
3.7×10^4	14	28	2	1	42	7	6	90
5×10^4	14	98	4	2	16	2	–	61

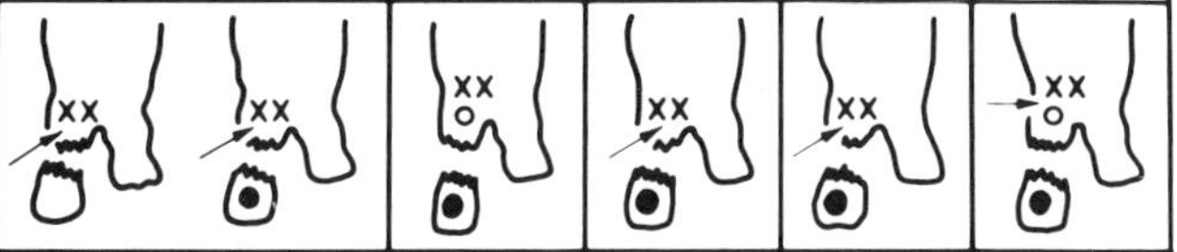

Fig. 10. *Corynebacterium parvum* (one injection) and RLNC cytotoxicity, primary tumor removed. Percent tumor-cell destruction (*).

	DAYS POST TREATMENT	TUMOR REMOVAL	SALINE		2nd TUMOR	C. PARVUM	BCG	2nd TUMOR + C. PARVUM
	7	21	7*	2	18	3	1	19
I	7	21	4	4	18	5	6	16
II	14	28	9	11	20	9	15	35
III	14	28	0	0	32	4	6	39
IV	14	28	1	0	19	1	0	44
V	14	98	2	3	3	4	–	23

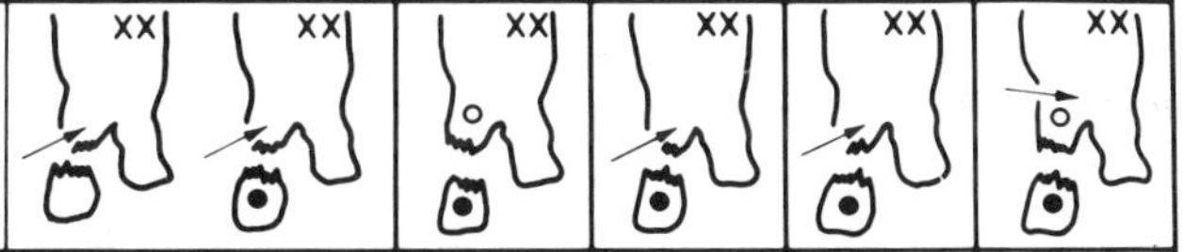

Fig. 11. *Corynebacterium parvum* (one injection) and NRLNC cytotoxicity, primary tumor removed. Percent tumor-cell destruction (*). NRLNCs $= 1 \times 10^5$.

cytotoxicity. The combination of *C. parvum* with a second tumor markedly and significantly enhanced cytotoxicity by RLNCs to a much greater extent than tumor alone. This was particularly evident when smaller numbers of RLNCs (3.7 $\times$ 10^4) were employed. When treatment was instituted 84 days after removal of the primary, the synergistic effect of *C. parvum* and a second tumor on RLNC cytotoxicity was demonstrated. Whereas, the presence of a second tumor for 14 days resulted in only a 16% destruction of tumor cells and *C. parvum* alone in a 2% destruction, the two together produced a 61% eradication of tumor cells.

The cytotoxic activity of NRLNCs was also found to be augmented when cells were evaluated 14 days after the inoculation of a second tumor plus *C. parvum* in proximity to nodes regional to a removed first tumor (Fig. 11). For example, in one experiment, two weeks after inoculation of a second tumor, the *in vitro* tumor destruction by 1 $\times$ 10^5 RLNCs was 19%, by *C. parvum,* 1%, and by cells exposed to both a second tumor and *C. parvum,* 44%. Seven days following treatment, no enhanced cytotoxicity was observed when *C. parvum* was given with a second tumor. When *C. parvum* plus tumor were inoculated 84 days following primary tumor removal (98 days at sacrifice), NRLNCs demonstrated cytotoxicity (23%), whereas neither *C. parvum* alone nor tumor alone had any such effect. When *C. parvum* plus tumor were implanted in the region of distant nodes (NRLNs) (not shown), the cytotoxicity of the nodes regional to the first tumor was increased. Cells from such nodes demonstrated greater cytotoxicity (30%) than cells directly exposed to a second tumor (16%).

Whereas a single injection of *C. parvum* in the area of nodes regional to a removed first tumor failed to significantly restore tumor cytotoxicity by

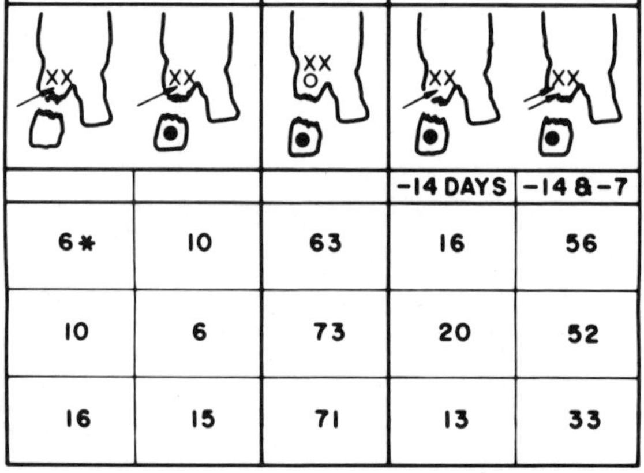

	SALINE		2nd TUMOR	C. PARVUM	
				−14 DAYS	−14 & −7
I	6*	10	63	16	56
II	10	6	73	20	52
III	16	15	71	13	33

Fig. 12. *Corynebacterium parvum* (two injections) and RLNC cytotoxicity, primary tumor removed. Percent tumor-cell destruction (*). RLNCs = 1 $\times$ 10^5.

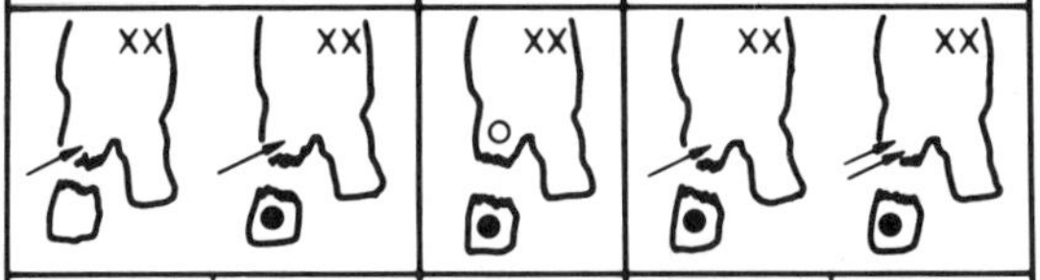

	SALINE		2nd TUMOR	C. PARVUM	
				−14 DAYS	−14 & −7
I	9*	10	32	9	30
II	8	10	29	6	28
III	11	10	27	12	20

Fig. 13. *Corynebacterium parvum* (two injections) and NRLNC cytotoxicity, primary tumor removed. Percent tumor-cell destruction (14 days post-treatment) (*). NRLNCs = 1×10^5.

RLNCs, 2 injections at weekly intervals did enhance tumor cytotoxicity by these cells (Fig. 12). Cells from NRLNs were similarly stimulated by 2 injections of *C. parvum*. The percent of tumor destruction by those cells was, in all experiments, almost identical to that resulting from the presence of a second tumor (Fig. 13).

Comment

It has been observed that following removal of a primary tumor, cytotoxicity of RLNCs and NRLNCs was rapidly lost (B. Fisher *et al.*, 1974) and that rechallenge with a tumor of the same type was progressively less effective in restoring cytotoxicity as the time between removal and re-exposure to tumor increased. These findings suggest that insofar as *in vitro* cytotoxicity is concerned, such LNCs had become immunologically "paralyzed" to that tumor antigen. It seems unlikely that the lack of a secondary response could be attributed to loss of immunologic memory by such cells, for in such circumstances, a response similar in magnitude to that obtained as a result of primary tumor exposure might be anticipated. The data indicate that the administration of *C. parvum* together with tumor overcomes this "paralysis." When that treatment regimen was employed at a time when neither tumor alone, nor a single dose of *C. parvum*, was capable of restoring the cytotoxicity, a magnitude of cytotoxicity was achieved which was equivalent to that occurring as a consequence of the initial tumor. Even at a time following primary tumor removal, when RLNCs and NRLNCs were still capable of responding to a second tumor challenge by demonstrating cytotoxicity similar to that achieved by a first tumor exposure, *C. parvum* inoculated with a second tumor synergistically augmented such cytotoxicity. It is of interest that under these circumstances, two doses of *C. parvum* given without tumor were able to restore cytotoxicity.

Since a variety of stimulating agents capable of inducing cell transformation are capable of producing nonspecific lymphocyte cytotoxicity (Butterworth, 1973; Holm *et al.,* 1964; Lundgren *et al.,* 1968), the possibility that the observed findings were nonspecific might be entertained. Failure to observe cytotoxicity by LNCs from non-tumor-bearing mice receiving *C. parvum* tends to diminish that possibility. Moreover, failure to observe nonspecific cytotoxicity after inoculating two doses of *C. parvum* into non-tumor-bearing animals weighs against the possibility that the first dose resulted in a sensitization enabling lymphocyte transformation and the production of nonspecific cytotoxicity by the second dose.

In all instances in which enhanced cytotoxicity of RLNCs was observed as a result of *C. parvum* administration, similar changes, but of considerably lesser magnitude, were observed in NRLNCs. Demonstration of such activity by the latter suggests that this phenomenon was a systemic one and was not restricted only to RLNCs. Further evidence for this effect was provided by the demonstration that inoculation of *C. parvum* together with tumor at a site remote from RLNs was able to synergistically augment cytotoxicity of RLNCs. Whether the lesser response by NRLNCs was due to insufficient *C. parvum* and/or tumor antigen reaching NRLNs, to a difference in the cell population capable of responding, or a preferential recruitment of immunocompetent cells by RLNs is speculative.

Whatever the mechanism(s) responsible for the findings, these investigations have provided information which may be of pertinence for the formulation of a scheme of therapy in the control of human malignancy. The observation that *C. parvum* given together with tumor can synergistically augment cytotoxicity, or restore it, when nonresponsiveness to tumor antigen exists, provides a possible rationale for the administration of *C. parvum* together with a tumor vaccine. Furthermore, the observation that two doses of *C. parvum* can restore cytotoxicity provides a basis for the repetitive administration of that agent.

Further investigations are being carried out in this laboratory to correlate these findings with the tumor-growth inhibition observed following the employment of *C. parvum* alone and in combination with chemotherapy (cyclophosphamide). Until such relationships can be established, the true significance of these *in vitro* findings remains speculative, despite their wide employment—both clinically and experimentally—as indices of immunologic reactivity.

Effect of Prolonged *C. parvum* and Cyclophosphamide Administration on the Growth of Established Tumors

Methods

The mice, tumors, *C. parvum,* and BCG were all similar to those described earlier. In all experiments, tumors approximately 5 mm in diameter, developing by 14 days, were used. The longest diameter of a tumor was measured, and the same diameter was used for all subsequent measurements during the course of the experiment.

C. parvum and BCG, unless otherwise stated, were administered once a week. Cyclophosphamide (CY) was injected i.p. once a week. Preliminary pilot studies indicated that 90 mg/kg, when given weekly, was well tolerated and produced almost no mortality. Larger doses (120 mg or 200 mg/kg) could be safely given on one occasion, but subsequent administration at weekly intervals resulted in a high incidence of drug-induced deaths.

When weekly *C. parvum* was given in combination with weekly CY, it was always given 4 days following CY. Thus, in the regimen employed, CY was given on days 0, 7, 14, etc., with *C. parvum* being administered on days 4, 11, 18, etc.

When BCG was employed in combination with CY, CY was administered initially and BCG was always given 4 days following CY.

Results

Treatment with C. parvum

The continued weekly administration of *C. parvum* alone to animals with tumors (Fig. 14) produced, in most instances, a limited, but significant, inhibitory effect on tumor growth. The consequence of giving *C. parvum* by different routes to animals bearing 3- to 4-mm tumors was ascertained. Subcutaneous administration of *C. parvum* failed to decrease the rate of tumor growth from that occurring in untreated animals. At no time during the treatment was there a significant difference between the two groups. Weekly i.p. *C. parvum* inoculation did, however, retard tumor growth. During the second, third, and fourth weeks of treatment, tumor sizes of treated animals were significantly less than those of untreated mice. This difference persisted for the duration of the experiment. One i.p. inoculation of *C. parvum* was also effective in decreasing tumor growth. Further evidence substantiating the tumor-growth depressive effect of *C. parvum* was obtained in an experiment where the initial injection of *C. parvum* was i.p. and subsequent doses were s.c. (Fig. 15).

Results from these experiments indicate that *C. parvum* administration prolongs the survival of tumor-bearing mice. In all experiments, at a time when every control animal had died, some of the members of *C. parvum*-treated groups were still alive. When a cumulative mortality curve utilizing all controls and all *C. parvum*-treated animals from five different experiments was prepared, the percentage of survival was significantly higher ($P < 0.01$) in the treated group at and following 63 days of tumor growth (Fig. 16).

Treatment with C. parvum and CY

Employing mice with tumors approximating 1 cm, CY was given in weekly doses (90 mg/kg) alone and in concert with *C. parvum,* which was administered

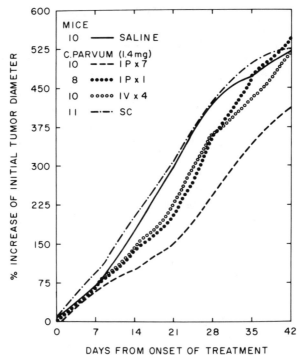

Fig. 14. Effect of *Corynebacterium parvum* on growth of established C_3H tumors.

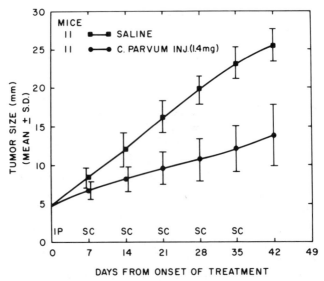

Fig. 15. Effect of *Corynebacterium parvum* on growth of established C_3H tumors.

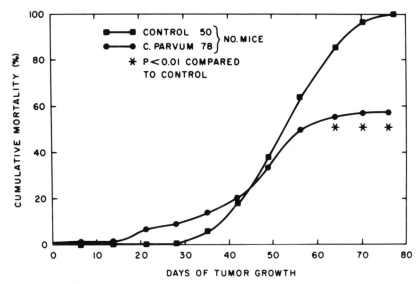

Fig. 16. Effect of *Corynebacterium parvum* in prolonging survival of C_3H tumor-bearing mice.

by various routes (Fig. 17). CY was administered prior to *C. parvum*. When i.p. *C. parvum* was employed in combination with CY (Group V), striking tumor-growth inhibition, not achieved with either agent alone, resulted. Tumor-growth rates were arrested for the duration of the experiment (90 days). When animals in that group were individually evaluated (Fig. 18), it was noted that total tumor-growth arrest occurred in every mouse. In one, a marked regression in tumor size occurred during treatment. The combination of s.c. *C. parvum* and CY likewise produced a greater effect than either agent alone, but was not as repressive as when CY was employed with i.p. *C. parvum*. Of considerable significance was the observation that when 100% of nontreated mice and 95% of those receiving *C. parvum* alone were dead, 90% of those getting combined therapy were still alive.

To confirm the findings in the above experiment, it was repeated, employing mice with smaller tumors (approximately 5 mm). Again (Fig. 19), i.p. *C. parvum* combined with CY resulted in greater tumor inhibition than when either agent was used alone. Total arrest of tumor growth was achieved. *C. parvum* alone was almost completely ineffective in suppressing tumor growth.

BCG was administered to tumor-bearing mice alone or in combination with CY in a dosage schedule similar to that employed with *C. parvum* and CY (Fig. 20). No effect on tumor growth was observed when BCG was repetitively administered as the only therapeutic modality. While BCG combined with CY did retard tumor growth, it was significantly less effective than *C. parvum* and CY.

GROUP	TREATMENT CY (90mg/Kg) ▪	C. PARVUM (1.4mg) ●	MICE	% SURVIVAL (DAYS OF TUMOR GROWTH) 14	21	28	35	42	49	56	90
I —··—	−	−	10	100	80	80	60	10	10	0	0
II ————	+	−	10	100	100	80	80	80	80	80	60
III —·—·—	−	I P	10	100	100	80	80	60	20	10	0
IV ●●●●●●●●	−	SC	10	100	80	60	40	20	0	0	0
V ————	+	I P	10	100	100	100	100	90	90	90	80
VI ··········	+	SC	10	100	100	90	90	90	90	90	90

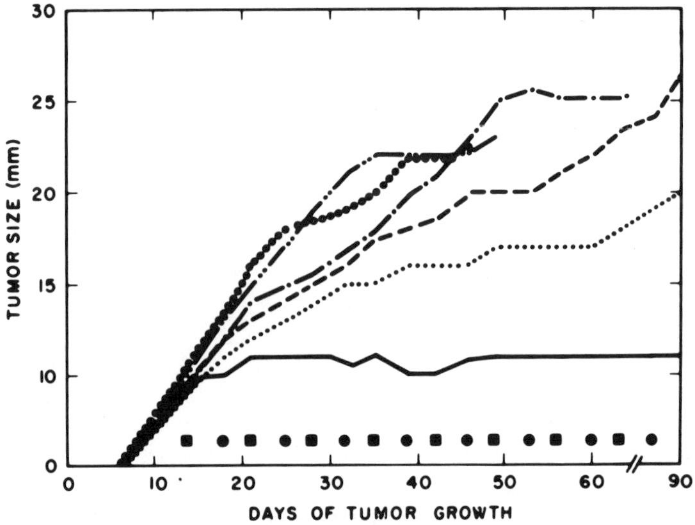

Fig. 17. Effect of *Corynebacterium parvum* and/or cyclophosphamide on C_3H tumor growth.

Tumors in all treatment groups exhibited varying degrees of necrosis (Fig. 21). Viable tumor cells in all treatment groups did not exhibit any distinguishing cytologic characteristics. Mitotic indices (average number of mitoses per high-power field, based upon examination of approximately 20 fields) were 1.4, 1.1, and 1.8 for mice in the CY only group, CY plus *C. parvum* i.p. group, and CY plus *C. parvum* s.c. group, respectively. The only difference in the growth pattern of the various groups was the more conspicuous desmoplastic stroma isolating tumor aggregates and islands in the mice treated with CY and *C. parvum* i.p. (Fig. 22). This was less evident in mice treated with CY and *C. parvum* s.c. (Fig. 23), although more so in the latter group than in animals receiving CY alone. In no tumors of any treatment group was there any significant lymphoid infiltrate present at the periphery or within the cell population of the tumors. The only inflammatory reaction noted was the presence of polymorphonuclar leukocytes in foci of tumor necrosis in all groups studied.

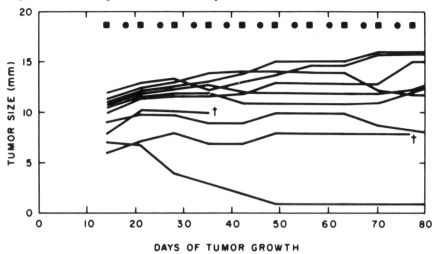

Fig. 18. Effect of *Corynebacterium parvum* and cyclophosphamide on C₃H tumor growth. CY ■; *C. parvum* ●.

GROUP	TREATMENT ■ CY (90 mg/kg)	TREATMENT ● C PARVUM (1.4mg)	MICE	% SURVIVAL DAYS OF TUMOR GROWTH 12	19	26	33	40	47	54	61
I —··—	—	—	10	100	100	100	100	100	60	20	10
II -----	+	—	10	100	100	100	100	100	100	100	100
III —·—·—	—	I P	10	100	100	100	100	100	60	40	20
IV ———	+	I P	10	100	100	100	100	100	80	70	60
V •••••••	+	SC	10	100	100	100	100	100	100	100	100

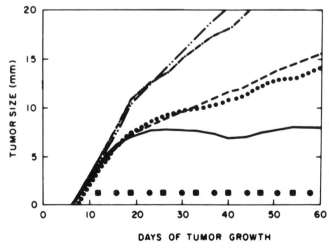

Fig. 19. Effect of *Corynebacterium parvum* and/or cyclophosphamide on C₃H tumor growth.

| GROUP | TREATMENT | | | MICE | % SURVIVAL DAYS OF TUMOR GROWTH | | | | | | | |
	CY (90 mg/Kg) ■	C. PARVUM (1.4 mg) ●	BCG 26×10⁶ VU ▲		10	17	24	31	38	45	52	5
I —··—	—	—	—	12	100	100	100	100	83	75	50	2
II ∘∘∘∘∘∘∘∘∘	+	IP	—	13	100	100	100	92	85	85	77	7
III —–––	+	—	IP	13	100	100	100	100	100	100	100	10
IV ●●●●●●●●	—	—	IP	12	100	100	100	92	92	67	33	

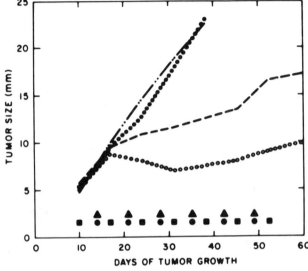

Fig. 20. Effect of *Corynebacterium parvum* or BCG and cyclophosphamide on C_3H tumor growth.

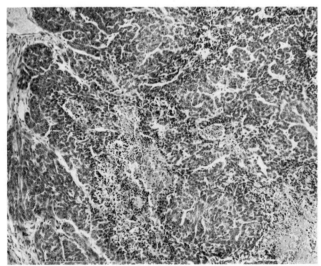

Fig. 21. Varying degrees of necrosis exhibited in the cells of all tumor groups.

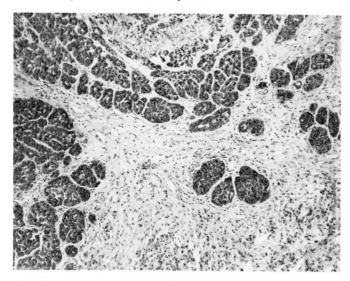

Fig. 22. Conspicuous desmoplastic stroma isolating tumor aggregates and islands in mice treated with CY and *Corynebacterium parvum.*

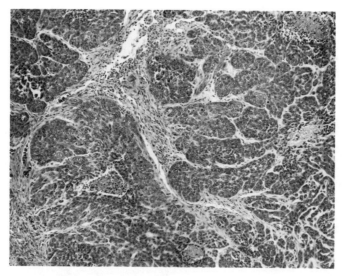

Fig. 23. The desmoplastic stroma seen in Fig. 22 is less evident in mice treated with CY and *Corynebacterium parvum* s.c.

Comment

The present results have demonstrated a growth-inhibitory effect when prolonged *C. parvum,* as the only therapeutic modality, was instituted on unequivocally established, measurable tumors. Better tumor inhibition was achieved when *C. parvum* was administered i.p. Subcutaneous administration was only slightly and sporadically effective. Such findings furnish evidence to justify consideration of the evaluation of *C. parvum* in clinical situations. Its limited effectiveness, however, suggests that it be used only in the presence of a minimal tumor burden.

When BCG in combination with CY was compared to *C. parvum* with CY, the latter proved more effective in retarding tumor growth. Whether this is a result of the conditions employed, or due to differences in the mechanism of action of the agents or to a difference in their immunopotentiating capacity, remains to be elucidated.

Experiments evaluating the effects of combining *C. parvum* with cytostatic agents are of vital importance, since such combinations have been suggested for use in patients with nonmetastatic cancers and are being currently employed in the treatment of advanced disease (Israel, 1973; Israel and Edelstein, 1973; Israel and Halpern, 1972).

The results presently reported differ from any as yet obtained (Currie and Bagshawe, 1970; Woodruff and Dunbar, 1973). The additive effect of *C. parvum* and CY was reproducible and was achieved in all experiments when this combination was repetitively employed. The results also provide evidence that prolonged, repeated, alternating administration of *C. parvum* and CY can be achieved with minimal toxicity and no increase in mortality.

When both CY and *C. parvum* were employed, a complete arrest in the rate of tumor-growth occurred. A reproducible, infinite tumor-doubling time was achieved. The rate of proliferation of clonogenic tumor cells seemingly equalled the rate of cell destruction. This "steady state" was maintained throughout the length of the experiment without tumor "escape." When similar treatment was administered to a 0.5-cm or a 1.0-cm tumor, the same balance was achieved, despite anticipation that the smaller tumor would be more readily affected by similar dosage schedules. No explanation for this phenomenon is currently available.

These results conclusively demonstrate that it is possible to administer CY, a potent B-cell depressor (Poulter and Turk, 1972; Stockman *et al.,* 1973), in combination with *C. parvum,* a B-cell-oriented immunopotentiator (Howard *et al.,* 1973a), on a prolonged basis with the continued maintenance of marked tumor suppression. Although CY may be theoretically capable of inhibiting immunocompetent cells activated by *C. parvum,* this phenomenon was not observed when tumor growth was employed as an index of inhibition.

Cytologically, tumors in all treatment groups appeared comparable with similar mitotic indices. On the other hand, a marked desmoplastic reaction characterized tumors exhibiting the greatest inhibition of tumor growth, i.e., tumors treated by CY and *C. parvum* i.p. Although the genesis and significance of this response is at present uncertain, nevertheless it may reflect a significant host response or defensive mechanism against tumor growth.

Recently, the results of utilizing *C. parvum* in combination with five-drug therapy in a variety of advanced cancers have been reported (Israel, 1973; Israel and Edelstein, 1973; Israel and Halpern, 1972). In patients so treated, a significant increase in prolongation of life was effected with no added undesirable sequellae. As a result of these findings, together with the present data, a rationale for investigation of such combined therapy in human malignancy is present. The use of such a regimen in preliminary clinical trials involving patients with early, as well as disseminated tumor growth, deserves serious consideration.

Continuing investigations on mechanism of action, dose schedules, and frequency of administration are currently in progress in this laboratory. Preliminary data indicate the prolonged effectiveness of a single administration of *C. parvum,* suggesting that it may need be less frequently administered.

Summary

Comparison of single inoculations of *C. parvum* and BCG into tumor- and non-tumor-bearing mice indicates that both agents are capable of rapidly and transiently stimulating bone-marrow macrophage-colony production to a similar extent. A second inoculation of *C. parvum,* administered at a time when the stimulation from the first injection was terminating, synergistically augmented bone-marrow macrophage-colony production. A repeated injection of BCG at a similar time failed to produce such a response. A single administration of *C. parvum* to tumor-bearing animals resulted in a greater augmentation of bone-marrow macrophage-colony production than did similar inoculations to non-tumor-bearing mice. It was observed that i.v. and i.p. *C. parvum* administration were more effective in stimulating and prolonging bone-marrow macrophage-colony production than s.c. inoculation.

C. parvum administered to tumor-bearing animals augmented *in vitro* cytotoxicity of regional and nonregional lymph-node cells (RLNCs and NRLNCs). Following primary tumor removal, RLNs and NRLNs became progressively less responsive to a second exposure to tumor. The administration of *C. parvum* together with a second tumor fully restored lymph-node cell cytotoxicity, even at a time when complete loss of that response to tumor alone existed. In animals whose LNCs were still capable of responding to a second tumor challenge, the administration of *C. parvum* and tumor produced a synergistic augmentation of cytotoxicity. Inoculation of two doses of *C. parvum* without tumor antigen restored cytotoxicity to levels achieved by a second tumor exposure. The administration of one or two doses of *C. parvum* to normal animals never exposed to tumor failed to result in cytotoxicity by lymph-node cells, indicating that a specific immune response is involved.

In studies investigating the effects of prolonged administration of *C. parvum* alone and in combination with cyclophosphamide (CY) for the treatment of established, measurable, C_3H tumors, the continued weekly administration of *C. parvum* by itself provided a limited, but significant, inhibitory effect on tumor growth and significantly prolonged survival. Intraperitoneal and intravenous administration was found to be more effective than the subcutaneous route. When *C. parvum* was administered asynchronously in combination with CY, a tumor growth-inhibitory effect was achieved which was greater than that resulting from either agent alone. Such an effect was consistently obtained. An arrest in the rate of tumor growth occurred, resulting in infinite tumor-doubling time for the duration of observation (> 90 days). The combination of *C. parvum* and CY produced a more effective inhibition of tumor growth than did BCG and CY. The importance of these findings relative to clinical application was considered. The significance and genesis of the marked desmoplastic reaction characterizing tumors from animals treated with *C. parvum* and CY is at present speculative.

Acknowledgment

We acknowledge with gratitude the technical assistance of Elizabeth Saffer, Jean Coyle, and Morton Levine in the accomplishment of these studies.

References

Baum, M. and Fisher, B. (1972). Macrophage production by the bone marrow of tumor-bearing mice. *Cancer Res.* 32:2813.

Biozzi, G., Howard, J. G., Mouton, D., and Stiffel, C. (1965). Modifications of graft-versus-host reaction induced by pretreatment of the host with *M. tuberculosis* and *C. parvum. Transplantation* 3:170.

Biozzi, G., Stiffel, C., Mouton, D., Bouthillier, Y., and Decreusfond, C. (1972). Importance of specific and nonspecific immunity in antitumor defense. *Ann. Inst. Pasteur, Paris* 122:685.

Bradley, T. R. and Metcalf, D. (1966). The growth of mouse bone-marrow cells *in vitro. Aust. J. Exp. Biol. Med. Sci.* 44:287.

Butterworth, A. E. (1973). Nonspecific cytotoxic effects of antigen-transformed lymphocytes, kinetics, cell requirements, and the role of recruitment. *Cell. Immunol.* 7:357.

Castro, J. E. (1973). In: *Immunopotentiation* (Ciba Foundation Symposium, New Series), p. 116.

Currie, G. A. and Bagshawe, K. D. (1970). Active immunotherapy with *Corynebacterium parvum* and chemotherapy in murine fibrosarcomas. *Br. Med. J.* 1:541.

Evans, R. and Alexander, P. (1972). Mechanism of immunologically specific killing of tumor cells by macrophages. *Nature (Lond.)* 236:168.

Fisher, B., Saffer, E., and Fisher, E. R. (1974). Studies concerning the regional lymph node cells. *Cancer* 33:631.

Fisher, B., Taylor, S., Levine, M., Saffer, E., and Fisher, E. R. (1974). Effect of *Myobacterium bovis* (strain bacillus calmette-guerin) on macrophage production by the bone marrow of tumor-bearing mice. *Cancer Res.* 34:1668.

Fisher, J. C., Grace, W. R., and Mannick, J. A. (1970). The effect of nonspecific immune stimulation with *Corynebacterium parvum* on patterns of tumor growth. *Cancer* 26:1379.

Frost, P. and Lance, E. M. (1973). The relation of lymphocyte trapping to the mode of action of adjuvants. In: *Immunopotentiation* (Ciba Foundation Symposium, New Series), p. 29.

Halpern, B. (1974). In: *Corynebacterium parvum and Its Application in Experimental and Clinical Oncology*, Edition Foundation Merieux, Paris.

Halpern, B., Biozzi, G., Stiffel, C., Mouton, D. (1966). Inhibition of tumour growth by administration of killed *Corynebacterium parvum*. *Nature (Lond.)* 212:853.

Halpern, B., Fray, A., Cripin, Y., Platica, O., *et al.* (1973). In: *Immunopotentiation* (Ciba Foundation Symposium, New Series), p. 217.

Holm, G., Perlmann, P., and Werner, B. (1964). Phytohemagglutinin-induced cytotoxic action of normal lymphoid cells on cells in tissue culture. *Nature (Lond.)* 203:841.

Howard, J. G., Christie, G. H., and Scott, M. T. (1973a). Biological Effects of *Corynebacterium parvum*. IV. Adjuvant and inhibitory activities on B lymphocytes. *Cell. Immunol.* 7:290.

Howard, J. G., Scott, M. T., and Christie, G. H. (1973b). Cellular mechanisms underlying the adjuvant activity of *Corynebacterium parvum:* interactions of activated macrophages with T and B lymphocytes. In: *Immunopotentiation* (Ciba Foundation Symposium, New Series), p. 101.

Israel, L. (1973). Preliminary results of nonspecific immunotherapy for lung cancer. *Cancer Chemother. Rep.* 4:283.

Israel, L. and Edelstein, R. (1973). Nonspecific immunostimulation with *C. parvum* in human cancer. In: *26th Annual M.D. Anderson Symposium on Fundamental Cancer Research* (in press).

Israel, L. and Halpern, B. (1972). Le *Corynebacterium parvum* dans les cancers avancees. *Nouv. Presse Med.* 1:19.

Lundgren, G., Collste, L., and Moller, G. (1968). Cytotoxicity of human lymphocytes: antagonism between inducing processes. *Nature (Lond.)* 220:289.

Poulter, L. W. and Turk, J. L. (1972). Proportional increase in O-carrying lymphocytes in peripheral lymphoid tissue following treatment with cyclophosphamide. *Nature (London) New Biol.* 238:17.

Scott, M. T. (1972). Biological effects of the adjuvant *Corynebacterium parvum*. I. Inhibition of pha mixed lymphocyte and gvh reactivity. *Cell. Immunol.* 5:459.

Scott, M. T. (1972b). Biological effects of the adjuvant *Corynebacterium parvum*. II. Evidence of macrophage T-cell interaction. *Cell. Immunol.* 5:469.

Smith, S. E. and Scott, M. T. (1972). Biological Effects of *Corynebacterium parvum*. III. Amplification of resistance and impairment of active immunity to murine tumors. *Br. J. Cancer* 26:361.

Stockman, G. D., Heim, R. L., South, M. A., and Trentin, J. J. (1973). Differential effects of cyclophosphamide on the B- and T-cell compartments of adult mice. *J. Immunol.* 110:277.

Woodruff, M. F. A. and Boak, J. L. (1966). Inhibitory effect of injection of *Corynebacterium parvum* on the growth of tumour transplants in isogenic hosts. *Br. J. Cancer* 20:345.

Woodruff, M. F. A. and Dunbar, N. (1973). In: *Immunopotentiation* (Ciba Foundation Symposium, New Series), p. 287.

Woodruff, M. F. A., Dunbar, N., and Ghaffar, A. (1973). The growth of tumours in T-cell deprived mice and their response to treatment with *Corynebacterium parvum*. *Proc. R. Soc. Lond.* 184:97.

22

Tumor-Specific Rejection Associated with Killed *Corynebacterium parvum*

VILAS V. LIKHITE

Introduction

Undoubtedly, the injection of immunostimulant adjuvants, such as the living attenuated strain of *Mycobacterium bovis* (commonly known as BCG) and killed *Corynebacterium parvum* vaccine, has been known to protect experimental animals against tumor growth subsequent to the inoculation of tumor cells. Subsequent studies by Zbar *et al.* (1970) revealed that BCG totally prevented tumor cells from growing in recipients, provided the BCG was admixed with the living tumor cells prior to their intradermal inoculation in the recipients. BCG was also observed to result in the destruction of tumor cells if it was infiltrated directly into established growing intradermal [at a site that promotes tumor growth, as well as rejection (Gross, 1943)] nodules (Zbar *et al.*, 1971). However, BCG was ineffective if the microorganisms were killed prior to injection or if they were injected into the host at sites other than the transplanted tumor itself. (Bartlett *et al.*, 1972). Reproducible results were obtained only in intradermal tumors which had not involved more deeply, nor formed metastases. Efficacy

VILAS V. LIKHITE, Thorndike Memorial Laboratory, Harvard Medical Unit, Present address: Rm. 336, Building E2, Harvard Medical School, 25 Shattuck St., Boston, Massachusetts, 02115.

also required well-functioning and responsive immune systems in the host (Zbar, 1972).

A quite different phenomenon was observed when tumor cells plus killed *C. parvum* were injected subcutaneously into syngenic animals (Likhite and Halpern, 1973). Contrary to the delayed cytotoxic effects reported previously, the malignant cells injected along with killed *C. parvum* exhibited normal rates of tumor growth (at injection site) for approximately two weeks, followed by complete rejection of growing tumors in all animals. Furthermore, this delayed, but complete, rejection of the growing tumor conferred a life-long tolerance to the malignant cells, even if repeated attempts to inoculate living tumor cells were made. Permeating injections of killed *C. parvum* into growing subcutaneous tumors (the subcutaneous site, unlike the intradermal site, allows a considerable potential for dissemination of these tumor cells) resulted in rapid rejection of the tumors in all animals; the rejection being completed within seven days thereafter (Likhite and Halpern, 1974). These later studies demonstrated that killed *C. parvum* was effective even when injected at sites remote from the growing tumor. These studies also revealed that following tumor rejection, an immunelike response was induced which was uniformly capable of preventing incipient metastases, as well as perhaps destroying any metastases present at the time of remote injection of killed *C. parvum*.

The experiments presented here were designed to investigate the nature of protection in mice following *C. parvum*-mediated tumor rejection associated with intratumor *C. parvum* compared to inoculation of tumor cells admixed with *C. parvum*.

Materials and Methods

Mice

Female DBA/2 mice (age 8–10 weeks) were obtained from the Jackson Laboratory, Bar Harbor, Maine, and were used throughout these experiments. They were kept under normal laboratory conditions and were fed laboratory chow and tap water *ad libitum*.

Tumors

The CAD_2 mammary adenocarcinoma (Jackson Laboratory) is a spontaneous tumor, originating in a DBA/2 female mouse, that has been serially transplanted in syngenic mice without loss of characteristics. The 100% subcutaneous lethal dose is 10^3 cells, and an injection of 10^7 cells will kill all recipients (with growing tumors and metastases) in 28–35 days. The tumor is weakly immunogenic and does not grow in allogenic mice. Spontaneous regressions of established tumors have never been observed.

The T1699 mammary adenocarcinoma (Jackson Laboratory) is also a spontaneous tumor that has been serially transplanted in syngenic DBA/2 mice. It is histologically similar to the CAD_2 tumor, but appears to be antigenically different. It is a slower-growing tumor and a subcutaneous injection of 10^7 T1699 cells results in death, usually in the range of 40–50 days.

C. parvum was obtained from Institut Mérieux, Lyon, France.

Tumor Implantation

Using aseptic technique, tumor tissue was removed from freshly killed donor animals. Suspensions of tumor cells in Hank's solution were obtained by mild manipulation on surgical tantalum gauze, washed three times (400 g; 10 min) using Hank's solution, and resuspended at concentrations of 5×10^7 cells/ml for inoculation.

Results

Tumor-Specific Protection Associated with Subcutaneous Injection of Tumor Cells Mixed with Killed C. parvum

One hundred mice were separated into ten groups of ten mice each. Each mouse in one group received a subcutaneous injection of 10^7 CAD_2 cells in the lateral posterior region. Similarly, 10^7 T1699 cells were injected into another group of mice. Two groups of mice received 10^7 CAD_2 cells mixed with killed C. parvum (400 µg), and two additional groups of mice received 10^7 T1699 cells admixed with killed C. parvum. The remaining four groups of mice received one of the following subcutaneous injections (volume: 0.2 ml Hank's): either (a) 10^7 killed* CAD_2 cells, (b) 10^7 killed T1699 cells, (c) 10^7 irradiated† CAD_2 cells, or (d) 10^7 irradiated-T1699 cells.

The results (Table I) revealed that the mice receiving tumor cells mixed with C. parvum developed tumors (at the injection site) that exhibited normal rates of tumor growth for approximately two weeks (CAD_2: 12 days; T1699: 16 days), followed by complete disappearance of tumors in all of the animals. The groups of animals receiving either killed or irradiated tumor cells did not exhibit tumor growth, and those animals grafted with tumor cells alone all died with growing tumors and metastases (ranges of death: T1699, 38–50 days; CAD_2, 25–40 days).

Sixty days after the beginning of the experiment, the surviving eight groups of mice and two groups (ten mice each) of unsensitized mice of similar ages were separated respectively into two subgroups of five mice each. Each mouse of the unsensitized group (5 mice) received subcutaneously 10^5 CAD_2 cells, and the other group received 10^8 CAD_2 cells. Two groups of sensitized mice similarly

---

*Heat-killed (56°C, 1 h), formalin-treated (24 h).
†4000 R

Table I. The Nature of Tumor-Specific Protection Following Administration of Tumor Cells Mixed with *Corynebacterium parvum*

Group	First injection (10 mice per group)	Second injection (5 animals per group)	Survival (percentage)
—	None	10^5 CAD$_2$ cells	0
—		10^8 CAD$_2$ cells	0
—	None	10^5 T1699 cells	0
—		10^8 T1699 cells	0
1	10^7 CAD$_2$ cells + *C. parvum*	10^5 CAD$_2$ cells	100
		10^8 CAD$_2$ cells	100
2	10^7 CAD$_2$ cells + *C. parvum*	10^5 T1699 cells	0
		10^8 T1699 cells	0
3	10^7 T1699 cells + *C. parvum*	10^5 T1699 cells	100
		10^8 T1699 cells	100
4	10^7 T1699 cells + *C. parvum*	10^5 CAD$_2$ cells	0
		10^8 CAD$_2$ cells	0
5	10^7 killed CAD$_2$ cells	10^5 CAD$_2$ cells	0
		10^8 CAD$_2$ cells	0
6	10^7 killed T1699 cells	10^5 T1699 cells	0
		10^8 T1699 cells	0
7	10^7 irradiated CAD$_2$ cells	10^5 CAD$_2$ cells	100
		10^8 CAD$_2$ cells	0
8	10^7 irradiated T1699 cells	10^5 T1699 cells	100
		10^8 T1699 cells	0

received either 10^5 or 10^8 T1699 cells. Five of each of the surviving groups of ten mice received either 10^5 or 10^8 cells of the tumor-cell lines (Table II).

The groups of mice exhibiting *C. parvum*-associated rejection of CAD$_2$ or T1699 tumors were protected only when reinjected with either 10^5 or 10^8 cells of the tumor line employed in the original sensitization (Table I). Animals rejecting tumors of one line died with growing tumors and metastases when injected with 10^5 or 10^8 cells of the antigenically different tumor. The groups of animals sensitized with irradiated tumor cells were protected when reinjected with 10^5 tumor cells of the same line, but died with growing tumors and metastases when the cell dose was 10^8 tumor cells. The groups of animals

Table II. Tumor-Specific Protection Following Intratumor _C. parvum_ (400 g)[a]

Group	First injection (12 animals per group)	Second injection (8 animals per group)	Survival (percentage)
—	None	10^5 CAD$_2$ cells	0
		10^8 CAD$_2$ cells	0
—	None	10^5 CAD$_2$ cells	0
		10^8 CAD$_2$ cells	0
1	CAD$_2$ tumor (intratumor _C. parvum_)	10^5 CAD$_2$ cells	100
		10^8 CAD$_2$ cells	66
2	CAD$_2$ tumor (intratumor _C. parvum_)	10^5 T1699 cells	0
		10^8 T1699 cells	0
3	T1699 tumor (intratumor _C. parvum_)	10^5 T1699 cells	100
		10^8 T1699 cells	50
4	T1699 tumor (intratumor _C. parvum_)	10^5 CAD$_2$ cells	0
		10^8 CAD$_2$ cells	0
5	Irradiated 10^8 CAD$_2$ cells	10^5 CAD$_2$ cells	100
		10^8 CAD$_2$ cells	0
6	Irradiated 10^8 T1699 cells	10^5 T1699 cells	100
		10^8 T1699 cells	0

[a]Mean tumor size: CAD$_2$ tumor, 0.090 cm; T1699 tumor, 0.82 cm.

sensitized with killed tumor cells, like the unsensitized groups of mice, did not exhibit any protection and also died with growing tumors and metastases following injections of 10^5 or 10^8 tumor cells.

Tumor-Specific Protection Following Intratumor Administration of Killed _C. parvum_

At the beginning of the previous experiment, 96 previously unsensitized mice were separated into eight groups of 12 mice each. A group of mice received subcutaneously 10^8 irradiated-CAD$_2$ cells, and another group received 10^8 irradiated T1699 cells. Three groups of mice received 10^7 CAD$_2$ cells, and another three groups received 10^7 T1699 cells. At sixteen days, the tumors formed at the injection site reached respective mean diameters of 0.90 cm (CAD$_2$) and 0.82 cm (T1699). At this time, a group of mice bearing, respectively, T1699 tumor and CAD$_2$ tumor received a single permeation (injections) of 0.9% saline (0.3 ml). All mice of the remaining four groups received a single intratumor permeation injection of killed *C. parvum* (600 μg).

The results (Table II) revealed that the tumors in the mice receiving intratumor *C. parvum* disappeared (in all animals), whereas the mice receiving intratumor saline died with growing tumors and metastases. The mice receiving irradiated tumor cells did not develop tumors. The groups of surviving mice were separated respectively into two subgroups of six mice each. Four groups (6 mice per group) of previously unsensitized animals, served as controls. These animals then received (60 days after the beginning of the experiment) subcutaneous injections of either 10^5 or 10^8 tumor cells (Table II). On reinjection, animals previously sensitized to a tumor of one antigenic line were protected against a second injection of tumor cells of the same line, but died with growing tumors and metastases following injection of cells of a different antigenic line. Of these, 50% (T1699 group) and 66% (CAD_2 group) of the mice (that had rejected tumors following intratumor *C. parvum*) survived when the injection cell dose was 10^8 tumor cells of the respective antigenic line. Animals presensitized with irradiated tumor cells exhibited protection to a second injection of 10^5 cells of the same line, but died with growing tumors and metastases when the injected dose was 10^8 cells.

Discussion

The experiments presented above revealed that there was tumor-specific protection in mice following (a) inoculation of tumor cells previously admixed with *C. parvum* or (b) intratumor permeation with killed *C. parvum*. The nature of the protection in these animals was markedly increased when compared to the protection conferred following sensitization with irradiated-tumor cells. Animals pretreated with killed-tumor cells failed to exhibit any protection to subsequent inoculation of tumor cells of the line initially used.

The studies presented here are comparable to those previously reported. Although the mechanisms associated with *C. parvum*-associated tumor rejection remain to be defined, animals receiving injections of *C. parvum* vaccine reflect an intense stimulation of the reticuloendothelial system and phagocytosis (Biozzi *et al.*, 1964; Halpern *et al.*, 1964), steps that appear to be essential not only for host resistance, but also for indication of the immune response (Claman *et al.*, 1967; Feldman and Gallily, 1968). We have obtained histological sections of 10- and 18-day-old tumors after inoculation of tumor cells mixed with *C. parvum*. Microscopic examination of these tumors at 10 days revealed an intense and organized infiltration of polymorphonuclear leukocytes and macrophages around tumor follicles. At 18 days, these tumors revealed some areas where tumor follicles were being replaced with endothelial cells. Other areas of these sections revealed an infiltration of tumor follicles (tumor cells) with small lymphocytes.

Although the immunopotentiative properties of BCG and *C. parvum* appear to be similar (Biozzi *et al.,* 1965), there are notable differences. Optimal tumor rejection mediated by BCG requires (a) living BCG, (b) intracutaneous (intradermal) tumor, (c) close contact between BCG and tumor cells, and (d) an intact host immune system of the delayed-hypersensitivity type. Optimal effects with *C. parvum* are also observed when there is close contact with tumor cells. However, inhibition of tumor growth and prolonged survival have been observed following injection near the tumor site or following intraperitoneal administration of this immunopotentiator (Likhite and Halpern, 1973; 1974). In these cases, injection of *C. parvum* near the tumor site may have resulted in tumor-cell–*C. parvum* contact, either directly or via lymphatic channels. We performed autopsies on the animals receiving subcutaneous tumor-cell grafts which were followed by twice weekly injections of *C. parvum* administered via the intraperitoneal route. The results revealed that there was a paucity of peritoneal metastases present after these injections. Preliminary studies at our laboratory also revealed that there was a paucity of pulmonary metastases following intravenous administration of *C. parvum* in animals receiving subcutaneous tumor-cell grafts.

The work presented here may offer additional information on the use of *C. parvum* in cancer immunotherapy in patients; it already has been employed (Mathé, 1971; Israel and Halpern, 1972) as a nonspecific immunostimulant. Whether the use of *C. parvum* in close contact with autochthonous cells affords additional benefits to nonspecific therapy remains to be studied.

References

Bartlett, G. L., Zbar, B., and Rapp, H. J. (1972). Suppression of murine tumor growth by immune reaction to the Bacillus Calmette-Guerin strain of *Mycobacterium bovis. J. Natl. Cancer Inst.* **48**:245.

Biozzi, G., Stiffel, C., Mouton, D., Bouthillier, Y., and Descreusefond, C. (1964). Survival of spleen cells transplanted into syngenic and allogenic mice during stimulation of the reticuloendothelial system induced by *Mycotuberculosis* (BCG) infection. *Br. J. Exp. Pathol.* **45**:357.

Biozzi, G., Howard, J. G., Mouton, D., and Stiffel, D. (1965). Modifications of graft-versus-host reaction induced by the pretreatment of the host with *M. tuberculosis* and *C. parvum. Transplantation* **3**:170.

Claman, H. N., Chaperon, E. A., and Triplett, R. F. (1967). Thymus-marrow cell combinations. Synergism in antibody production. *Proc. Soc. Exp. Biol. Med.* **122**:1167.

Feldman, M. and Gallily, R. (1968). Cell interactions in the inductions of antibody formation. *Cold Spring Harbor Symp. Quant. Biol.* **32**:415.

Gross, L. (1943). Intradermal immunization of C_3H mice against a sarcoma that originated in an animal of the same line. *Cancer Res.* **3**:326.

Halpern, B. N., Prévot, A. R., Biozzi, G., Stiffel, C., Mouton, D., Morad, J. C., Bouthillier, Y., and Decreusefond, C. (1964). Stimulation de l'activité phagocytaire du système réticuloendothélial provoquée par *Corynebacterium parvum. J. Reticuloendothel. Soc.* **1**:77.

Israel, L. and Halpern, B. (1972). Le *Corynebacterium parvum* dans les cancers avancés. Première evaluation de l'activité thérapeutique de cette immunostimuline. *Nouv. Presse Med.* 1:19.

Likhite, V. V. (In preparation.) Cellular mechanisms associated with *Corynebacterium parvum*-mediated tumor rejection in experimental animals.

Likhite, V. V. and Halpern, B. (1973). The delayed rejection of tumors formed from the administration of tumor cells mixed with killed *C. parvum. Int. J. Cancer* 12:699.

Likhite, V. V. and Halpern, B. (1974). Lasting rejection of mammary adenocarcinoma-cell tumors in DBA/2 mice with intratumor injection of killed *C. parvum. Cancer Res.* 34:341.

Mathé, G. (1971). Immunotherapy in the treatment of acute lymphoid leukemia. *Hosp. Pract.* 6:43.

Zbar, B. (1972). Tumor regression mediated by *Mycobacterium bovis* (strain BCG). *Natl. Cancer Inst. Monog.* 35:341.

Zbar, B., Bernstein, I. W., Tanaka, T., and Rapp, H. J. (1970). Tumor immunity produced by the intradermal inoculation of living tumor cells and living *Mycobacterium bovis* (strain BCG). *Science* 170:1217.

Zbar, B., Bernstein, I. W., and Rapp, H. J. (1971). Suppression of tumor growth at the site of infection with living *Bacillus Calmette-Guerin. J. Natl. Cancer Inst.* 46:931.

23

An Analysis of the
Antitumor Effects of
Corynebacterium parvum

J. E. CASTRO and T. E. SADLER

In defined situations *Corynebacterium parvum* has an inhibitory effect on tumor growth. In our experiments, 0.2 ml of intraperitoneal *C. parvum*, given on two consecutive days, caused inhibition of Ehrlich's ascitic tumor (Fig. 1) and similar effects were observed in CBA mice given S.37 ascites sarcoma (Fig. 2). The growth of subcutaneous Lewis lung tumor in male mice was inhibited by intravenous or intraperitoneal *C. parvum,* but contralateral subcutaneous *C. parvum* was ineffective (Fig. 3). Intravenous and intraperitoneal *C. parvum* decreased pulmonary metastases from the tumor (Table I).

Intraperitoneal *C. parvum* also inhibited growth of ascitic Meth. A tumors in male Balb/c mice (Fig. 4). This effect was studied in detail. Meth. A tumor is a methylcholanthrene-induced sarcoma which was obtained from and described by Old *et al.* (1962).

We confirmed that it is syngenic for Balb/c mice, antigenic, and, on electron-microscopic examination, it does not contain virus particles. The *C. parvum* (Wellcome Research Laboratories, batch EZ.174) was given as two daily doses of 0.2 ml of a 7 mg/ml solution immediately before inoculation of tumor cells.

J. E. CASTRO and T. E. SADLER, Urology and Transplant Unit, Royal Postgraduate Medical School, London, W.12, U.K. Supported by the Cancer Research Campaign.

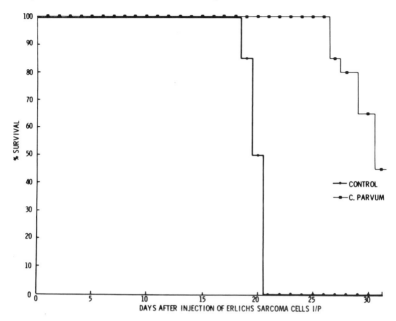

Fig. 1. The effect of *Corynebacterium parvum* on death from 1×10^5 Ehrlich's sarcoma cells given intraperitoneally. *C. parvum*, 0.2 ml, was given on two consecutive days before tumor inoculation. Controls were untreated.

The effects of *C. parvum* on increasing tumor dose were studied. Six groups of at least eight mice were given *C. parvum*, and two weeks later, each of these groups and equal numbers of controls were given graded doses of (3.5×10^2, 10^4, 10^6, 10^7, 10^8) tumor cells. At high tumor doses, *C. parvum* had slight protective effects, but increasing protection was afforded with decreasing tumor challenge (Fig. 5). In further experiments (to be described) 3.5×10^3 intraperitoneal cells were used.

C. parvum increased spleen mass (Fig. 6), but splenectomy did not significantly affect the antitumor effects of the drug (Fig. 7). This was studied in four groups of 20 mice; two groups were splenectomized (Castro, 1974a), two were not. One splenectomized and one control group were given *C. parvum*, and two weeks later, these and the untreated groups were injected with tumor. An increased number of macrophages in other organs (Halpern *et al.*, 1964) might account for the minimal effects of splenectomy on the antitumor effects of *C. parvum*, and changes of cytotoxic antibodies could account for the effects of splenectomy on tumor growth in control mice.

Changes of cell-mediated immunity may affect the growth of some tumors (Balner and Dersjant, 1969; Castro, 1974b; Nehlsen, 1971; Penn and Starzl,

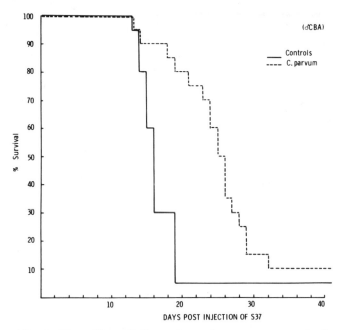

Fig. 2. The effect of *Corynebacterium parvum* on death from 1×10^5 S.37 tumor cells given intraperitoneally. *C. parvum*, 0.2 ml, was given on two consecutive days before tumor inoculation.

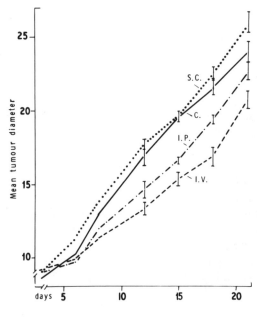

Fig. 3. The effect of *Corynebacterium parvum* on the growth of a 0.1 ml homogenate of Lewis lung carcinoma given subcutaneously. *C. parvum*, 0.1 ml, was injected at the same time as the tumor inoculation, either intravenously, intraperitoneally, or subcutaneously. The controls were untreated. Each point represents the mean tumor diameter from 9 mice; the standard error is shown.

Table I. The Effect of *Corynebacterium parvum* on Pulmonary Metastases from Lewis Lung Tumor[a]

Treatment	Number of mice	Average number of metastases	Range of metastases
Controls, untreated	9	24	10–37
0.1 ml *C. parvum* i.v.	9	4	0–11
0.1 ml *C. parvum* i.p.	9	4	0–8
0.1 ml *C. parvum* s.c.	9	18	7–36

[a]Lewis lung carcinoma was inoculated subcutaneously as a 0.1-ml homogenate at the same time that 0.1 ml *C. parvum* was given. The mice were killed 21 days later, and the number of pulmonary metastases was counted.

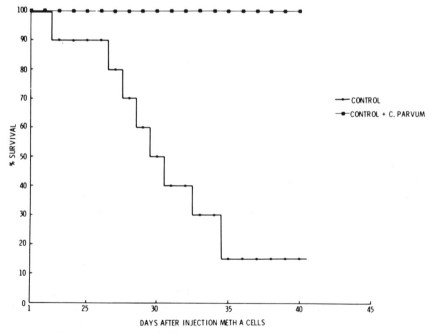

Fig. 4. Effect of *Corynebacterium parvum* on death from 3.5×10^3 Meth. A tumor cells given intraperitoneally. *C. parvum*, 0.2 ml, was given on two consecutive days before tumor inoculation.

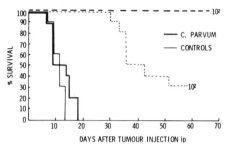

Fig. 5. Effect of *Corynebacterium parvum* on death from high (1 × 10⁸) and low (1 × 10²) doses of Meth. A cells. *C. parvum* was injected intraperitoneally on two consecutive days, and tumor was given intraperitoneally two weeks later to all mice.

1969). The relationship between the antitumor activity of *C. parvum* and cell-mediated immunity was investigated in adult thymectomized mice and mice given antilymphocyte serum (ALS), which has an inhibitory effect upon cell-mediated immunity (Gray *et al.*, 1966).

The effect of thymectomy was studied in four groups of 20 mice (Table II). *C. parvum* was given two weeks after thymectomy, and tumor was injected two weeks afterward. Thymectomy had only a slight, late inhibitory effect on the antitumor activity of *C. parvum* (Fig. 8). These data suggest that the effects of *C. parvum* are not mediated through the thymus, although the late inhibitory effect could be explained if a subpopulation of thymus-derived cells, which are long lived (> 3 weeks), were required for the protective effects of *C. parvum*. Alternatively, thymectomized mice may be at a disadvantage when the antitumor effects of *C. parvum* decline (Castro, 1974c).

Five groups of mice were used in the study with ALS (Table III). *C. parvum* was given immediately after the initial course of ALS (sheep anti-mouse-thymocyte serum, 0.25 ml subcutaneously for 3 days and 0.25 ml weekly thereafter), and tumor cells were injected one day later. The slight inhibition of antitumor activity of *C. parvum* produced by ALS (Fig. 9) probably resulted from a nonspecific toxicity of ALS in *C. parvum*-treated mice. Despite ALS, *C. parvum* was still a very active antitumor agent, for mice treated this way survived significantly longer than those given ALS alone. These results, while not excluding the need for a small number of thymus-derived cells, suggest that the tumor-protective effects of *C. parvum* do not result from increased cell-mediated immunity.

There is evidence that *C. parvum* may depress cell-mediated immunity, for when given to CBA mice, it caused atrophy of the thymus (Fig. 10). This could result from a nonspecific effect of stress, but findings of T-cell depression *in vitro* (Scott, 1972) make a specific effect more likely.

The content of thymus-processed cells in thymuses of *C. parvum*-treated mice were studied by the trypan-blue exclusion method with antitheta serum

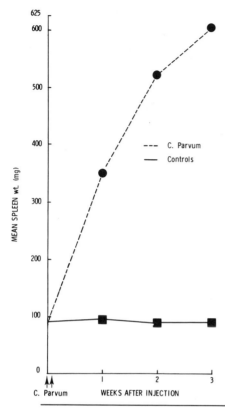

Fig. 6. Effect of two doses of 0.2 ml *Corynebacterium parvum* on mean spleen weight of CBA mice.

Source	Sum squares	°Freedom	F-ratio	Significance
Treatment				
Time	1907994	5	140	$P < 0.001$
Interaction				
Treatment	1684402	1	621	$P < 0.001$
Time	110353	2	20	$P < 0.001$
Interaction	113238	2	20	$P < 0.001$
Error	97627	36		

prepared in AKR mice (Raff, 1969). The percentage of theta-positive cells in mice given *C. parvum* was similar to untreated controls (Table IV), but because of the much smaller thymuses of *C. parvum*-treated mice, the total number of theta-positive cells was less in these animals. The percentage of theta-positive cells in spleens from *C. parvum*-treated mice was less than controls, but this could be explained by either a real decrease of theta-positive cells or, more

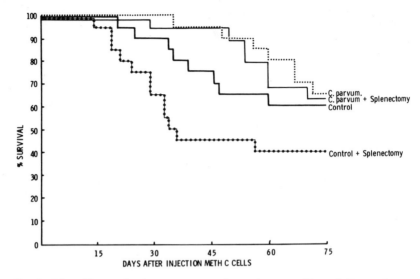

Fig. 7. The effects of splenectomy on the antitumor effect of *Corynebacterium parvum*. Splenectomy slightly inhibited the protective effects of *C. parvum*, but splenectomized mice given *C. parvum* survived much longer than untreated controls.

Table II. Experimental Groups for the Investigation of the Effect of Thymectomy on the Antitumor Activity of *Corynebacterium parvum*[a]

No. mice	Thymectomy	C. parvum	Tumor cells
20	+	+	+
20	+	+	
20		+	+
20			+

[a]Treatment received = +.

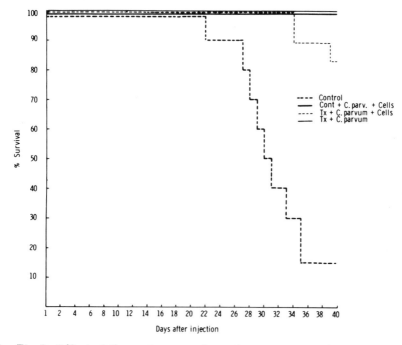

Fig. 8. Effect of thymectomy on the antitumor activity of *Corynebacterium parvum*. Control mice given tumor died rapidly, and *C. parvum* given to control mice had a protective effect. Thymectomy only slightly inhibited this protective effect.

Table III. Experimental Groups for the Study of the Effect of ALS on the Antitumor Activity of *Corynebacterium parvum*[a]

No. mice	ALS	*C. parvum*	Tumor cells
20			+
11	+		+
15		+	+
17	+	+	+
11	+	+	

[a]Treatment received = +.

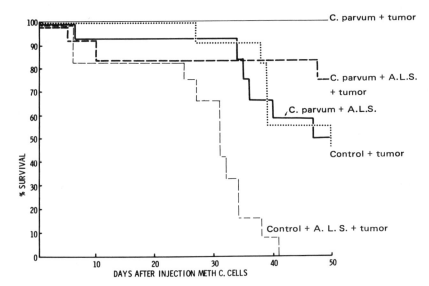

Fig. 9. The effect of A.L.S. on antitumor activity of *Corynebacterium parvum.*

Table IV. Percentage Cells Lysed by Antitheta Serum in Thymus and Spleen of Control or *Corynebacterium parvum*-Treated Mice

	Thymus		Spleen	
	Control	C. parvum	Control	C. parvum
Untreated	2	2	2	1
NMS	3	10	10	6
Antitheta	87	98	55	22

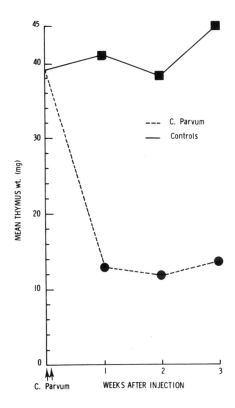

Fig. 10. Effect of two 0.2-ml doses of *Corynebacterium parvum* on mean thymus weight of CBA mice aged 6 weeks.

Source	Sum squares	°Freedom	F-ratio	Significance
Treatment ⎫ Time ⎬ Interaction ⎭	8724	5	38	$P < 0.001$
Treatment	8677	1	189	$P < 0.05$
Time	13	2	$\phi 148$	0
Interaction	33	2	$\phi 364$	0
Error	1655	36		

likely, by dilution with a theta-negative cellular population which caused spleno-megaly.

Functional depression of cell-mediated immunity accompanied these cellular changes. *C. parvum* given one week before, or on the day of skin allografting, prolonged graft survival (Castro, 1974d).

Interaction of macrophages with other cell types makes it difficult to study the effects of *C. parvum* on antibody production, and the small increase of response to sheep erythrocytes (Castro, 1974e) could be explained by altered antigen processing. Certainly, there was no increase of anti-H-2 cytotoxic anti-body in *C. parvum*-treated mice after the first and second sets of allografts, as measured by a ^{51}Cr-release method (Wigzell, 1965).

In the tumor system described, the antitumor activity of *C. parvum* is not mediated by changes of cell-mediated immunity, and it most likely results from increased macrophage activity, but in the situation where tumor cells and *C. parvum* make contact intraperitoneally, a direct toxic effect cannot be excluded. However, there is no doubt that intraperitoneal *C. parvum* does affect immuno-logical reactivity. Currently we are studying the effects of *C. parvum* on different tumor models.

In summary, (1) *C. parvum* had powerful antitumor activity in defined situations. (2) Splenectomy did not inhibit the tumor-protective effects of *C. parvum*. (3) The antitumor activity of *C. parvum*, in the tumor system described, was not effected by increased cell-mediated immunity. (4) *C. parvum* caused atrophy of the thymus and a loss of theta-positive cells. (5) *C. parvum* did not affect the production of anti-H-2 cytotoxic antibody.

References

Balner, H. and Dersjant, H. (1969). Increased oncogenic effect of methylcholanthrene after treatment with antilymphocyte serum. *Nature (Lond.)* **224**:376.

Castro, J. E. (1974a). Surgical procedures in small laboratory animals. *J. Immunol. Methods* (in press).

Castro, J. E. (1974b). Orchidectomy and the immune response. I. Effect of orchidectomy on lymphoid tissues of mice. II. Response of orchidectomized mice to antigens. *Proc. R. Soc. London B.* **185**:425–437.

Castro, J. E. (1974c). Orchidectomy and immune response. III. The effect of orchidectomy on tumor induction and transplantation in mice. *Proc. R. Soc. London B.* **186**:387.

Castro, J. E. (1974d). Antitumor effects of *Corynebacterium parvum. Eur. J. Cancer* **10**:121.

Castro, J. E. (1974e). The effect of *Corynebacterium parvum* on the structure and function of the lymphoid system in mice. *Eur. J. Cancer* **10**:115.

Gray, J. G., Monaco, A. P., Wood, M. L., and Russell, P. S. (1966). Studies on heterologous antilymphocyte serum in mice. *J. Immunol.* **96**:217.

Halpern, B. N., Prévot, A. R., Biozzi, G., Stiffel, C., Mouton, D., Morard, J. C., Bouthillier, Y., and Decreusefond, C. (1964). Stimulation de l'activité phagocytaire du système réticuloendothélial provoquée par *Corynebacterium parvum. J. Reticuloendothel. Soc.* **1**:77.

Nehlsen, S. L. (1971). Prolonged administration of antithymocyte serum in mice. *Clin. Exp. Immunol.* **9**:63.

Old, L. J., Boyse, E. A., Clarke, D. A., and Carswell, E. A. (1962). Antigenic properties of chemically-induced tumors. *Ann. N.Y. Acad. Sci.* **101**:80.

Penn, I. and Starzl, T. E. (1969). Immunosuppression and cancer. *Transplant. Proc.* **5**:943.

Raff, M. C. (1969). The isoantigen as a marker of thymus-derived lymphocytes in mice. *Nature (Lond.)* **224**:378.

Scott, M. T. (1972). Biological effects of the adjuvant *Corynebacterium parvum*. I. Inhibition of PHA, mixed lymphocyte, and GVH activity. *Cell Immunol.* **5**:459.

Wigzell, H. (1965). Quantitative titrations of mouse anti-H-2 iso-antibodies using [51] Cr-target cells. *Transplantation* **3**:423.

DISCUSSION

ADLAM: Perhaps I could raise a note of caution about the interpretation of some of the experiments which we have heard today. I am concerned about those tests where intraperitoneally injected *Corynebacterium parvum* was followed by a tumor challenge via the same route. It is well-known that intraperitoneal injection of, for example, saline or broth, may stimulate the peritoneum to produce various cell types which may alter the subsequent outcome of intraperitoneal challenge.

One way around this problem might be to use a negative-control bacterium, such as an inactive strain of *C. parvum* or *Corynebacterium diphtheriae*. This control would ensure that any antitumor effects seen are really due to *C. parvum* stimulation.

PARAF: Has anyone checked whether *C. parvum* has a direct effect on tumor cells? Is there any substance synthesized by the *C. parvum* which is possibly active at the cell-membrane level?

Recently, we carried out experiments with plasmacytomas synthesizing an immunoglobulin with antibody activity. It is possible to stop tumor growth by the specific antigen using doses close to the tolerogenic dose of this antigen.

HALPERN: We are all aware, and I emphasized this point, of the care which should be taken in interpreting the results from the experiments in which tumor inoculum and *C. parvum* were both injected intraperitoneally. There is no doubt, as emphasized by Dr. Adlam, that the i.p. inoculation of any foreign substance—be it as physiological as isotonic saline or cell broth media—will induce an inflammatory reaction, attracting a variety of blood- or tissue-borne cells. In our hands, control experiments performed by intraperitoneal adminis-tration of saline or, better, of the supernatant of *C. parvum* showed that although producing inflammatory-type reactions, these inoculants were ineffec-tive. I also attempted to obviate this objection by spacing the time interval between *C. parvum* injection and the tumor inoculum by a week. The effects on tumor repression were similar. Finally, experiments were performed in which the tumor inoculum was given intraperitoneally and *C. parvum* intravenously. As could be seen from the data reported, the results—although not so spectacular—are nevertheless highly significant.

As to Dr. Paraf's question concerning the possible role of immune factors in the process of tumor rejection in animals treated with *C. parvum,* such a hypothesis cannot be eliminated. It is difficult to prove it in our system, as the YC8 tumor seems to be very weakly antigenic in the isogenic Balb/c recipients, a dose of less than 100 tumor cells killing almost 100% of the animals. The only evidence of an immunological reaction was proven *in vitro* by the cytotoxicity of lymphocytes obtained from tumor-bearing animals. However, very large tumor inocula were required to obtain a cytotoxicity rate surpassing 20–30%.

WRBA: We all investigate *C. parvum* because we want to improve the treatment of cancer and because it is an intriguing organism. I think Dr. Fisher's work is very important in experimental terms, inasmuch as everybody talks about adjuvant therapy with *Corynebacterium.* We need to find a combination which improves a potential therapy with the adjuvant, *Corynebacterium.* We should elaborate schedules for experimental research in this context.

REED: In reference to Dr. Fisher's experiment on macrophage-colony stimulation in which he found that the second dose of *C. parvum* enhanced the effect of the first dose, was that timing important? More specifically, did it have to be given toward the end of the effect of the first dose, and what would have happened if the second dose had been given before then?

FISHER: The temporal relationships were that the time interval between the two doses was seven days, the marrow being taken a week after the second dose. We have not done this experiment on a whole spectrum of time intervals, so I cannot be more specific than that.

COHEN: We know that the doses of *C. parvum* do not cause death of the mice; was there any other nonspecific toxicity, such as weight loss, of the mice during these experiments?

FISHER: In our experiments in which weekly doses of 1.4 mg *C. parvum* had been given for a 90-day period, the animals were completely healthy. Deaths after *C. parvum* administration have occurred, sometimes early in the treatment, for no obvious reason. I cannot explain these deaths.

The animals receiving the cytoxan and *C. parvum* for as long as three months, on a weekly basis, were absolutely healthy and gained weight.

COHEN: Have any dose-response curves to cytoxan been done to see whether it would be possible to get more cytoxan into animals?

FISHER: This is now being done. We found that 120 mg cytoxan in the normal animal, or in the *C. parvum*-treated animal, was lethal after the first, or second injections; 60 mg of cytoxan had no tumor-controlling effect, but all the animals were healthy. A dose of 90 mg worked well; this dose of cytoxan is nontoxic and has a tumor effect, but not sufficient to cause inhibition of tumor growth.

FELDMAN: Dr. Halpern described how *C. parvum* confers cytostatic properties on macrophages, and many have reported here that *C. parvum* prevents tumor growth under certain conditions. Has anyone tested the macrophages from animals manifesting resistance to tumor following the application of *C. parvum* to determine whether they also manifest either cytostatic or cytotoxic properties *in vitro?* Can any capacity to resist tumor growth be transferred by such macrophages to other recipients?

MILAS: We tried to transfer resistance against artificial pulmonary metastases of a murine fibrosarcoma by intravenous inoculation of tumor-cell recipients with peritoneal cells from mice previously treated with *Corynebacterium granulosum.* The data of this preliminary experiment showed that only a moderate reduction in the number of lung metastases was achieved when a large number of cells (about 3.8×10^7) was transferred.

HALPERN: I may mention an observation we made in *C. parvum*-treated animals, although this is not relevant to Dr. Feldman's question. When the number of peritoneal macrophages was numerated in animals receiving an intravenous injection of *C. parvum,* it was found that the macrophage population was increased for the following days by about 50%. The cells were obtained by a simple washing of the peritoneal cavity with warm Hank's equilibrated medium.

WHITE: Were any effects observed on the bone-marrow or blood macrophages in those animals?

HALPERN: I did not mean to infer that, but merely to allude to the results, which agree with those presented by Prof. Dimitrov, who showed that *C. parvum* induces an increase in colony-forming cells. As it is accepted that monocytes which are macrophage precursors originate from the bone-marrow stem cells, this may be relevant to the increase in the peritoneal cavity macrophage population—to which I was referring—following the intravenous injection of *C. parvum.*

FELDMAN: I realize that, but all these experiments—which are indeed beautiful—were performed on animals which had been challenged only with *C. parvum* and not a tumor. Have animals similarly treated with a tumor, and in which the tumor was rejected, been shown to have macrophages which have any effect on tumor cells, either cytostatic or cytotoxic? The main question is whether under these conditions, the macrophages are perhaps not only cyto-static, but are indeed cytotoxic—as has been shown in some other cases.

HALPERN: This is an interesting suggestion.

OETTGEN: The question of the best time to administer *C. parvum* has been raised. In experiments with a methylcholanthrene-induced sarcoma in syngenic hosts, we found that there can be complete regression of the tumor graft—even when *C. parvum* is given (intradermally) one day after inoculation.

We tested a number of different strains of BCG, and we were unable to induce tumor regression with any of them when they were injected one day after inoculation of the tumor.

As to the timing in relation to chemotherapy, we repeated Currie's experiments and confirmed his observation that when *C. parvum* is given on day 6 and cytoxan on day 18 after tumor inoculation, the therapeutic effect is small. When the schedule is reversed, however, a complete regression of a larger proportion of the grafted tumors occurs.

HALPERN: Are the results mentioned already published?

OETTGEN: Not yet.

HALPERN: Results recently reported [M. F. A. Woodruff and N. Dunbar (1973). In: *Immunopotentiation,* Ciba Foundation Symposium, Elsevier, North Holland] by Woodruff of Edinburgh showed similar time relationships concerning *C. parvum* treatment and cyclophosphamide.

FISHER: In our particular animal system, however, I am not so sure that this is some magic number. Certainly, in our system, it worked whether *C. parvum* or cytoxan was given first. I am not even convinced that the time intervals we used were necessary; other time intervals might work just as well.

24

Inhibition by *Corynebacterium parvum* of Lung-Nodule Formation by Intravenously Injected Fibrosarcoma Cells

R. BOMFORD and M. OLIVOTTO

INTRODUCTION

Immunotherapy of cancer is likely to be most efficacious for the elimination of disseminated deposits of tumor cells remaining after the surgical removal of a primary solid tumor, or after a chemotherapeutically-induced remission of leukemia. It is, therefore, important to develop procedures for strengthening systemic immunity, specifically or nonspecifically, and to understand the mechanisms of tumor-cell destruction at favored sites of metastasis, such as the lung or the liver.

Milas and Mujagić (1972) reported that subcutaneous injection of 1 mg of

R. BOMFORD, Department of Experimental Immunobiology, Wellcome Research Laboratories, Beckenham, Kent BR3 3BS, England and M. OLIVOTTO, Department of Experimental Immunology, Wellcome Research Laboratories, Beckenham, Kent, England. Present address: Istituto di Patologia Generale della Università di Firenze, Viale Morgagni 50, Firenze, Italy.

Corynebacterium parvum into C_{57} Bl mice before or after the intravenous injection of syngenic fibrosarcoma cells reduced the number of lung nodules detectable 25 days after tumor-cell injection.

This paper reviews the results of our experiments designed to elucidate the mechanisms whereby treatment with *C. parvum* might increase resistance to the establishment and growth of lung nodules. *C. parvum* (Wellcome strain CN6134, batch PX289) was supplied by Wellcome Reagents Ltd., Beckenham, Kent, England. In all experiments, the dose was 350 μg, injected intravenously in 0.2 ml saline.

Activation of Lung Macrophages by Intravenous Injection of *C. parvum*

The idea that activated macrophages may be responsible for the antitumor action of *C. parvum* arises from the classical observations by Halpern *et al.* (1964) of reticuloendothelial stimulation and histiocytic infiltration of spleen and liver after *C. parvum* injection, and also from the later observations that the inhibition of PHA responsiveness of spleen cells of *C. parvum*-treated mice

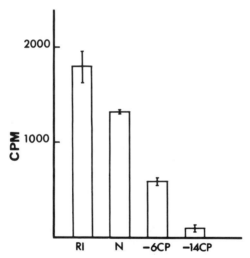

Fig. 1. [^{3}H]-TdR incorporation (cpm) into syngenic leukemia cells alone (RI), with normal lung macrophages (N), and with lung macrophages 6 and 14 days after *Corynebacterium parvum* injection (−6 CP and −14 CP). (Reproduced with permission, from Olivotto and Bomford, 1974.)

(Scott, 1972a) may be reversed by the removal of macrophages (Scott, 1972b). The macrophage hypothesis has also been advanced by authors who have shown that the antitumor action of *C. parvum* is still demonstrable in T-cell-depleted mice (Woodruff *et al.,* 1973; Castro, 1974) and, therefore, probably does not depend, in these systems, on the potentiation of the specific T-cell response to tumor-specific transplantation antigens.

The antitumor activity of macrophages from normal and *C. parvum*-treated CBA mice was studied *in vitro* (Olivotto and Bomford, 1974). Syngenic leukemia or fibrosarcoma cells were added to monolayers of macrophages, and tumor-cell DNA synthesis was measured by the incorporation of [^{3}H]-TdR. Both peritoneal and lung macrophages from *C. parvum*-treated mice were inhibitory. The time course of development of inhibitory potential by lung macrophages is shown in Fig. 1. Activated peritoneal macrophages, able to inhibit tumor-cell DNA synthesis *in vitro,* which appear after *C. parvum* injection, have also been demonstrated by Halpern *et al.* (see Chapter 13).

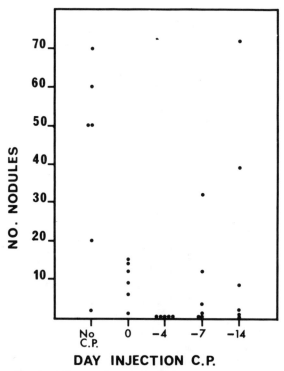

Fig. 2. Effect of *Corynebacterium parvum* injected at various times before T3 cells on numbers of lung nodules. (Reproduced with permission, from Bomford and Olivotto, 1974.)

Inhibition of Lung-Nodule Formation by *C. parvum*

The effect of *C. parvum* on lung-nodule formation by syngenic T3 fibrosarcoma cells has been studied (Bomford and Olivotto, 1974). Injection of *C. parvum* before 1.5×10^5 T3 cells inhibited nodule formation, maximally when *C. parvum* was given between 1 and 4 days before the T3 cells (Fig. 2). This did not correspond to the time course of the appearance of activated macrophages detectable *in vivo*. However, this does not invalidate the hypothesis that activated macrophages mediate protection, since the lung macrophages for the *in vitro* experiments, although obtained by mincing the lungs, probably comprise a large proportion of true alveolar macrophages not encountered by tumor cells in blood vessels. Protection could also be brought about by an influx of macrophages into the lung.

C. parvum given 2, 6, or 10 days after T3 cells did not reduce nodule numbers, and was usually without effect on survival (significant prolongation occurred in only one experiment out of three). This is at variance with the work of Milas and Mujagić (1972) and with Milas's later results (see Chapter 26 this volume) showing a therapeutic effect of *C. parvum* given after intravenous tumor cells. It is not clear what factor is responsible for this difference.

C. parvum Is Specific as a Protective Agent

An experiment was performed to discover if the ability to inhibit lung-nodule formation is restricted to those strains of coryneform bacteria which stimulate the RES and induce splenomegaly. A strain of *C. parvum* and of *Corynebacterium diphtheriae,* both previously shown to be inactive for these characteristics (Adlam and Scott, 1973), were compared with active-strains of *C. parvum*. All bacteria (350 μg) were injected intravenously 4 days before 10^5 T3 cells, and the lungs were examined 14 days after T3-cell injection (Table I). Only the active *C. parvum* strains caused nodule inhibition.

Distribution of Intravenously Injected Tumor Cells in Normal and *C. parvum*-Treated Mice

The fate of intravenously injected T3 cells in normal and *C. parvum*-treated mice was studied with ^{51}Cr-labeled T3 cells (Fig. 3). It is clear that the majority of T3 cells were initially trapped in the lungs in both types of mice. There is a more rapid elimination of radioactivity from the lungs of treated mice and a more rapid accumulation in the bladder; this indicates that at least part of the loss from the lung is due to cell death. Accelerated elimination of radioactivity from the lung is evident 24 h after *C. parvum* injection, suggesting that the protective mechanism is already operative at this time. (The assumption must be

Table I. Effect of *Corynebacterium parvum* (Active and Inactive Strains) and *Corynebacterium diphtheria* on Nodule Formation by T3 Cells[a]

Strain	ATCC[b]	Pasteur	Wellcome	Number of nodules	Spleen weight (mg) mean	range
C. diphtheriae	296	—	CN2000	>100, >100, >100, 53	93	(80–110)
C. parvum	11829	—	CN5888	>100, >100, >100, 4	75	(60–80)
C. parvum	—	4685	CN6134	0, 0, 0, 0	592	(540–690)
Untreated control				>100, >100, >100	100	(80–140)

[a]Bacteria were injected i.v. 4 days before T3 cells.
[b]American Type Culture Collection, Rockville, Md., USA.

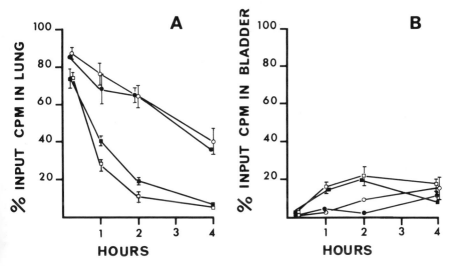

Fig. 3. (A) Percentage of radioactivity in lungs and (B) urinary bladders of normal and *Corynebacterium parvum*-treated mice at various times after injection of ⁵¹Cr-labeled T3 cells. Experiment 1: ○———○ normal, □———□ 4 days post *C. parvum;* Experiment 2: ●———● normal, ■———■ 1 day post *C. parvum*. (Reproduced, with permission, from Bomford and Olivotto, 1974).

made that the very small proportion, about 1 in 5×10^3, of the injected cells destined to grow into nodules in normal mice, and whose fate cannot be followed by radioactive methods, are more rapidly eliminated in treated mice in the same way as the majority of cells.) This rules out any mechanism of protection based on an immune response to the tumor cells, or to *C. parvum*, unless the mice are already naturally sensitized to *C. parvum*.

The Radiosensitivity of the Protective Effect

Mice were injected with *C. parvum* 1 day before 5×10^4 T3 cells. Irradiation (800 R) was applied at various times: 4 h before T3-cell injection, or 4 h, 24 h, or 6 days before *C. parvum* injection (Table II). Highly significant protection was still obtained in the groups irradiated 4 h before T3-cell or *C. parvum* injection, although these mice were totally immunosuppressed as judged by the absence of agglutinating antibodies against *C. parvum*. (The titer in the group injected with *C. parvum* without irradiation was 1/256). This confirms the conclusion from the ⁵¹Cr-labeled T3-cell experiment that the protective effect does not require an immune response to *C. parvum* or T3 antigens.

However, irradiation administered 24 h before the *C. parvum* destroyed the protective effect; and even when the interval between irradiation and *C. parvum*

Table II. Effect of 800 R Whole-Body, Sublethal Irradiation on Protection
against Lung-Nodule Formation by *Corynebacterium parvum*[a]

Irradiation (day relative to CP)[b]	Number of nodules		
	Control	C. parvum	P
None	1, 2, 6, 7, 8	0, 0, 0, 0, 0	0.004
−6	5, 10, 18, 30, 88	3, 5, 7, 17	0.08
−1	15, 54, 83, 86, >100	66, 68, 75, 95, >100	0.38
0	>100, >100, >100, >100, >100	5, 14, 17, 24, 36	0.004
+1	23, 36, 62, 72, 86	3, 5, 5, 17, 35	0.008

[a]Reproduced, by permission, from Bomford and Olivotto (1974).
[b]*C. parvum* = CP.

was 6 days, there was no significant protection. These results could be explained
by the destruction of radiosensitive precursors of a population of rapidly
turning-over cells needed for the mediation of *C. parvum* protection. Very
similar results were obtained by Milas (see Chapter 26 this volume).

Concluding Remarks

C. parvum protects against nodule formation by intravenously injected T3
cells, and this probably does not require an immune response to *C. parvum* or T3
cells. The cellular or pharmacological mechanism of protection is not yet clear.
It has not been possible to provide positive evidence for the role of the activated
macrophage, insofar as the kinetics of protection do not coincide with those of
the appearance of activated macrophages in the lung, and silica treatment does
not abolish the protective effect (Bomford and Olivotto, 1974). However,
neither is it possible to exclude the activated macrophage. It seems unlikely that
macrophages activated immunologically by the mechanism proposed by Mackaness (1970) can be responsible, since this would require an immune response to
C. parvum, but it is still feasible for activation to be induced by a direct action
of *C. parvum* on macrophages, perhaps via the macrophage-chemotactic factor of
Wilkinson *et al.* (1973) (see also Chapter 16 this volume).

References

Adlam, C. and Scott, M. T. (1973). Lymphoreticular stimulatory properties of *Corynebacterium parvum* and related bacteria. *J. Med. Microbiol.* **6**:261.

Bomford, R. and Olivotto, M. (1974). The mechanism of inhibition by *Corynebacterium parvum* of the growth of lung nodules from intravenously injected tumor cells. *Int. J. Cancer* **14**:226.

Castro, J. E. (1974). Antitumor effects of *Corynebacterium parvum* in mice. *Eur. J. Cancer* **10**:121.

Halpern, B. N., Prévot, A. R., Biozzi, G., Stiffel, C., Mouton, D., Morard, J. C., Bouthillier, Y., and Decreusefond, C. (1964). Stimulation de l'activité phagocytaire du système réticuloendothélial provoquée par *Corynebacterium parvum. J. Reticuloendothel. Soc.* **1**:77.

Mackaness, G. B. (1970). Cellular immunity. In: *Mononuclear Phagocytes,* p. 461 (R. V. Furth, ed.), Blackwell Scientific Publications, Oxford and Edinburgh.

Milas, L. and Mujagić, H. (1972). Protection by *Corynebacterium parvum* against tumor cells injected intravenously. *Rev. Eur. Etud. Clin. Biol.* **18**:498.

Olivotto, M. and Bomford, R. (1974). *In vitro* inhibition of tumor-cell growth and DNA synthesis by peritoneal and lung macrophages from mice injected with *Corynebacterium parvum. Int. J. Cancer* **13**:478.

Scott, M. T. (1972a). Biological effects of the adjuvant, *Corynebacterium parvum.* I. Inhibition of PHA, mixed lymphocyte, and GVH reactivity. *Cell. Immunol.* **5**:459.

Scott, M. T. (1972b). Biological effects of the adjuvant, *Corynebacterium parvum.* II. Evidence for macrophage T-cell interaction. *Cell. Immunol.* **5**:469.

Wilkinson, P. C., O'Neill, G. J., and Wapshaw, K. G. (1973). Role of anaerobic coryneforms in specific and nonspecific immunological reactions. II. Production of a chemotactic factor specific for macrophages. *Immunology* **24**:997.

Woodruff, M., Dunbar, N., and Ghaffar, A. (1973). The growth of tumor in T-cell deprived mice and their response to treatment with *Corynebacterium parvum. Proc. Roy. Soc. London B* **184**:97.

25

Regression of
Hamster Melanoma by
Corynebacterium parvum

NIKOLAI V. DIMITROV, IVAN CHOUROULINKOV, LUCIEN ISRAEL, and JOHN J. O'RANGERS

Introduction

The antitumor effect of *Corynebacterium parvum*, first demonstrated by Halpern *et al.* (1966) and Woodruff and Boak (1966), has led to the development of a major research effort into the use of bacterial products of corynebacteria as immunostimulants and antitumor agents (Halpern *et al.*, 1964; Smith and Woodruff, 1968; Paslin *et al.*, 1974; Proctor *et al.*, 1973; Adlam *et al.*, 1972; Likhite and Halpern, 1973; Milas *et al.*, 1974; Wilkinson *et al.*, 1973).

It has been shown that inoculation with *C. parvum* alone or in combination with irradiated hepatoma cells after the development of the tumor reduced the incidence and number of lung metastases in rats with hepatoma implanted into the leg (Proctor *et al.*, 1973). However, in another study (Milas *et al.*, 1974),

NIKOLAY V. DIMITROV, Department of Medicine, Division of Hematology and Medical Oncology, Hahnemann Medical College, Philadelphia, Pennsylvania, IVAN CHOUROULIN-KOV, LUCIEN ISRAEL, and JOHN J. O'RANGERS, CNRS, Villejuif, France; and Centre Hospitalier Universitaire Lariboisiere, Paris, France.

The work reported in this paper was undertaken during the tenure (N.V.D.) of an American Cancer Society Eleanor Roosevelt–International Cancer Fellowship awarded by the International Union Against Cancer.

pretreatment with *Corynebacterium granulosum* before inoculation of syngenic fibrosarcoma in C_3H mice reduced the number of lung metastases and prolonged the survival of the animals.

Previous work in our laboratory with intralesional injection of *C. granulosum* in hamster melanoma showed regression of the tumor and reduction in the number of lung metastases. Inoculation of *C. granulosum* prior to or concurrently with tumor injection did not significantly affect tumor rejection or the metastatic rate (Paslin *et al.*, 1974).

Similar results were obtained in mice using intralesional injections of *C. parvum* into other experimental tumors (Likhite and Halpern, 1973). It appears that in some experiments, the treated animals rejecting the tumor became resistant to repeated challenges with the same quantities of tumor cells (Likhite and Halpern, 1973).

The immunological effect of *C. parvum* has been studied extensively during the last decade (Halpern *et al.*, 1964; Wilkinson *et al.*, 1973). In addition to the antitumor effect, simultaneous injections with *C. parvum* and tumor cells significantly increased the lymphocyte cytotoxicity against the autochthonous malignant cells, which is regarded as an effect of the vaccine on cell-mediated immunity (Halpern, 1973).

Administration of *C. parvum* and *C. granulosum* to patients with neoplastic diseases appears to alter the immune status of the patients (Israel and Halpern, 1972; Israel and Edelstein, 1973).

Recent experimental work with *C. parvum* has been directed toward the determination of the best method of administration, the time of inoculation relative to tumor development, and the optimum dosage, both singly and in combination with other chemotherapeutic agents (Paslin *et al.*, 1974; Proctor *et al.*, 1973; Woodruff and Inchley, 1971).

Materials and Methods

Animals

Three- to five-month-old female golden hamsters were used for all experiments.

Tumors

Fortner's melanotic melanoma #1 has been maintained by serial subcutaneous (s.c.) injection of 10^8 tumor cells in a colony of golden hamsters, as previously described (Paslin *et al.*, 1974). A piece of tissue from the periphery of the tumor was fragmented and passed through an 80-μm sieve. Viability of the tumor cells was verified by the trypan-blue exclusion technique. The cells were suspended in medium 199 to a concentration of 10×10^8 cells/ml. Hamsters were inoculated s.c. in the upper right dorsal quadrant with 0.1 ml of suspension containing 1×10^8 tumor cells (transplantation generation No. 167).

Vaccine

C. parvum was obtained from the Institut Mérieux, Lyon, France, 1 ml containing 2 mg of heat-killed, formalin-fixed material in normal saline; BCG (Glaxo strain) from batch B-61 containing $4.8–6.1 \times 10^6$ live organisms/ml (Eli Lilly Co., Indianapolis, Indiana, USA).

Corynebacterium or BCG was injected subcutaneously before implantation of the tumor or intralesionally after the development of palpable tumor 0.6–1 cm in diameter.

Experimental Groups

The animals were divided into five experimental groups. Each group consisted of six hamsters: *Group 1,* five consecutive subcutaneous injections of 0.5 ml 0.9% NaCl (one injection weekly); *Group 2,* 0.2 ml of BCG (Glaxo), five consecutive intralesional injections after the formation of palpable tumor (0.6–1 cm diameter); *Group 3,* 0.5 ml of *C. parvum,* five consecutive intralesional injections after the formation of palpable tumor (0.6–1 cm diameter); *Group 4,* 0.2 ml of BCG (Glaxo), five consecutive intralesional injections after the formation of palpable tumor (0.6–1 cm diameter); *Group 5,* 0.5 ml of *C. parvum,* five consecutive intralesional injections after the formation of palpable tumor (0.6–1 cm diameter).

Procedures

The tumors were evaluated weekly by measuring the length, width, and depth of each tumor using calipers with a millimeter scale. Tumor volumes were calculated as ellipsoids: $V = 4abc/3.6$. The survival time of each experimental animal was recorded on a weekly basis. Cell-dead animals underwent post-mortem examination. The number of pulmonary metastases (hamster) was counted, and a mean value for each experimental group was obtained.

The spleen, liver, and both lungs underwent additional histological examination.

Results

The survival time of the experimental animals was similar in groups 1, 2, and 3 when *C. parvum* or BCG was administered before the implantation of the tumor (5–14 weeks). Significant differences were noted in groups 4 and 5, which represented animals with intratumoral injection of BCG and *C. parvum.* The survival time of the hamsters injected with BCG was longer than the control group (Fig. 1). However, the most significant results were obtained from the group of animals receiving intratumoral injections of *C. parvum.* All animals were alive at day 25, when reinoculation of the tumor was performed. This attempt for transplantation of the tumor failed. The second reinoculation of the

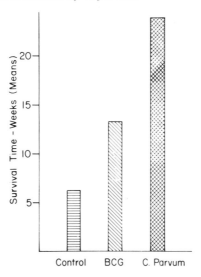

Fig. 1. Means of survival time in
animals that received intratumoral
injections of BCG and *Corynebacterium parvum.*

tumor was also rejected, after which the animals were killed two weeks later for
examination of the lungs and the site of tumor inoculation.

The growth of the tumor was delayed in the group of animals which received
intratumoral injections of BCG, but regression and complete disappearance of
the tumor was registered only in the animals treated with *C. parvum* intralesionally (Fig. 2). In all groups, the growth was identical up to the third week. During
the fourth week, the control group and BCG group continued growing, and the
group receiving *C. parvum* maintained the same level. After the fourth week,
there was continued development of the tumor, whereas the group of *C. parvum*
showed fast regression and disappearance of the tumor at the end of the ninth
week. The other two groups showed very rapid tumor growth, causing the death
of the animals.

One of the features of Fortner's melanoma is development of early pulmonary metastasis (Hanna *et al.,* 1972). Our experiments showed that all
untreated animals developed metastases during the second and third weeks, and
at the time of death, the number of metastases averaged twenty-five (Fig. 3).
There was no significant difference in the number of metastases between the
control group and the group injected with BCG. The animals from the *C. parvum*
group remained free of metastases. No metastases were noted after the reinoculation of the tumor.

Discussion

Treatment with immunostimulants is still a relatively new subject of experimental medicine. The antitumor effect of certain vaccines, including *C. parvum*, is a new field of investigation and most of the available information has been published during the last five years (Paslin *et al.,* 1974; Wilkinson *et al.,* 1973; Halpern, 1973; Woodruff and Inchley, 1971). The variety of tumors and species of animals used in the experimental designs produced a great deal of controversy due to the dose of the vaccine and the routes of administration. This requires a thorough investigation using different doses and schedules.

In our experiments, we chose the intralesional injection in order to evaluate the direct effect of *C. parvum* on the tumor growth and the dissemination of the

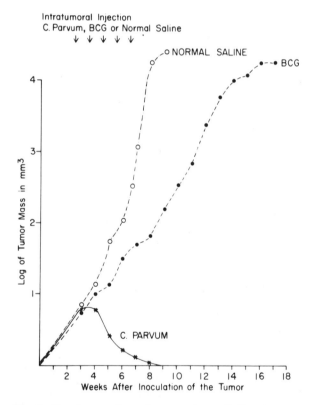

Fig. 2. Development and regression of the tumor after intratumoral injections with BCG and *Corynebacterium parvum*, expressed as means of the log of the tumor mass.

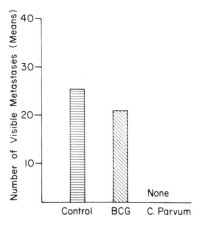

Fig. 3. Number of lung metastases (means).

disease. Fortner's melanoma develops early pulmonary metastasis and appears to be a suitable model for such experiments.

The results of this study indicate that only the group of animals receiving intratumoral injections of *C. parvum* after the development of measurable tumors showed regression and disappearance of the lesion. In this group, no visible or histological metastases were found.

On the contrary, the experimental animals from the other two groups developed progressive tumors and developed pulmonary metastases. The metastatic lesions in this tumor usually occur 2–3 weeks after the tumor inoculation, which coincides with the development of measurable tumor (Paslin *et al.*, 1974). The relationship between the time of the vaccine administration and antitumor effect has been extensively discussed (Paslin *et al.*, 1974; Proctor *et al.*, 1973; Milas *et al.*, 1974). The results from our study indicate that pretreatment with *C. parvum* does not significantly affect the growth of tumors. An obvious antitumor effect was obtained only when the vaccine was given intralesionally after the development of the tumor. Similar results have been obtained by Milas *et al.* (1974) and are reported elsewhere in these proceedings (see Chapter 26). Proctor *et al.* (1973), reported the disappearance of already developed pulmonary metastases in rats with hepatoma using *C. parvum* after removal of the primary tumor. Injections with BCG did not affect the development of the metastatic lesions in the lung.

The intratumoral administration of vaccines has been considered necessary for the regression of the tumor (Paslin *et al.*, 1974; Woodruff and Inchley, 1971). This applies much more for the melanoma, where in many cases, the primary tumor could be determined. The mechanism of the local effect of *C. parvum* at this time is not clear. However, the successful use of heat-killed

Corynebacteria in experimental melanoma further supports the concept that living organisms are not essential for inhibition of tumor growth or for the destruction of the tumor cells.

Regression of hepatocarcinoma has been demonstrated by Hanna *et al.* (1972) using intratumoral injections of BCG. The authors attributed the regression of the tumor and its regional metastases to the granulomatous reaction occurring at both skin and lymph node. The results obtained in our experiments suggest that the role of regional lymph nodes is not as essential as these authors suggest. The metastatic lesions in our model are considered to be blood-borne.

Since *C. parvum* is involved in the clearance of the colloids, its effect could be related to the clearance of some tumor antigens. Finally, the mixture of *C. parvum* and denatured melanoma cells may act both as immunizing agents and as stimulants of the reticuloendothelial system. This action could activate the macrophages which may take part in the destruction of the tumor cells.

References

Adlam, C., Broughton, E. S., and Scott, M. T. (1972). Enhanced resistance of mice to infection with bacteria following pretreatment with *Corynebacterium parvum. Nature (Lond.)* **235**:219–220.

Halpern, B. N. (1973). Inhibition of malignant tumor growth by *Corynebacterium parvum* and its mechanism. *International Research Communication System, April, 1973* (73–74), 1–3.

Halpern, B. N., Prévot, A. R., Biozzi, G., Stiffel, C., Mouton, D., Morard, J. C., Bouthillier, Y., and Decreusefond, C. (1964). Stimulation de l'activité phagocytaire du système réticuloendothélial provoquée par *Corynebacterium parvum. J. Reticuloendothel. Soc.* **1**:77–96.

Halpern, B. N., Biozzi, G., Stiffel, C., and Mouton, D. (1966). Inhibition of tumor growth by administration of killed *Corynebacterium parvum. Nature (Lond.)* **212**:853–854.

Hanna, M. G., Jr., Zbar, B., and Rapp, H. J. (1972). Histopathology of tumor regression after intralesional injection of *Mycobacterium bovis*. I. Tumor growth and metastases. *J. Natl. Cancer Inst.* **48**:1441–1445.

Israel, L. and Edelstein, R. (1973). Nonspecific immunostimulation with *C. parvum* in human cancer. *Symposium on Immune Mechanisms in Neoplasia*, M. D. Anderson and Tumor Institute, (in press).

Israel, L. and Halpern, B. N. (1972). Le *Corynebacterium parvum* dans les cancers avancés. Première évaluation de l'activité thérapeutique de cette immunostimuline. *Nouv. Presse Med.* **1**:19–23.

Likhite, V. V. and Halpern, B. N. (1973). The lasting of mammary adenocarcinoma cell tumors in DBA/2 mice with intratumor injection of killed *Corynebacterium parvum. Int. J. Cancer* **12**:699–704.

Milas, L., Hunter, N., and Withers, H. R. (1974). *Corynebacterium granulosum*-induced protection against artificial pulmonary metastases of a syngenic fibrosarcoma in mice. *Cancer Res.* **34**:613–620.

Paslin, D. A., Dimitrov, N. V., and Heaton, C. (1974). Regression of a transplantable hamster melanoma by intralesional injections of *Corynebacterium granulosum. J. Natl. Cancer Inst.* **52**:571–573.

Proctor, J., Rudenstam, C. M., and Alexander, P. (1973). Increase of lung metastasis following treatments of rats bearing hepatomas with irradiated tumor cells and the beneficial effect of *C. parvum* in this system. *Biomedicine* **19**:248–252.

Smith, J. H. and Woodruff, W. A. (1968). Comparative effects of two strains of *C. parvum* on pathogenic activity and tumor growth. *Nature (Lond.)* **219**:197–198.

Wilkinson, R. C., O'Neill, G. J., and Wapshaw, K. G. (1973). Role of anaerobic coryneforms in specific and nonspecific immunological reactions. II. Production of a chemotactic factor specific for macrophages. *Immunology* **24**:997–1006.

Woodruff, M. F. A. and Boak, J. F. (1966). Inhibitory effects of injection of *Corynebacterium parvum* on the growth of tumor transplants on isogenic hosts. *Br. J. Cancer* **20**:345–355.

Woodruff, M. F. A. and Inchley, M. P. (1971). Synergistic inhibition of mammary carcinoma transplants in A-strain mice by antitumor globulin and *C. parvum*. *Br. J. Cancer* **25**:584–593.

26

Corynebacterium granulosum-Induced Prophylaxis and Therapy of Artificial Pulmonary Metastases of Syngenic Murine Tumors

LUKAS MILAS, NANCY HUNTER, IVAN BAŠIĆ,
KATHY MASON, and H. RODNEY WITHERS

Introduction

There has recently been significant interest in the antitumor activity of anaerobic corynebacteria, potent nonspecific stimulators of the reticuloendothelial system (RES). *Corynebacterium parvum* was found to be effective against many syngenic and allogenic tumors of experimental animals (for more details, see Milas, 1974). Fewer tumor takes, delay of tumor appearance, and retarded

LUKAS MILAS, NANCY HUNTER, IVAN BAŠIĆ, KATHY MASON, and H. RODNEY
WITHERS, Section of Experimental Radiotherapy, The University of Texas System Cancer
Center, 6723 Bertner Ave., Houston, Texas 77025.

This investigation was supported by US Public Health Service Research Grant No. CA
11138-06 and CA 06294-13 from the National Cancer Institute.

growth were common observations following transplantation of tumor cells in mice treated with this bacterium. Another strain of anaerobic corynebacteria, *Corynebacterium granulosum*, also proved capable of exerting a strong antitumor adjuvant activity (Milas *et al.*, 1974f; Milas *et al.*, 1974c; Paslin *et al.*, 1974). *C. parvum* and *C. granulosum* were found to be potent adjuncts to chemotherapy (Currie and Bagshawe, 1970) and to radiotherapy (to be published) of murine fibrosarcomas. It has recently been observed that complete and lasting regressions of established tumors can be achieved with the intratumor injection of *C. parvum* (Likhite and Halpern, 1974) or with systemic application of *C. parvum* or *C. granulosum* (Milas *et al.*, 1974b; Milas *et al.*, 1974d; Milas *et al.*, 1974a,f).

In this paper, we describe the various aspects of the antitumor response induced by *C. granulosum* against artificial pulmonary metastases of a syngenic murine fibrosarcoma, as well as two syngenic murine mammary carcinomas. The assay of pulmonary metastases (colonies, nodules) is a suitable quantitative test for transplantability of tumors (Hill and Bush, 1969; Milas *et al.*, 1974e). As a model for nonspecific immunotherapy for tumor metastases, the assay was first used in mice by one of us (Milas and Mujagić, 1972) and subsequently for similar studies in rats by Baldwin and Pimm (1973).

Animals, Tumors, and Anaerobic Corynebacteria

Specific-pathogen-free mice of the inbred C_3Hf/Bu strain were used. Mice of both sexes were 3 months old at the initiation of each experiment. The tumors were syngenic fibrosarcoma (FSA), originally induced by methylcholanthrene (Suit and Suchato, 1967) and 2 syngenic mammary carcinomas. For purposes of simplification, the carcinomas will be designated mammary carcinoma 1 and 2 (MCA-1 and MCA-2). MCA-1 arose spontaneously in a multiparous C_3H/He mouse (Silobrčić and Suit, 1967), and MCA-2 in a C_3H/Bu female mouse that had been irradiated 26 months earlier in the cervical area with 2100 rads of γ rays. This tumor developed outside the radiation field. The FSA was in its 5th isotransplant generation, and MCA-1 in its 3rd, and MCA-2 in its 7th isotransplant generation when used in the present study. The FSA contains strong tumor-specific antigens (Suit and Kaštelan, 1970; Milas *et al.*, 1974e), MCA-1 weak antigens (Silobrčić and Suit, 1967), and MCA-2 fairly strong antigens (to be published). Single-cell suspensions from the FSA were prepared by trypsin digestion of tumor tissue containing no visible regions of necrosis or hemorrhage (Milas *et al.*, 1974e,f). Viability of these cells was regularly more than 95%, as determined by observing trypan-blue exclusion and phase contrast microscopy. Suspensions of cells from both mammary carcinomas were prepared by a mechanical method as described previously (Milas *et al.*, 1974f). The viability of cells from MCA-1 was about 30%, and from MCA-2 about 60%. The method used for counting the lung colonies that developed after intravenous (i.v.)

inoculation of FSA cells has been elsewhere described (Milas *et al.*, 1974e,f). Formalin-killed *C. granulosum* were generously supplied by Professor M. Raynaud, Institute Pasteur, France. Intravenous (i.v.), intraperitoneal (i.p.), and subcutaneous (s.c.) injections of mice with the bacterium were also described earlier (Milas *et al.*, 1974f).

Results

Protection against FSA Metastases

Mice were given s.c. or i.v. injections of 0.25 mg of *C. granulosum*, and 7 days later, were injected with 10^5 or 10^6 viable FSA cells i.v. The number of lung metastases was determined 11 days after tumor-cell inoculation (Table I). The number of tumor nodules generated by 10^5 FSA cells was reduced from 76.5 ± 8.5 in control mice to 2.5 ± 0.6 and to less than 1 in mice that were protected with *C. granulosum* s.c. and i.v., respectively. In control mice that received 10^6 FSA cells, colonies were confluent (more than 250). The number of colonies in some mice treated s.c. with this immunostimulant was reduced below 250 and could therefore be counted. Intravenous treatment with *C. granulosum* was more efficient; it reduced the number of metastases to 13.3 ± 2.9.

C. parvum (batch No. EZ 174 from Borroughs Wellcome Company, London)

Table I. *Corynebacterium granulosum*-Induced Protection against FSA Metastases in Lung[a,b]

| Treatment of tumor-cell recipients | Metastases in lung generated by FSA cells | | | |
| | 10^5 | | 10^6 | |
	Mean ± S.E.	Range	Mean ± S.E.	Range
None	76.5 ± 8.5	32–119	Confluent[c]	
C. granulosum s.c.	2.5 ± 0.6	0–6	Confluent (3 mice) 70, 116, 128, 152, 175, 180[d]	
C. granulosum i.v.	< 1	0–1	13.3 ± 2.9	1–26

[a]Data from Milas *et al.* (1974a).
[b]*C. granulosum* (0.25 mg), was given 7 days before i.v. inoculation of tumor cells. Number of metastases was determined 11 days after tumor-cell inoculation. Each group consisted of 9 or 10 mice.
[c]More than 250 colonies.
[d]Individual values.

protected mice against FSA metastases in a similar manner to that just described for *C. granulosum* (Milas *et al.*, 1974a).

Further studies (to be published) showed that a single i.p. injection with *C. granulosum* was more efficient in reducing FSA metastases than 2 or 3 injections, and that animals treated i.p. with this bacterium were resistant to tumor cells, even if the cells were injected i.v. 82 days later.

Therapy for FSA Metastases

C. granulosum was also effective in reducing the number of FSA metastases if given to mice after tumor cells. Mice were injected i.v. with 10^5 FSA cells, and 2 or 7 days later, treated i.p. with 0.5 mg of *C. granulosum*. Some animals were killed 14 days after inoculation of tumor cells to determine the number of lung metastases, and the remainder were kept to check the effect of *C. granulosum* on survival of mice (Table II). All normal and treated mice had metastases. The number of metastases in control mice was 99.3 ± 15. This number was significantly reduced in mice treated with the immunostimulant 2 days (39.7 ± 7.2), but not 7 days (82.0 ± 8.0), after tumor-cell inoculation. The effect of *C. granulosum* was more pronounced on the survival of mice. While all mice receiving only tumor cells died in 22.7 ± 0.8 days, a proportion of those treated with *C. granulosum* survived the duration of the experiment (Table II). This implies that *C. granulosum* induced complete regressions of the established pulmonary metastases. Also, mice that were not cured by *C. granulosum* survived significantly longer than untreated controls. Given after tumor cells, both *C. granulosum* (Milas *et al.*, 1974a,b,d) and *C. parvum* (Milas *et al.*, 1974a) also induced complete, lasting regressions of a proportion of established s.c.-growing FSAs.

Protection against Irradiation-Induced Enhancement of FSA Metastases

Irradiation may facilitate the development of metastases in the treated area. When the whole body or thoracic area alone of mice was irradiated one day before i.v. injection of tumor cells, an increased incidence of pulmonary metastases occurred (Brown, 1973; Van den Brenk *et al.*, 1973; Withers and Milas, 1973; Milas *et al.*, 1974e). Stimulation of mice with *C. granulosum* before the administration of radiation can abolish this enhancing effect of irradiation on metastases. Animals injected i.p. with 0.5 mg of *C. granulosum* were whole-body irradiated 6 days later with 200, 400, 600, or 800 rads of γ rays. The day following irradiation, they were injected i.v. with 2.5×10^4 FSA cells; 14 days thereafter (11 days for mice receiving 800 rads), they were sacrificed. The number of lung metastases (Table III) was increased in irradiated mice and reduced in those treated with *C. granulosum*. The irradiation, however, did not influence this antitumor effect exerted by the immunostimulant.

C. granulosum protected the mice against radiation-induced enhancement of

Table II. Effect of *Corynebacterium granulosum* (0.5 mg, i.p.) Given after FSA Cells on Tumor Metastases in Lung and Survival of Mice[a,b]

Days given after tumor cells	Metastases in lung[c]			Survival of recipients		
	Mice with metastases/ total mice	Mean number of metastases[b] S.E.	Range	Mice died/ total mice	Mean survival in days ± S.E.	Range
No treatment	7/7	99.3 ± 15.0	37–142	11/11	22.7 ± 0.8	21–27
2	7/7	39.7 ± 7.2[d]	16–60	4/7	38.8 ± 7.4[d]	24–58
7	7/7	82.0 ± 8.0	44–105	5/7	30.6 ± 3.6[e]	24–44

[a]Data from Milas *et al.* (1974f).
[b]Viable FSA cells (10^5) were inoculated i.v.
[c]Number of metastases was determined 14 days after tumor-cell inoculation.
[d]$P < 0.005$.
[e]$P < 0.01$.

Table III. Protection by *Corynebacterium granulosum* against Radiation-Induced Enhancement of FSA Metastases in Lung[a,b]

Radiation dose, rads	Lung metastases			
	Normal mice		Mice treated with *C. granulosum*	
	Mean number of metastases ± S.E.	Range	Mean number of metastases ± S.E.	Range
None	11.4 ± 2.0	3–17	<1	0–2
200	34.3 ± 5.9	18–58	1.7 ± 0.8	0–6
400	31.3 ± 6.0	12–55	<1	0–1
600	75.0 ± 6.3	60–97	<1	0–1
800	87.5 ± 7.0	51–111	<1	0–1

[a]Data from Milas *et al.* (1974f).

[b]Irradiation was delivered to the whole body of mice 1 day before i.v. inoculation of 2.5×10^4 FSA cells. *C. granulosum* (0.5 mg, i.p.) was administered 6 days before irradiation and 7 days before inoculation of tumor cells. Number of metastases was determined 14 days (11 days for mice receiving 800 rads) following tumor-cell inoculation. Each group consisted of 6–10 mice.

lung metastases if applied between 2 weeks before and 3 h after irradiation. However, radiation-induced enhancement of pulmonary metastases was not influenced if the immunostimulation with *C. granulosum* was applied 27 days before or 1 or 2 days after irradiation (Milas *et al.*, 1974c).

Effect on Concomitant Immunity to FSA Metastases

The number of pulmonary metastases generated by i.v.-injected FSA cells was reduced in mice bearing this tumor in their legs (Milas *et al.*, 1974e). Immunostimulation with *C. granulosum* can increase the efficiency of this concomitant immunity. FSA cells (2.4×10^5 per mouse) were implanted into the right hind legs of mice, and tumors were allowed to grow for 8 days. At this time, the mice were treated i.p. with 0.25 mg of *C. granulosum,* and 2 days later, were injected i.v. with 10^5 tumor cells. Fourteen days following tumor-cell inoculation, the number of colonies in the lungs was determined (Table IV). The presence of tumor growing in the legs reduced the number of colonies generated in the lung by cells injected i.v.: 12.8 ± 3.8 colonies as compared to 39.9 ± 6.3 colonies in controls. This number of metastases in tumor-bearing mice was further reduced by treatment with *C. granulosum* (1.0 ± 0.4 colonies). In contrast, active immunization of tumor-bearing mice with 10^7 heavily irradiated

Table IV. Effect of *Corynebacterium granulosum* on Concomitant Immunity to FSA Metastases in Lung

Recipients of 10^5 FSA cells inoculated i.v.	Metastases in lung[a]	
	Mean ± S.E.	Range
Normal mice	39.9 ± 6.3	15–72
Normal mice injected with *C. granulosum*[b]	4.5 ± 3.0	0–31
Mice bearing FSA in legs[c]	12.8 ± 3.8	1–32
Mice bearing FSA in legs and injected with *C. granulosum*	1.0 ± 0.4	0–4

[a]Number of metastases was determined 14 days after i.v. inoculation of tumor cells. Each group consisted of 10 mice.
[b]*C. granulosum* (0.25 mg) was given i.p. 2 days before i.v. inoculation of tumor cells.
[c]Tumors in legs were produced by injection of 2.4×10^5 viable FSA cells 10 days before i.v. inoculation of tumor cells. At this time, the tumors were between 7 and 8 mm in diameter.

FSA cells (10,000 rads of γ rays) 2 days before i.v. injection of viable tumor cells did not influence the already existing concomitant immunity; the number of tumor nodules in mice treated in this way was 11.3 ± 3.7. The immunization with heavily irradiated-tumor cells was, however, efficient in normal mice, reducing the number of colonies to 9.1 ± 4.1 (control had 39.9 ± 6.3 colonies).

Protection against Pulmonary Metastases of Mammary Carcinomas

Three or 6×10^5 viable cells from MCA-1 were injected i.v. into mice treated i.p. with 0.5 mg of *C. granulosum* a week earlier. Approximately one-half of the recipients were sacrificed 28 days after tumor-cell inoculation to determine the number of lung colonies, and the remaining half of the recipients was kept to check the effect of the immunostimulation on their survival (Table V). Treatment with *C. granulosum* significantly reduced the number of colonies in mice that were given i.v. injections of 6×10^5 tumor cells, but the reduction in mice receiving 3×10^5 tumor cells was not significant. Immunostimulation also prolonged the survival of recipients; the effect now being greater against 3×10^5 tumor cells.

Treatment of mice with 0.5 mg i.p. of *C. granulosum* induced a significant protection against 2.5×10^5 viable cells from MCA-2 that were injected i.v. 7 days later. The number of lung metastases, determined 28 days following tumor-cell inoculation, was 1.8 ± 0.4, as opposed to 20.4 ± 4.2 colonies in untreated mice.

Discussion

C. granulosum exerted strong antitumor activity against pulmonary metastases of a syngenic FSA, when given to mice before or after tumor cells. It also induced protection against i.v.-injected cells from two syngenic mammary carcinomas, which are less immunogenic than the FSA. In some instances, *C. granulosum* was capable of inducing complete regressions of established pulmonary metastases (Table II), as well as established, subcutaneously-growing FSAs (Milas *et al.,* 1974a,b,d).

The mechanism(s) by which *C. granulosum* exerts its antitumor activity is not completely understood. Like other immunostimulants, this bacterium induces an extensive proliferation of lymphoid tissues which then respond more efficiently against foreign antigens, including tumor-specific antigens. That the activity goes primarily through the immune system of the recipients is suggested by the inability of *C. granulosum* to induce antitumor response against FSA-lung nodules in mice exposed to whole-body irradiation 1 or 2 days before the immunostimulant was administered (Milas *et al.,* 1974c). In addition, FSAs regressing in mice treated with this bacterium are diffusely infiltrated with lymphocytes, histiocytes, and macrophages (Milas, 1974; Milas *et al.,* 1974d).

Proliferation of lymphoid tissues was more extensive after i.v. than s.c.

Table V. Effect of *Corynebacterium granulosum* on Tumor Metastases and Survival of Mice Injected i.v. with MCA-1 Cells [a,b]

Treatment of tumor cell recipients	Number of MCA-1 cells injected (× 10⁵)	Metastases in lung			Survival of recipients		
		Mice with metastases/ total mice	Mean number of metastases ± S.E.	Range	Mice died/ total mice	Mean survival in days ± S.E.	Range
None	3	6/7	3.3 ± 0.9	0–7	7/7	55.9 ± 2.8	47–65
	6	7/7	6.3 ± 1.4	2–13	7/7	53.1 ± 4.6	39–72
C. granulosum	3	5/7	2.0 ± 0.8	0–5	7/7	76.9 ± 5.6 [c]	59–98
	6	5/6	2.3 ± 0.5 [d]	0.3	5/5	64.4 ± 3.7	56–73

[a] Data from Milas *et al.* (1974f).
[b] *C. granulosum* (0.5 mg) was given 7 days before i.v. inoculation of tumor cells. Number of metastases was determined 28 days after tumor-cell inoculation.
[c] $P < 0.005$.
[d] $P < 0.025$.

injection of *C. granulosum* or *C. parvum* (Milas *et al.*, 1974a). This correlates well with the strength of resistance expressed against FSA cells injected i.v. (Milas *et al.*, 1974a), and it also suggests that the immune system stimulated with anaerobic corynebacteria plays a crucial role in the antitumor response.

The response to FSA was stronger than to MCA-2 and—in particular—to MCA-1, which is poorly immunogenic. This indicates that the strength of antigenicity of a tumor is important in the antitumor response of recipients treated with *C. granulosum*. Other possible mechanisms that may be involved in expression of antitumor activity by *C. granulosum*, *C. parvum*, or other immunostimulants are discussed in more detail elsewhere (Weiss, 1973; Milas, 1974).

Thymus-derived lymphocytes are presently considered to play a dominant role in the destruction of tumor cells (Freedman *et al.*, 1972; Goldstein *et al.*, 1972). These cells seem to be suppressed in mice treated with *C. granulosum* or *C. parvum*. Animals treated with *C. granulosum* tolerate skin grafts from allogenic donors much longer than normal mice, and their peripheral-blood lymphocytes, lymph nodes, and spleen cells exhibit *in vitro* a decreased response to stimulation by phytohemagglutinin (PHA) (to be published). A decreased responsiveness to PHA by lymphocytes from mice treated with *C. parvum* was recently reported by Scott (1972). Woodruff and Dunbar (1973) reported that mice deficient in T-lymphocytes (deficiency was induced by thymectomy, irradiation, and bone-marrow reconstitution) can resist tumor if treated with *C. parvum*. This also indicates that the antitumor effect of anaerobic corynebacteria may be independent of T-cell function.

It appears reasonable to suppose that thymus-independent lymphocytes (B cells) and/or macrophages might be involved in the destruction of tumor cells. Anaerobic corynebacteria, used in nonviable form, profoundly augment humoral immune response (Raynaud *et al.*, 1972; Adlam and Scott, 1973; Howard *et al.*, 1973; O'Neill *et al.*, 1973), the function of B-cells. These cells have recently been found to be able to destroy tumor cells *in vitro* (Lamon *et al.*, 1972; O'Toole *et al.*, 1973).

Macrophages are capable of destroying tumor cells in both an immunologically specific (Bennett, 1965) and nonspecific manner (Hibbs *et al.*, 1972). Several observations in our studies with *C. granulosum* suggested that these cells might largely participate in the antitumor immunity exerted by anaerobic corynebacteria: (a) animals treated with *C. granulosum* resisted immunosuppression induced by irradiation (Table III); (b) mice treated with *C. granulosum* were more resistant to tumor cells injected i.p. than s.c. or i.v. (Milas *et al.*, 1974f). Stimulation with this bacterium induced extensive proliferation of macrophages in the peritoneal cavity (Bašić *et al.*, 1974; Milas *et al.*, 1974c); (c) numerous macrophages were present in tumors undergoing rejection in mice treated with *C. granulosum* (Milas, 1974; Milas *et al.*, 1974d); and (d) peritoneal macrophages from mice treated with this immunostimulant could, in an immunologically nonspecific manner, destroy *in vitro* Chinese hamster ovary cells (Bašić *et al.*, 1974), cells from syngenic FSA, mouse L-P59 cells—which are tumorogenic in

C_3Hf/Bu mice, and cells from two melanomas of human origin (to be published). Olivotto and Bomford (1974) reported similar *in vitro* destruction of tumor cells by macrophages from mice treated with *C. parvum.*

The observation that irradiation did not affect the antitumor-immune response in mice treated with *C. granulosum,* but that the treatment with *C. granulosum* was ineffective in irradiated recipients, seems to be important for clinical tumor therapy. This suggests that nonspecific immunotherapy should be applied before surgery, radiotherapy, or chemotherapy—the forms of therapy for cancer that might impair, to some extent, the immunologic reactivity of patients, presuming only that the nonspecific immunologic activity of the tumor host is not altered by the presence of the tumor. The *C. granulosum*-induced increase in concomitant immunity against pulmonary metastases in the presence of subcutaneously growing FSA supports this conclusion. However, if the tumors are removed by conventional means, enough time should be allowed to permit recovery of the immune system before nonspecific immunotherapy is initiated.

Summary

We have described the prophylactic and therapeutic effectiveness of killed *Corynebacterium granulosum* against artificial pulmonary metastases of syngenic murine tumors. Treatment of mice with *C. granulosum* before intravenous injection of a fibrosarcoma or two mammary carcinomas greatly reduced the number of metastases in the lung. The effect was greater if the immunostimulant was given intravenously rather than subcutaneously. Also, mice were less protected against mammary carcinomas than against the antigenically stronger fibrosarcoma.

C. granulosum given to mice after fibrosarcoma cells reduced the number of pulmonary metastases and induced complete regressions of established pulmonary tumors. Furthermore, this immunostimulant increased the efficiency of concomitant immunity to metastases and also protected mice against radiation-induced enhancement of growth of fibrosarcoma deposits in the lung.

We have discussed possible immunological mechanisms by which *C. granulosum* may exert the antitumor effect, giving emphasis to the role of macrophages.

References

Adlam, C. and Scott, M. T. (1973). Lymphoreticular stimulatory properties of *Corynebacterium parvum* and related bacteria. *J. Med. Microbiol.* **6**:261.

Baldwin, R. W. and Pimm, M. V. (1973). BCG immunotherapy of pulmonary growth from intravenously transferred rat-tumor cells. *Br. J. Cancer* **27**:48.

Bašić, I., Milas, L., Grdina, D. J., and Withers, H. R. (1974). Destruction of hamster ovarian cells cultures by peritoneal macrophages from mice treated with *Corynebacterium granulosum. J. Natl. Cancer Inst.* **52**:1839.

Bennett, B. (1965). Specific suppression of tumor growth by isolated peritoneal macrophages from immunized mice. *J. Immunol.* **95**:656.

Brown, J. M. (1973). The effect of lung irradiation on the incidence of pulmonary metastases in mice. *Br. J. Radiol.* **46**:613.

Currie, G. A. and Bagshawe, K. D. (1970). Active immunotherapy with *Corynebacterium parvum* and chemotherapy in murine fibrosarcomas. *Br. Med. J.* **1**:541.

Freedman, L. R., Cerottini, J. C., and Brunner, K. T. (1972). *In vivo* studies of the role of cytotoxic T cells in tumor-allograft immunity. *J. Immunol.* **109**:1371.

Goldstein, P., Wigzell, H., Blomgren, H., and Svedmyr, E. A. J. (1972). Cell-mediating specific *in vitro* cytotoxicity. II. Probable autonomy of thymus-processed lymphocytes (T cells) for the killing of allogenic target cells. *J. Exp. Med.* **135**:890.

Hibbs, J. B., Jr., Lambert, L., Jr., and Remington, S. J. (1972). Possible role of macrophage-mediated nonspecific cytotoxicity in tumor resistance. *Nature (London) New Biol.* **235**:48.

Hill, R. P. and Bush, R. S. (1969). A lung-colony assay to determine the radiosensitivity of the cells of a solid tumor. *Int. J. Radiat. Biol.* **15**:435.

Howard, J. G., Scott, M. T., and Christie, G. H. (1973). Cellular mechanisms underlying the adjuvant activity of *Corynebacterium parvum:* interactions of activated macrophages with T and B lymphocytes. In: *Immunopotentiation* (Ciba Foundation Symp. 18) p. 101, (J. Knight, ed.), Associated Scientific Publishers, Amsterdam.

Lamon, E. W., Skurzak, H. M., Klein, E., and Wigzell, H. (1972). *In vitro* cytotoxicity by a nonthymus-processed lymphocyte population with specificity for a virally-determined tumor cell-surface antigen. *J. Exp. Med.* **136**:1072.

Likhite, V. V. and Halpern, N. B. (1974). Lasting rejection of mammary adenocarcinoma-cell tumors in DBA/2 mice with intratumor injection of killed *Corynebacterium parvum.* *Cancer Res.* **34**:341.

Milas, L. (1974). Tumor immunotherapy with anaerobic corynebacteria: Assessment with lung colony assay. In: *Interaction of Radiation and Host Immune Mechanisms in Malignancy* (Rep. 50418), Brookhaven National Laboratory, Upton, N.Y., p. 293.

Milas, L. and Mujagić, H. (1972). Protection by *Corynebacterium parvum* against tumor cells injected intravenously. *Eur. J. Clin. Biol. Res.* **17**:498.

Milas, L., Gutterman, J. U., Hunter, N., Bašić, I., Mavligit, G., Hersh, E. M., and Withers, H. R. (1974a). Immunoprophylaxis and immunotherapy for a murine fibrosarcoma with *C. granulosum* and *C. parvum. Int. J. Cancer* **14**:439.

Milas, L., Hunter, N., Bašić, I., and Withers, H. R. (1974b). Immunotherapy of a murine fibrosarcoma with *Corynebacterium granulosum. Proc. Am. Assoc. Cancer Res.* **15**:95.

Milas, L., Hunter, N., Bašić, I., and Withers, H. R. (1974c). Protection by *Corynebacterium granulosum* against radiation-induced enhancement of artificial pulmonary metastases of a murine fibrosarcoma. *J. Natl. Cancer Inst.* **52**:1875.

Milas, L., Hunter, N., Bašić, I., and Withers, H. R. (1974d). Complete regression of an established murine fibrosarcoma induced by systemic application of *Corynebacterium granulosum. Cancer Res.* **34**:2470.

Milas, L., Hunter, N., Mason, K., and Withers, H. R. (1974e). Immunological resistance to pulmonary metastases in C_3 Hf/Bu mice bearing syngenic fibrosarcoma of different sizes. *Cancer Res.* **34**:61.

Milas, L., Hunter, N., and Withers, H. R. (1974f). *Corynebacterium granulosum*-induced protection against artificial pulmonary metastases of a syngenic fibrosarcoma in mice. *Cancer Res.* **34**:613.

Olivotto, M. and Bomford, R. (1974). *In vitro* inhibition of tumor-cell growth and DNA synthesis by peritoneal and lung macrophages from mice injected with *Corynebacterium parvum. Int. J. Cancer* **13**:478.

O'Neill, G. J., Henderson, D. C., and White, R. G. (1973). The role of anaerobic coryneforms on specific and nonspecific immunological reactions. I. Effect on particle clearance and humoral and cell-mediated immunological responses. *Immunology* 24:377.

O'Toole, C., Perlman, P., Wigzell, H., Unsgaard, B., and Zetterlund, C. G. (1973). Lymphocyte cytotoxicity in bladder cancer. No requirement for thymus-derived effector cells? *Lancet* 1:1085.

Paslin, D., Dimitrov, N. V., and Heaton, C. (1974). Regression of a transplantable hamster melanoma by intralesional injections of *Corynebacterium granulosum. J. Natl. Cancer Inst.* 52:571.

Raynaud, M., Kouznetzova, B., Bizzini, B., and Cherman, J. C. (1972). Etude de l'effect immunostimulant de diverses especes de corynebacterie anaerobie et de leurs fractions. *Ann. Inst. Pasteur, Paris* 122:695.

Scott, M. T. (1972). Biological effects of the adjuvant *Corynebacterium parvum*. I. Inhibition of PHA, mixed lymphocyte and GVH reaction. *Cell. Immunol.* 5:459.

Silobrčić, V. and Suit, H. D. (1967). Tumor-specific antigen(s) in a spontaneous mammary carcinoma of C_3H mice. I. Quantitive cell transplants into mammary-tumor-antigen-positive and free mice. *J. Natl. Cancer Inst.* 39:1113.

Suit, H. D. and Kaštelan, A. (1970). Immunologic status of host and response of methylcholanthrene-induced sarcoma to local X-irradiation. *Cancer* 26:232.

Suit, H. D. and Suchato, D. (1967). Hyperbaric oxygen and radiotherapy of fibrosarcoma and squamous-cell carcinoma of C_3H mice. *Radiology* 89:713.

Van den Brenk, H. A. S., Burch, W. M., Orton, C., and Sharpington, C. (1973). Stimulation of clonogenic growth of tumor cells and metastases in the lungs by local X-irradiation. *Br. J. Cancer* 27:291.

Weiss, D. (1973). Current aspects of tumor immunology. *Israel J. Med. Sci.* 9:205.

Withers, H. R. and Milas, L. (1973). Influence of preirradiation of lung on development of artificial pulmonary metastases of fibrosarcoma in mice. *Cancer Res.* 33:1931.

Woodruff, M. F. A. and Dunbar, N. (1973). The effect of *Corynebacterium parvum* and other reticuloendothelial stimulants on transplanted tumours in mice. In: *Immunopotentiation* (Ciba Foundation Symp. 18) p. 287, (J. Knight, ed.), Associated Scientific Publishers, Amsterdam.

DISCUSSION

HALPERN: The fibrosarcoma tumor is isogenic to which strain?

MILAS: The tumor is syngenic to specific pathogen-free C_3Hf/Bu mice.

27

A Possibility of Synergism between *Corynebacterium parvum* and Lentinan, Serotonin, or Thyroid Hormone in Potentiation of Host Resistance against Cancer

KAZUKO ISHIMURA, YUKIKO Y. MAEDA,
and GORO CHIHARA

Introduction

There is some reliable evidence that shows the presence of a resistance to cancer intrinsic in a human body, such as the correlation between senility and cancer incidence, the low metastatic rate against the number of tumor cells in blood flow, and the spontaneous cure of cancer observed in some cases. To clarify the mechanism of this resistance and to find a substance that would increase this

KAZUKO ISHIMURA, YUKIKO Y. MAEDA, and GORO CHIHARA, National Cancer Center Research Institute, Tokyo, Japan.

resistance seems to be one of the important means in opening a way for new therapy in the treatment of cancer.

There have been several excellent studies made on immunopotentiators for cancer, such as *Corynebacterium parvum* (Halpern *et al.*, 1966), BCG (Biozzi *et al.*, 1959; Halpern *et al.*, 1959; Old *et al.*, 1959), and others. These are all interesting and important materials, and their future development is anticipated. On the other hand, the mode of action of such immunopotentiators and immunopotentiation methods is extremely varied, and the action includes macrophage activation, T-oriented adjuvants, B-oriented adjuvants, hormone-mediated immunopotentiation, etc. Consequently, there is a possibility of making a concerted attack on cancer by a suitable combination of these various immunopotentiators or methods for potentiating the host's resistance against cancer.

The present report gives the most recent progress of some of our studies made on the antitumor polysaccharide, lentinan (Maeda and Chihara, 1971; 1973a,b; Maeda *et al.*, 1973), the host-mediated antitumor action of 5-hydroxytryptophan and serotonin (Maeda *et al.*, 1973), and the effect of thyroid hormone on immune responses. In addition, a discussion will be presented on the possibility of further extending the antitumor activity of *C. parvum* by using the above materials in combination.

Lentinan and Antitumor Polysaccharides

Antitumor Activity of the Hot-Water Extract of Basidiomycetes

The fundamental principle behind oriental medicine practiced in Japan and China from olden times is to "adjust homeostasis of the whole body, rather than directly attack the disease source, and thus bring the patient to a normal state." Beginning with that concept, we re-examined numerous home remedies known from olden times in Japan as being effective against cancer. As a result, we found that the hot-water extract of several basidiomycetes of the Polyporaceae family and edible mushrooms showed a strong antitumor activity against solid tumors of sarcoma-180 transplanted subcutaneously in Swiss albino mice (Ikekawa *et al.*, 1968, 1969) (Table I). Some of these mushrooms had been used as a remedy for cancer since olden times.

Recently, Tsukagoshi *et al.* (1973) reported that protein-bound polysaccharide (PS-K) extracted from *Coriolus versicolor* (FR.) QUÉL. was effective against rat ascites hepatoma AH-13 and nitrogen mustard-resistant Yoshida sarcoma, besides sarcoma-180, especially by oral administration.

Antitumor Activity of Lentinan, the Polysaccharide from *Lentinus edodes*

The hot-water extract of *Lentinus edodes* (BERK.) SING., one of the most popular edible mushrooms in Japan, was submitted to fractional precipitation

Table I. Antitumor Effect of Hot-Water Extracts from Some Basidiomycetes against Sarcoma-180 Transplanted Subcutaneously in Swiss Albino Mice[a]

Samples	Tumor-inhibition ratio, %	Complete regression of tumor
(Polyporaceae)		
Ganoderma applanatum (PERS.) PAT.	69.4	5/10
Phelinus linteus (BERK. and CURT) AOSHIMA	96.7	7/8
Coriolus versicolor (FR.) QUÉL.	77.5	4/8
Coriolus hirsutus (FR.) QUÉL.	65.0	2/10
Daedaleopsis tricolor (FR.) BOND. and SING.	70.2	4/7
(Edible mushrooms)		
Lentinus edodes (BERK.) SING.	80.7	6/10
Agaricus bisporus (LANGE) SING. (mushroom)	12.7	0/10

[a]Sarcoma-180 (8×10^6 cells) were subcutaneously inoculated in the groin of mice. Each sample was injected intraperitoneally at a dose of 200 mg/kg daily for ten days from a day after inocuation. Tumor-inhibition ratios were determined at five weeks after tumor transplantation.

Table II. Antitumor Activity of Lentinan against Various Tumors on Various Strains of Mice[a]

Tumors	Mice	Dose, mg/kg $\times$ days	Tumor-inhibition ratio, %	Complete regression of tumor
Sarcoma-180	SWM/Ms	5×10	44.0	0/5
Sarcoma-180	SWM/Ms	1×10	100	10/10
Sarcoma-180	SWM/Ms	0.5×10	94.7	8/10
Sarcoma-180	SWM/Ms	0.1×10	19.1	0/9
Sarcoma-180	ICR-JCL	1×10	100	10/10
Sarcoma-180	C3H/He	1×10	36.8	0/9
Ehrlich's carcinoma	SWM/Ms	1×10	2.7	0/5
CCM-adenocarcinoma	SWM/Ms	1×10	65.2	0/10
558-adenocarcinoma	SWM/Ms	1×10	9.5	0/4
MM-102 carcinoma	C3H/Arima	1×10	40.3	0/5
NTF-reticulocell sarcoma	SWM/Ms	1×10	27.3	0/9
FM3 A carcinoma	C3H/He	1×10	7.0	0/7
SR-C3H/He sarcoma[b]	C3H/He	1×10	47.5	0/9

[a]Antitumor activity was assayed by the same method described in Table I.
[b]The data given by cooperation with Dr. H. Mitsui.

with ethanol and cetyltrimethylammonium hydroxide, fractional solubilization with acetic acid, Sevag method, and column chromatography over diethylamino-ethylcellulose, and six polysaccharide preparations were isolated: lentinan, LC-11, LC-12, LC-13, EC-11, and EC-14. Lentinan is a β-(1→3)-glucan with a certain amount of β-(1→6) branching, having a molecular weight of ca. 1,000,000; LC-11 is a β-(1→6), (1→4)-glucan; LC-12 is α-(1→6)-glucan; LC-13 is a β-(1→4), (1→6)-glucan containing a small amount of β-(1→4) branching; EC-11 is a mannofucogalactan; and EC-14 is a polysaccharide with glucose and galactose as the major components. None of these polysaccharides showed any antitumor activity, except lentinan and LC-11 (Chihara *et al.*, 1970a,b).

Antitumor activity of lentinan was examined in detail with various tumors and under a variety of conditions, using several strains of mice (Table II).

Lentinan has a strong antitumor activity, as evidenced by the complete regression of a solid tumor of sarcoma-180 transplanted subcutaneously in Swiss or ICR mice by intraperitoneal administration in a dose of 1 mg/kg for 10 days. An interesting fact is that there is a conspicuous optimal dose in the antitumor activity of lentinan against sarcoma-180; a dose of 0.5–1 mg/kg for 10 days has stronger antitumor activity than a dose of 5 mg/kg or 0.1 mg/kg for 10 days. The antitumor activity of lentinan is also affected by the strain of host mice, and it is completely inactive against sarcoma-180 transplanted in C3H/He mice.

The antitumor spectrum of lentinan is not very broad. The tumors in which lentinan has been found effective to date are CCM-adenocarcinoma, MM-102 carcinoma, and SR-C3H/He sarcoma, a viral tumor.

Nakahara and his collaborators reported that lentinan is ineffective against autochthonous tumor (Tokuzen and Nakahara, 1971), but they succeeded in complete regression of a spontaneous autochthonous tumor in mice, at a high rate of 23 out of 37, when the autochthonous graft of the spontaneous mammary tumor was implanted with sarcoma-180, utilizing the local cellular reaction induced by lentinan (Tokuzen, 1971; Tokuzen and Nakahara, 1973).

Lentinan is also ineffective against the ascitic tumor of sarcoma-180. Lentinan has no direct cytotoxicity against tumor cells, and its antitumor activity is host-mediated. Viability of sarcoma-180 cells cultured in a medium containing various concentrations of lentinan is almost 100% after 24 h.

Characteristics of Lentinan as an Immunopotentiator

Lentinan has several interesting characteristics different from the mechanisms of the known immunopotentiators.

Participation of Thymus or T Cells

Antitumor activity of lentinan disappears completely in neonatally thymectomized mice, and decreases markedly after the administration of antilymphocyte serum (Maeda and Chihara, 1971, 1973a,b). This fact does not prove that lentinan directly activates T cells, but does indicate that the thymus function, or the T cells, take part in some way in tumor regression by lentinan.

Several reports have recently been published from various institutes that lentinan is a T-oriented adjuvant or is a T-helper cell stimulator or restorer. Kitagawa and his colleagues (Takatsu *et al.,* 1972a; Haba *et al.,* 1973) revealed that the tumor-bearing mice transplanted with transplantable tumors, such as sarcoma-180 and Ehrlich's carcinoma, or mice intraperitoneally injected with Ehrlich's carcinoma ascites, showed lowered function of antihapten-memory cells (B cells) and anticarrier-memory cells (T cells) when hapten-carrier was used as the antigen, and that the activity of T cells (helper cells) collected from the tumor-bearing mice at the early period of immunization was practically nil. They also showed that lentinan restores the lowered activity of T-helper cells to the normal level. Dresser and Phillips (1973) classified the adjuvants into T-oriented and B-oriented adjuvants in their experiment using thymectomized mice, and proposed that *Bordetella pertussis* is both a T- and B-oriented adjuvant, the lipopolysaccharide from *Shigella typhosa* is B-oriented, and lentinan is a T-oriented adjuvant. Dennert and Tucker (1973) reported that lentinan stimulated the antibody-dependent cell-mediated immunity and antibody synthesis, and they consider that this effect is due to the stimulation of T-helper cells, but not T-killer cells, by lentinan.

On the other hand, Howard *et al.* (1973) reported that *C. parvum* inhibited the T-cell-mediated immunity, but exerted a strong adjuvant effect on B cells, and that this phenomenon was mediated by activated macrophages. The importance of activated macrophages on the antitumor activity of *C. parvum* has been emphasized in this conference. We would like to point out the value of experimenting with the combination of *C. parvum* and lentinan as a T-helper cell adjuvant.

Effect of Lentinan on Various Conventional Immune Responses

In addition to the strong antitumor activity on transplanted tumors and stimulation of T-helper cells, lentinan has another feature of having almost no effect on several conventional immune responses, which differs from *C. parvum* (Maeda and Chihara, 1973a).

Mice were given various doses of lentinan, and blood was drawn from the retro-orbital venous plexus after various periods. Peripheral leukocyte count in these blood samples showed that the number of circulating leukocytes in the lentinan-administered group was no different from the control group. The action of lentinan differs in this point from that of *B. pertussis* (Morse, 1965), dextran sulfate, or heparin (Sasaki, 1967; Sasaki and Suchi, 1967), which stimulate the flow of a large number of lymphocytes from the spleen.

Lentinan does not stimulate the reticuloendothelial system, as does *C. parvum* (Halpern *et al.,* 1964), BCG (Biozzi *et al.,* 1954), and several other adjuvants. Carbon clearance activity, as measured by the conventional method of

Biozzi *et al.* (1953), is no different between the lentinan-administered group and the control group. On this point, the adjuvant action mechanism of lentinan differs from that of BCG (Biozzi *et al.*, 1954), endotoxin (Benaceraff and Sebestyen, 1957), and zymosan (Riggi and Di Luzio, 1961). Measurement of the number of plaque-forming cells in the mouse spleen against sheep erythrocytes, by the conventional method of Jerne (Jerne *et al.*, 1963) showed that there was no significant difference between the lentinan-administered and control groups.

Lentinan does not accelerate the reaction of skin-graft rejection [(C3H/H X DDD)F_1→C3H/He or AKR→C3H/He], which is considered to be a typical immune response mediated by thymus-derived cells. Lentinan also does not affect delayed cutaneous hypersensitivity (Uhr *et al.*, 1957; Salvin, 1958), such as the skin reaction.

Lentinan has entirely no toxicity, and its acute toxicity, LD_{50}, is over 1600 mg/kg. The antigenicity of lentinan itself—examined by various methods, including passive cutaneous anaphylaxis and precipitin test—has not been observed. Table III summarizes the immunological characteristics of lentinan.

Antitumor Action of 5-Hydroxytryptophan and Serotonin

Increased Histamine or Serotonin Sensitivity of Mice by Antitumor Polysaccharide and Anticomplementary Activity

As has been stated above, lentinan has several characteristics which are considerably different from numerous known immunopotentiators, and it seems necessary to study its action from an entirely different standpoint. In this sense, the study of Homma and Kuratsuka (1973) is of interest, because they found that lentinan markedly increases the sensitivity of mice to histamine, as does *B. pertussis* (Table IV). They found that while 6 mg/mouse or more of histamine hydrochloride does not kill normal mice, all 10 mice of ddY strain given 6 mg/mouse of histamine hydrochloride died of shock when it was given 4 days after administration of 50 μg/mouse of lentinan. This phenomenon is observed only when an antitumor polysaccharide is given and does not occur if the polysaccharide has no antitumor activity. We observed that administration of lentinan, as with administration of serotonin or histamine, in adrenalectomized mice (ICR) resulted in death of almost all the animals from shock within 8–10 days from the beginning of administration, but that only 1 out of 7 mice died when given pachyman, a β-(1→3)-glucan without antitumor activity.

On the other hand, antitumor polysaccharides, including lentinan, have strong anticomplementary activity and an activity of releasing anaphylatoxin (Okuda *et al.*, 1972) (Table V).

Lentinan inactivates 96% of the hemolytic activity of C3, the third component of the complement, without affecting C1 at all, *in vitro*. This phenomenon is also only observed when using polysaccharides with an antitumor activity, and not with those lacking such activity. Recently, Adlam *et al.* (1972) showed

Table III. The Effects of Lentinan on Various Immune Reponses

Immune responses	Method	Result	References	Remarks
Lymphocytes promoting activity	Numbers of peripheral lymphocytes	−	Maeda and Chihara (1973a)	Difference from dextran-sulfate, heparin
Antibody production	Number of plaque-forming spleen cells	−	Maeda and Chihara (1973a)	
Phagocytic activity	Carbon clearance	−	Maeda and Chihara (1973a)	Difference from BCG, *C. parvum,* and zymosan
Delayed-cutaneous hypersensitivity	Skin reaction	−	Maeda and Chihara (1973a)	
Homograft rejection	Skin-graft test	−	Maeda and Chihara (1973a)	
Peritoneal cell activation	Cytotoxicity of PE-cells	+	Maeda and Chihara (1973b)	
Early local cellular reaction	Historogical observation	++	Tokuzen (1971)	
Helper T-cell restoration	Hapten-carrier	++	Takatsu *et al.* (1972); Haba *et al.* (1973)	
Helper T-cell stimulation		++	Dennert and Tucker (1973)	
T-oriented adjuvant		++	Dresser and Phillips (1973)	
Anticomplementary activity and anaphylatoxin release		++	Okuda *et al.* (1972)	
Histamine-serotonin sensitizing effect	Histamine shock and skin test	+	Homma and Kuratsuka (1971)	

Table IV. Histamine-Sensitizing Activity of Lentinan[a]

Samples	Dose, μg/mouse X days	Histamine treatment Dose, mg/mouse	Days[b]	Death/total
Lentinan	50 X 5	6	4	10/10
Lentinan	50 X 5	–	–	0/10
Pachyman[c]	25 X 10	6	4	1/10
Control		6	–	0/10

[a]Mice: ddY strain, 5-week-old females. Data from Homma *et al.* (1972).
[b]Interval between the last administration of lentinan or pachyman and histamine challenge.
[c]A polysaccharide without antitumor activity from *Poria cocos* (SCHW ex FR.) WOLF.

that *C. parvum* also had the ability to increase the susceptibility of mice to histamine. Although there is a great difference between lentinan and *C. parvum* in their mode of action, they are identical in increasing the susceptibility of mice to histamine. It is entirely obscure whether such a phenomenon has any implication on tumor inhibition *in vivo,* but the fact should be kept in mind as one of the important elements in studying the mechanism of the antitumor activity of *C. parvum* and lentinan. Adrenalectomized mice have high susceptibility to serotonin and histamine, as well as higher immunological reactivity. Since epinephrine is concerned with histamine sensitivity (Munoz and Bergman,

Table V. Anticomplementary Activity of Antitumor Polysaccharides[a]

Samples	Loss in C3 hemolytic activity, %	Skin reaction	Antitumor activity Dose, mg/kg X day	Inhibition ratio, %
Lentinan	96	+++	1 X 10	100
Pachymaran	68	+++	5 X 10	86
Screloglucan	73	++	3 X 10	89
Dextran T-2000	6	±	Not effective	
GVB[b]	0			

[a]Data from Okuda *et al.* (1972).
[b]Gelatin-Veronal buffer (0.1%).

1968), we should consider the important role of the adrenal medulla, as well as the adrenal cortex, in the host's defense against cancer, because it is difficult to produce experimental cancer in guinea pigs having both high sensitivity to histamine and a high immunological susceptibility.

Antitumor Activity of 5-Hydroxytryptophan and Serotonin

In connection with the increase of susceptibility of mice to histamine and serotonin by lentinan, we found that some antihistamine agents slightly inhibited the antitumor activity of lentinan (Maeda *et al.*, 1973). We reexamined the antitumor activity of numerous biogenic amines and found that 5-hydroxytryptophan and serotonin had strong antitumor activity against sarcoma-180 solid tumor (Table VI).

The antitumor activity of serotonin has been reported by Pukhalskaya (1964) as one of the active ingredients in a Russian plant. The presence of an antitumor activity in serotonin is very interesting because serotonin itself does not show any effect on the ascitic tumor of sarcoma-180, and the viability of sarcoma-180 cells after 24 h of culture in a medium containing serotonin is no different from that of the control. Thus, this antitumor activity is host-mediated and not due to direct cytotoxic action on cancer cells. Serotonin itself is not a mediator of any of the cell-mediated immune responses.

It is still obscure what mechanism lies in the antitumor activity of serotonin, but since serotonin has a protective effect against radiation and also against acute stress—which acts as immunosuppressive (Gisler *et al.*, 1971; Gisler and Schenkel-Hulliger, 1971), it may be possible to consider that various hormones, especially of the adrenal–pituitary system and nervous secretion system, are taking part in the antitumor activity of serotonin. Reserpine, a pituitary-oriented drug, has a tumor-inhibitory effect (Dukor *et al.*, 1966). It seems to be of value to carry out experiments on the combination of *C. parvum* with serotonin or 5-hydroxytryptophan.

A Possibility of Concerted Attack on Cancer by the Combined Use of Various Immunopotentiators and Various Immunopotentiation Methods

Effect of Hormones on Various Immune Responses

From our studies on the mode of action of antitumor polysaccharides, we came to entertain the idea that various hormones derived from the pituitary and adrenal functions are in close cooperation with the regression mechanism of allogenic tumors, besides the thymus-derived cellular immunity. The effect of hormones on immune responses has been studied by the coworkers of Medawar, Lance, Castro (Medawar and Russell, 1958; Gunn *et al.*, 1970; Lance and Cooper, 1970; Castro, 1974a,b), and Pierpaoli and Sorkin (Pierpaoli *et al.*, 1970;

Table VI. Antitumor Effect of Various Biogenic Amines and Related Compounds, Especially Serotonin and 5-Hydroxytryptophan[a]

Samples	Dose, mg/kg $\times$ days	Tumor inhibition ratio, %
5-Hydroxytryptophan	50 $\times$ 27	44.6
	100 $\times$ 27	50.1
	150 $\times$ 27	61.2
Serotonin	10 $\times$ 10	15.5
	20 $\times$ 10	40.4
	25 $\times$ 29	63.7
	50 $\times$ 29	76.6
Histamine	25 $\times$ 10	18.0
	100 $\times$ 10	42.6
Compound 48/80	1 $\times$ 12	−18.7
Dopamine	50 $\times$ 10	24.1
DOPA	50 $\times$ 10	−19.7
5-Hydroxyindoleacetic acid	50 $\times$ 10	21.5
Spermine	25 $\times$ 10	3.4
Spermidine	25 $\times$ 10	3.4

[a]Sarcoma-180 (6 $\times$ 10^6 cells) were transplanted subcutaneously into 5-week-old female ICR mice, and the sample was injected intraperitoneally daily after transplantation. The inhibition ratios of tumors were determined at the end of the fifth week after transplantation.

Pierpaoli and Sorkin, 1972). In his review article, Dougherty (1952) stated that growth hormone and thyroid hormone increased the weight of the thymus and lymphoid tissue and increased the immunological capability of animals, but various sex hormones and adrenocortical hormones worked immunosuppressively. He also emphasized the correlation between the hormone and immunity. Antihormonal therapy for cancer is, at present, limited chiefly to tumors of the hormone-dependent organs, such as breast carcinoma and prostatic carcinoma. However, it may be necessary to extend the use of this therapy to tumors other than those of hormone-dependent organs. In this sense, the recent reports of Castro (1974a,b) that orchidectomy increases cellular immune reactions, in general, is of interest. We examined the effect of various hormones on antitumor activity, using lentinan as an index.

Inhibition of Antitumor Activity of Polysaccharides by Hydrocortisone

The fact that hydrocortisone or cortisol is an immunosuppressor (Lance and Cooper, 1970) and that the antitumor activity of zymosan is inhibited by cortisone has already been reported by Bradner *et al.* (Bradner and Clarke, 1959; Bradner *et al.*, 1958). The antitumor activity of lentinan is also slightly suppressed by hydrocortisone (Table VII).

Bradner *et al.* reported that the antitumor activity of zymosan was almost completely suppressed by a single administration of 4 mg/mouse of hydrocortisone 7 days after transplantation of sarcoma-180, but no such effect could be seen with lentinan under the same conditions as theirs. Daily administration of 50 mg/kg of hydrocortisone for 10 consecutive days resulted in about a 20–30% lowering of the antitumor effect of lentinan.

Blocking of the Antitumor Activity of Lentinan by Thyroxine

Based on the report that a growth hormone or thyroid hormone increases the immunological capability of a human body (Marx *et al.*, 1942; Reinhaldt and Wainman, 1942) and expecting the loss of the antitumor activity of lentinan by antithyroid agents, such as 6-propyl-2-thiouracil (as in neonatally thymectomized mice), we carried out some experiments. Contrary to our expectations, however, antithyroid agents had no effect at all on the antitumor activity of

Table VII. The Effect of Hydrocortisone Acetate on the Antitumor Activity of Lentinan[a]

Samples	Dose, mg/kg × days	Average tumor weight, g	Tumor inhibition ratio, %	Complete regression
Lentinan	1 × 10	0.1	99.0	7/10
Hydrocortisone acetate Lentinan	50 × 10 1 × 10	1.7	54.9	2/9
Control		4.8		0/10
Lentinan	1 × 10	0.5	95.5	5/10
Hydrocortisone acetate Lentinan	50 × 10 1 × 10	2.8	73.0	1/10
Hydrocortisone acetate	50 × 10	6.1	42.2	0/10
Control		10.5		0/10

[a]Mice: female ICR, 5 weeks old; Tumor: Sarcoma 180, subcutaneously injected, 6 × 10^6 cells; Lentinan or hydrocortisone acetate, intraperitoneally injected.

Table VIII. Effect of L-Thyroxine or Antithyroides on the Antitumor Activity of Lentinan[a]

Samples	Dose, mg/kg $\times$ days	Number of mice	Body-weight change, g	Average tumor weight, g	Tumor-inhibition ratio, %
Lentinan	1 $\times$ 10	9	+5.85	0.23	96.9
Lentinan Thyroxine[b]	1 $\times$ 10 10 $\times$ 10	8	+7.08	3.22	56.0
Thyroxine	10 $\times$ 10	9	+9.34	10.17	−39.1
Control		10	+8.29	7.31	
Lentinan Thyroxine	1 $\times$ 10 10 $\times$ 10	8	+4.87	4.88	42.2
Control		9	+4.47	7.75	
Lentinan	1 $\times$ 10	10	+6.85	0.25	97.3
Lentinan Propylthiouracil[c]	1 $\times$ 10 20 $\times$ 10	10	+3.76	0.14	98.4
Control		10	+6.71	8.79	

[a]Mice: ICR; Tumor: Sarcoma-180, subcutaneously injected; Lentinan or thyroxine: intraperitoneally injected. Determination of tumor-inhibition ratio was done at the end of fifth week after transplantation.
[b]L-Thyroxine sodium-salt pentahydrate.
[c]6-Propyl-2-thiouracil.

lentinan, but, inversely, administration of thyroxine was found to markedly block this antitumor activity (Table VIII). The strong antitumor activity of lentinan (inhibition ratio, 86.9–96.9%) was markedly reduced to 42.2–56% by the administration of thyroxine, though thyroxine itself tended to enhance the growth of tumor.

The action of hormones is generally reversed in physiological dose and pharmacological dose. The dose of the hormone we used for mice was extremely large, and the result was entirely contrary to our expectations. This fact indicates that there is a close correlation between immune responses and the action of the thyroid and adrenal medulla, and fully suggests the possibility that the attempted increase in immunological capability of the hormone is one way

Table IX. Activation of Various Biological Systems by Various Immunopotentiators

| Materials | T cells | | B cells | Macro-phages | Immune capability | Pituitary-adrenal | Antitumor effect |
	Killer	Helper					
Lentinan	−	+++	−	−	−	++	+++
C. parvum	−	−	+	+++		++	+++
LPS	−	−	+++	+			+
Endotoxine	−	−	+	++			++
Poly(I) poly(C)	−	−	+	++			+
Poly(A) poly(U)	+	−					
B. pertussis	+		++				++
Serotonin						++	++
Reserpine			−	−		++	++
Thyroxine					++		−
Growth hormone					++		−
Cortisol	−	−	−	−	−		−

of effecting immunopotentiation against cancer. It is generally known that there is little cancer in hyperthyroid patients and that cancers are prevalent in myxo-edema patients.

Conclusion

Many and varied characteristics of *C. parvum* were reported at this conference. One of the most important was the role of activated macrophages in their antitumor mechanism. The mechanisms of various immunopotentiators and immunopotentiation methods are many and varied. Centered around our own studies, Table IX summarizes these various mechanisms.

We believe that the range of antitumor activity of *C. parvum* can be extended by a suitable combination, or combinations, of these varied immunopotentiation methods, because we are certain that the physiological defense against cancer consists of pharmacological functions that bind various hormones with hypothalamus–adrenal medulla, as well as various immune mechanisms.

Acknowledgments

We thank Mrs. Yoko Yamada and Mrs. Asayo Takasuka for their excellent assistance and Dr. J. Hamuro, Prof. Tomoko Okuda, Dr. Reiko Homma, and Dr. H. Mitsui for their cooperation in experimental work and valuable discussion. We are deeply indebted to Drs. Waro Nakahara and Fumiko Fukuoka for their heartfelt encouragement.

References

Adlam, C., Broughton, E. S., and Scott, M. T. (1972). Enhanced resistance of mice to infection with bacteria following pretreatment with *Corynebacterium parvum*. *Nature (Lond.) New Biol.* 235:219.

Benacerraf, B. and Sebestyen, M. M. (1957). Effect of bacterial endotoxins on the reticulo-endothelial system. *Fed. Proc.* 16:860.

Biozzi, G., Benacerraf, B., and Halpern, B. N. (1953). Quantitative study of the granulopectic activity of the reticuloendothelial system. II. A study of the kinetics of the granulopectic activity of the RES in relation to the dose of carbon injected. Relationship between the weight of the organs and their activity. *Br. J. Exp. Pathol.* 34:441.

Biozzi, G., Benacerraf, B., Grumbach, F., Halpern, B. N., Levaditi, J., and Rist, N. (1954). Etude de l'activité granulopexique du systeme réticuloendothelial au cours de l'infection tuberculeuse experimentale de la souris. *Ann. Inst. Pasteur, Paris* 87:291.

Biozzi, G., Stiffel, C., Halpern, B. N., and Mouton, D. (1959). Effet de l'inoculation du *Bacille de Calmette-Guérin* sur le devéloppement de la tumeur ascitique d'Ehrlich chez la souris. *C. R. Soc. Biol.* 153:987.

Bradner, W. T. and Clarke, D. A. (1959). Stimulation of host defense against experimental cancer. II. Temporal and reversal studies of the zymosan effect. *Cancer Res.* 19:673.

Bradner, W. T., Clarke, D. A., and Stock, C. C. (1958). Stimulation of host defense against experimental cancer. I. Zymosan and sarcoma 180 in mice. *Cancer Res.* 18:347.

Castro, J. E. (1974a). Orchidectomy and immune response. I. Effect of orchidectomy on lymphoid tissues of mice. *Proc. R. Soc. (Lond.) B.* 185:425.

Castro, J. E. (1974b). Orchidectomy and immune response. II. Response of orchidectomized mice to antigens. *Proc. R. Soc. (Lond.) B.* 185:437.

Chihara, G., Hamuro, J., Maeda, Y. Y., and Arai, Y. (1970a). Antitumor polysaccharides lentinan and pachymaran. *Saishin Igaku* 25:1043.

Chihara, G., Hamuro, J., Maeda, Y. Y., Arai, Y., and Fukuoka, F. (1970b). Fractionation and purification of the polysaccharides with marked antitumor activity, especially lentinan, from *Lentinus edodes* (BERK.) SING. (an edible mushroom). *Cancer Res.* 30:2776.

Dennert, G. and Tucker, D. (1973). Antitumor polysaccharide lentinan, a T cell adjuvant. *J. Natl. Cancer Inst.* 51:1727.

Dougherty, T. F. (1952). Effect of hormones on lymphatic tissue. *Physiol. Rev.* 32:379.

Dresser, D. W. and Phillips, J. M. (1973). The cellular targets for the action of adjuvants: T adjuvants and B adjuvants. In: *Immunopotentiation* (Ciba Foundation Symposium, New Series 18), p. 3, (G. E. W. Wolstenholme and J. Knight, eds.), Associated Scientific Publishers, Amsterdam.

Dukor, P., Salvin, S. B., Dietrich, F. M., Gelzer, R., Hess, R., and Loustalot, P. (1966). Effect of reserpine on immune reactions and tumor growth. *Eur. J. Cancer* 2:253.

Gisler, R. H., Bussard, A. E., Mazié, J. C., and Hess, R. (1971). Hormonal regulation of the immune response. I. Induction of an immune response *in vitro* with lymphoid cells from mice exposed to acute systemic stress. *Cell. Immunol.* 2:634.

Gisler, R. H. and Schenkel-Hulliger, L. (1971). Hormonal regulation of the immune response. II. Influence of pituitary and adrenal activity on immune responsiveness *in vitro. Cell. Immunol.* 2:646.

Gunn, A., Lance, E. M., Medawar, P. B., and Nehlsen, S. L. (1970). Synergism between cortisol and antilymphocyte serum. Part I. Observation in murine allograft systems. In: *Hormones and the Immune Response* (Ciba Foundation Study Group No. 36), p. 66, (G. E. W. Wolstenholme and H. Knight, eds.), Churchill, London.

Haba, S., Takatsu, K., Masaki, H., and Kitagawa, M. (1973). Immunosuppression by cancerous ascites and the restoration with antitumor agent. *Proc. Jap. Cancer Assoc.* 32:249.

Halpern, B. N., Biozzi, G., Stiffel, C., and Mouton, D. (1959). Effet de la stimulation du système réticuloendothélial par l'inoculation du *Bacille de Calmette-Guérin* sur le développement de l'épithelioma atypique T-8 de Guérin chez le rat. *C. R. Soc. Biol.* 153:919.

Halpern, B. N., Prévot, A. R., Biozzi, G., Stiffel, C., Mouton, D., Morard, J. C., Bouthiller, Y., and Decreusefond, C. (1964). Stimulation de l'activité phagocytaire du système réticuloendothélial provoquée par *Corynebacterium parvum. J. Reticuloendothel. Soc.* 1:77.

Halpern, B. N., Biozzi, G., Stiffel, C., and Mouton, D. (1966). Inhibition of tumor growth by administration of killed *Corynebacterium parvum. Nature (Lond.)* 212:853.

Homma, R. and Kuratsuka, K. (1973). The histamine-sensitizing activity of lentinan, an antitumor polysaccharide. *Experientia* 29:290.

Howard, J. G., Scott, M. T., and Christie, G. H. (1973). Cellular mechanisms underlying the adjuvant activity of *Corynebacterium parvum:* interactions of activated macrophages with T and B lymphocytes. In: *Immunopotentiation* (Ciba Foundation Symposium, New Series 18), p. 101, (G. E. W. Wolstenholme and J. Knight, eds.), Associated Scientific Publishers, Amsterdam.

Ikekawa, T., Nakanishi, M., Uehara, N., Chihara, G., and Fukuoka, F. (1968). Antitumor action of some basidiomycetes, especially *Phellinus linteus. Gann* 59:155.

Ikekawa, T., Uehara, N., Maeda, Y. Y., Nakanishi, M., and Fukuoka, F. (1969). Antitumor activity of aqueous extracts of edible mushrooms. *Cancer Res.* 29:734.

Jerne, N. K., Nordin, A. A., and Henry, C. (1963). The agar-plaque technique for recognizing antibody-producing cells. In: *Cell Bound Antibody,* p. 109 (B. Amos and H. Koprowski, eds.), Wistar Institute Press, Philadelphia.

Lance, E. M. and Cooper, S. (1970). Synergism between cortisol and antilymphocyte serum. Part II. Effect of cortisol and antilymphocyte serum on lymphoid populations. In: *Hormones and the Immune Response,* (Ciba Foundation Study Group No. 36), p. 73, (G. E. W. Wolstenholme and J. Knight, eds.), Churchill, London.

Maeda, Y. Y. and Chihara, G. (1971). Lentinan, a new immuno-accelerator of cell-mediated responses. *Nature (Lond.)* 229:634.

Maeda, Y. Y. and Chihara, G. (1973a). The effects of neonatal thymectomy on the antitumor activity of lentinan, carboxymethylpachymaran, and zymosan, and their effects on various immune responses. *Int. J. Cancer* 11:153.

Maeda, Y. Y. and Chihara, G. (1973b). Periodical consideration on the establishment of antitumor action in host and activation of peritoneal exudate cells by lentinan. *Gann* 64:351.

Maeda, Y. Y., Hamuro, J., and Chihara, G. (1971). The mechanisms of action of antitumor polysaccharides. I. The effect on antilymphocyte serum on the antitumor activity of lentinan. *Int. J. Cancer* 8:41.

Maeda, Y. Y., Hamuro, J., Yamada, Y. O., Ishimura, K., and Chihara, G. (1973). The nature of immunopotentiation by the antitumor polysaccharide, lentinan, and the significance of biogenic amines in its action. In: *Immunopotentiation* (Ciba Foundation Symposium, New Series 18), p. 259, (G. E. W. Wolstenholme and J. Knight, eds.), Associated Scientific Publishers, Amsterdam.

Marx, W., Simpson, M. E., Reinhaldt, W. O., and Evans, H. M. (1942). Response to growth hormone of hypophysectomized rats when restricted to food intake of controls. *Am. J. Physiol.* 135:614.

Medawar, P. B. and Russell, P. S. (1958). Adrenal homografts in mice, with special reference to immunological adrenalectomy. *Immunology* 1:1.

Morse, S. I. (1965). Studies on the lymphocytosis induced in mice by *Bordetella pertussis. J. Exp. Med.* **121:**49.

Munoz, J. and Bergman, R. K. (1968). Histamine-sensitizing factors from microbial agents, with special reference to *Bordetella pertussis. Bacteriol. Rev.* **32:**103.

Okuda, T., Yoshioka, Y., Ikekawa, T., Chihara, G., and Nishioka, K. (1972). Anticomplementary activity of antitumor polysaccharides. *Nature (Lond.) New Biol.* **238:**59.

Old, L. J., Clarke, D. A., and Benacerraf, B. (1959). Effect of *Bacillus Calmette-Guérin* infection on transplanted tumors. *Nature (Lond.)* **184:**291.

Pierpaoli, W., Fabris, N., and Sorkin, E. (1970). Developmental hormones and immunological maturation. In: *Hormones and the Immune Response* (Ciba Foundation Study Group No. 36), p. 126 (G. E. W. Wolstenholme and J. Knight, eds.), Churchill, London.

Pierpaoli, W. and Sorkin, E. (1972). Hormones, thymus and lymphocyte functions. *Experientia* **28:**1385.

Pukhalskaya, E. Ch. (1964). Mechanism of antimitotic and antitumor action of 5-hydroxytryptamine (serotonin). *Acta Unio. Int. Contra Cancrum* **20:**131.

Reinhaldt, W. O. and Wainman, P. (1942). Effect of thyroidectomy, castration, and replacement therapy on thymus, lymph nodes, and spleen in male rats. *Proc. Soc. Exp. Biol. Med.* **49:**257.

Riggi, S. J. and Di Luzio, N. R. (1961). Identification of a reticuloendothelial-stimulating agent in zymosan. *Am. J. Physiol.* **200:**297.

Salvin, S. B. (1958). Occurrence of delayed hypersensitivity during the development of arthus-type hypersensitivity. *J. Exp. Med.* **107:**109.

Sasaki, S. (1967). Production of lymphocytosis by polysaccharide polysulfates (heparinoids). *Nature (Lond.)* **214:**1041.

Sasaki, S. and Suchi, T. (1967). Mobilization of lymphocytes from lymph nodes and spleen by polysaccharide polysulfates. *Nature (Lond.)* **216:**1013.

Takatsu, K., Hamaoka, T., and Kitagawa, M. (1972a). Suppressed activity of thymus-derived cell in tumor-bearing host. *Proc. Jap. Cancer Assoc.* **31:**209.

Takatsu, K., Hamaoka, T., Yamashita, U., and Kitagawa, M. (1972b). Suppressed activity of thymus-derived cell in tumor-bearing host. *Gann* **63:**273.

Tokuzen, R. (1971). Comparison of local cellular reaction to tumor graft in mice treated with some plant polysaccharides. *Cancer Res.* **31:**1590.

Tokuzen, R. and Nakahara, W. (1971). Die Wirkung einiger pflanzlicher Polysaccharide auf das spontane Mamma-Adenocarcinom der Maus. *Arzneim.-Forsch.* **21:**269.

Tokuzen, R. and Nakahara, W. (1973). Suppression of autochthonous grafts of spontaneous mammary tumor by induced allogenic graft rejection mechanism. *Cancer Res.* **33:**645.

Tsukagoshi, S., Sakurai, Y., Otsuka, S., Ueno, S., Yoshikuni, C., and Fujii, T. (1973). Antitumor activity of protein-bound polysaccharide, PS-K, isolated from basidiomycetes. *Abst. 8th International Congress of Chemotherapy,* **B:**156.

Uhr, J. W., Salvin, S. B., and Pappenheimer, A. M., Jr. (1957). Delayed hypersensitivity. II. Induction of hypersensitivity in guinea pigs by means of antigen—antibody complexes. *J. Exp. Med.* **105:**11.

28

Comparative Effects of Various Strains of *Corynebacterium parvum* and Other Prophylactic Agents on Tumor Development in Animals

HEINRICH WRBA

After the publication by Halpern *et al.* (1966) of an article on the tumor-inhibiting effect of *Corynebacterium parvum* (Cp), we undertook a large series of similar experiments. At that time, a strain of Cp from the American Type Culture Collection (ATCC) was at our disposal.* An exact repetition of the experiments as published produced negative results in our laboratory. It was therefore decided to investigate growth inhibition on a spectrum of tumors.

The first series of experiments was conducted with 10^9 Cp bacteria after heat denaturation and treatment with 1% formalin. The administration of Cp was started before transplantation, until the day specified on the chart, in a regular biweekly rhythm of two injections—either intraperitoneally or sub-

HEINRICH WRBA, Institute for Cancer Research of the University of Vienna, Austria.

*We are grateful to Dr. Eibl of the Österreichische Immuno A.G. for supplying us with this strain, and for other assistance.

Table I. Results of Application of 10⁹ Heat Denatured *Corynebacterium parvum* in Relation to the Transplantation of Various Tumors

Tumor	Application	Schedule: twice a week	Animals treated		Control	Bouillon only	Effect
Ehrlich's ascites	s.c.	−24 0	10 ♀ 1 month	Swiss	10	10	0
Krebs ascites	s.c.	−24 0	10 ♀ 2 month	Swiss	10	10	0
Lewis lung tumor	i.p.	−23 ..... +16	10 ♀ 7 months	BDF₁	10	10	0
Harding-Passey melanoma	i.p.	−25 ..... +13	15 ♀ 10 months	Swiss	15	15	Mean survival time increased from 80 to 90 days
Friend's leukemia	s.c.	−24 0	10 ♀ 2 months	Swiss	10	10	0
Nemeth-Kellner lymphoma	i.p.	−21 ..... +10	15 ♀ 7 months	Swiss	15	15	0
Sarcoma 180	i.p.	−25 ..... +10	35 ♀ 6 months	Swiss	35	15	Mean survival time increased from 50 to 60 days
Plasmocytoma KG13	i.p.	−28 ..... +10	10 ♂ 3 months	hamsters GP	10	10	0
Walker carcinoma	i.p.	−23 ..... +19	10 ♀ 3 months	Swiss	10	10	0
Yoshida sarcoma	i.p.	−23 ..... +19	10 ♂ 3 months	rats Wistar	10	10	Mean survival time increased from 70 to 80 days

cutaneously. Sterile, culture bouillon was used for the control animal. Table I lists the methods of application, types, number, and ages of animals used, as well as the varieties of transplantation tumor.

Where specific strains were used, experimental animals were drawn from inbred strains of the Institute. The Swiss albino mice were from an outbred strain kept at the Institute. The animals received water and pellets *ad libitum.* Throughout this experimental series, which started in 1968, no significant tumor suppression could be demonstrated. A minimal increase in the mean survival rate was apparent in the Harding-Passey melanoma, in the apparently very sensitive sarcoma-180, and in the Yoshida sarcoma of the rat. It seems to us of note that this method evoked no response in 7 different varieties of transplantation tumor.

In the second experimental series (Table II), four mouse tumors and one rat carcinoma were investigated in order to determine the optimal time for application of the inhibitor. From two days before till two days after tumor inoculation, a single 2-ml dose of the same preparation was administered per animal. On this occasion, the Cp was adjusted against 0.5 mg nitrogen/ml. Intravenous injection of Cp in single doses respectively for AKR leukemia, Ehrlich's ascitic tumor, and the Krebs ascites showed no response. No reaction was apparent in the Walker carcinoma of the rat.

In contrast, we found an improvement in survival time at each treatment day with Cp against sarcoma-180, application on day 0—that is the day of transplantation—producing a healing rate of 50% of animals. 100 days after the injection, half the animals who had received Cp were tumor-free.

It seems worthy of note that the strain used by us was quite obviously sensitive to the effect of Cp. In agreement with the literature, the best effect was against sarcoma-180, as against a whole series of other transplantation tumors which showed no suppression.

Table II. Experiments on Timing of Intravenous Application of Heat-Denatured *Corynebacterium parvum* (0.5 mg/ml) in Reference to Transplantation[a]

Tumor	Animals treated		Effect
AKR leukemia	♂ 2 months	AGF_1 mice	No effect
Ehrlich's ascites	♀ 2 months	Swiss	No effect
Krebs ascites	♀ 2 months	Swiss	No effect
Sarcoma-180	♀ 2 months	Swiss	Good results: 50% cured on day 0
Walker carcinoma	♀ 4 months	Wistar rats	No effect

[a]On day −2, −1, 0, +1, +2, a single 0.2-ml dose was injected into 10 animals per each dose. Control: 20 animals.

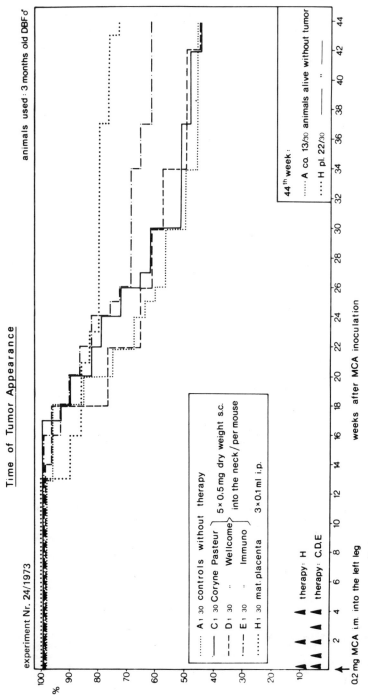

Fig. 1. Long-term investigation to determine the best time for the application of a prophylactic agent for tumors. The comparative action of a placenta preparation having a suppressive effect on methylcholanthrene-tumor production.

The important question here would seem to be, why, under conditions of immune stimulation, tumor inhibition was not achieved in a large number of cases. Factors to explain this question should be sought in an examination of the relationship between effect and factors such as species of bacterium, animal strain, dose, age, and, possibly, also nutritional condition of the animal.

Since 1973 we have had at our disposal, in addition to the Cp from the American Tissue Type Collection, Cp from the Institut Pasteur and a strain from Burroughs Wellcome. At this point, an experimental series was started which could throw light on the mechanisms of tumor suppression in respect of the effect of prophylactic measures. The application of a single dose of 0.2–0.5 mg methylcholanthrene i.m. per mouse produced tumors 9–10 weeks later with 100% regularity. If no suppressive mechanism was introduced, death from tumor generally occurred in all animals within 50 weeks.

A large number of such investigations with prophylactic preparations are now being conducted. The major problem, however, lies in the wide range of variability possible between application of the prophylactic and the carcinogen. The crucial question is, naturally, the optimal time of application, i.e., the moment of critical confrontation between the action of the carcinogen and the prophylactic agent. One such long-term investigation is illustrated in Fig. 1. It shows the comparative action of a placenta preparation developed by us (proven in a large series of investigations to have a significant suppressive effect on methylcholanthrene-tumor production) against three lines of Cp. From this, it is apparent that the effect of our original line of Cp from the American Tissue Type Collection is just on the border of significance. It will therefore also be necessary to undertake a systematic testing of Cp in this investigation.

On the whole, it would appear that nonspecific stimulation through Cp is most effective on slow-growing tumors, the optimal effect being reached by simultaneous application of tumor and Cp. The use of Cp as a protective agent against carcinogens seems to be promising, and will be the subject of further investigations. Similarly, it seems worthwhile to investigate the effect of combinations of Cp and other effective substances.

Undoubtedly, in addition to the question of timing, we still have the important problems of correlating the routes of administration and the effect of sex, age, and type of animal, and other factors, on unspecific immune stimulation. In particular, experiments demonstrating negative action could have an important significance in such experiments.

Reference

Halpern, B. N., Biozzi, G., Stiffel, C., and Mouton, D. (1966). Inhibition of tumor growth by administration of killed *Corynebacterium parvum*. *Nature (Lond.)* **212**:853–854.

DISCUSSION

CHOUROULINKOV: I have had the opportunity of analyzing the histology of Professor Dimitrov's experiments with *Corynebacterium parvum, Corynebacterium granulosum,* and BCG. The local tissue reaction is the same as that described by M. G. Hanna *et al.* [(1972). *J. Natl. Cancer Inst.* 48:1441–1445] with BCG in guinea pigs with hepatocarcinoma. In the first stage, this reaction is an acute inflammatory one with polynuclear, mononuclear, and some poorly-defined cells which could be histiocytes or macrophages (Fig. 1). Ten to 15 days later, there remains almost only a histiocytic reaction, which may present a tumorlike aspect (Fig. 2). Finally, after tumor regression, all that remains is some macrophages with phagocytosed melanin, as Professor Dimitrov showed earlier.

The evolution of the reaction after *C. parvum* inoculation is interesting, since the polynuclear and mononuclear (in lower level) cells appear first, in the few hours following inoculation. The macrophages appear, as shown previously, four or five days later.

The later morphology of the reaction by itself is not so important. It is more important to know the correlation between this morphology and the mechanism of the corynebacteria activity.

If the modality of inoculation is considered, we know now that when *C. parvum* is inoculated prior to the tumor grafting—or at the same time, but in another site, there is a strong reaction and stimulation of the reticuloendothelial system. This is a nonspecific reaction, having a cytostatic effect, as Professor Halpern reported. The consequences are a higher immunological resistance of the animals, an inhibition of tumor growth, and protection against lung metastasis.

When *C. parvum* is inoculated with the tumor cells or into the tumors (especially in the hamster's melanoma), 7, 9, or 14 days after grafting, the reaction is in some ways different. At first, there is a cell stimulation. The tumor cells alone, allogenic or isogenic—all antigenic—induce cell sensitization and antibodies (complete or incomplete) in the sera, the two being detectable

319

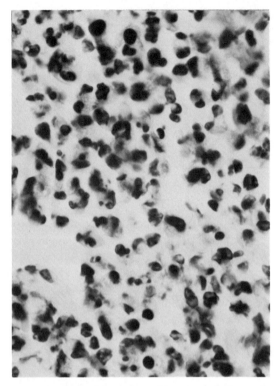

Fig. 1. Polymorphic cells infiltration, 7 days after intratumor *Corynebacterium parvum* inoculation. (Dimitrov's experiments) (1200 ×).

four or five days after the tumor inoculation. In the case of the allograft, a rejection generally follows. In the case of the isograft, the tumor continued to grow. By its nonspecific activity, the *C. parvum* inoculated with the tumor cells increased quantitatively the cell population which was susceptible to sensitization in contact with tumor cells. When *C. parvum* was inoculated in the tumor, there was not only an increase but also a stimulation of the sensitized cells. The second role of *C. parvum* here is probably the activation of the tumor antigen, water soluble or not, as Dimitrov mentioned. If the *C. parvum* is not injected in contact with the melanoma cells, inhibition rather than total regression results. Only a stimulation of the reticuloendothelial system occurs.

If we come back to the morphology and try to define when the macrophages interfere, it seems to me that they enter into play after the polynuclear and mononuclear cells—at the moment of the appearance of the sensitized cells and antibodies. This hypothesis is confirmed by the fact that the macrophages are observed 5–6 days after *C. parvum* inoculation, similarly to the results observed in an experiment carried out with RC_{19} ascitic tumor in mice treated with interferon. [I. Gresser *et al.* (1970). *Ann. N.Y. Acad. Sci.* **173**:694–707]. Twenty-four hours after tumor inoculation, the peritoneal cavity is rich in polynuclear and mononuclear cells and macrophages. If there is no treatment, all these cells disappear and the Ehrlich's tumor cells develop. When interferon is inoculated, the persistence of the poly- and mononuclear cells and a specific phagocytosis of the tumor cells result. We emphasize that this phagocytosis is never observed before the sixth day of the tumor inoculation. In other words, it appears to be linked to the immunologic response. In this case too, the polynuclear and mononuclear (lymphocytes) cells react first and the macrophages later.

In conclusion, *C. parvum* inoculated in contact with the tumor cells induces a local concentration and stimulation of immunologically active cells and

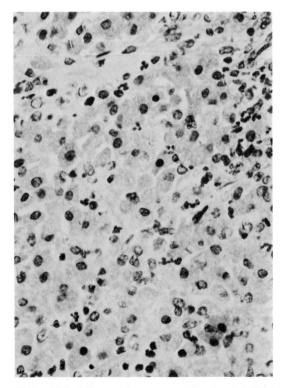

Fig. 2. Histiocytes with some polynuclear cells, 14 days after *Corynebacterium parvum* inoculation. Case of a complete tumor regression. (Dimitrov's experiments) (480 ×).

activates the antigenicity of the tumor cells. The intervention of macrophages, probably stimulated by *C. parvum*, follows the acute inflammatory reaction and occurs after the first immunologic reaction.

HALPERN: In Dr. Wrba's experiment, 3-methylcholanthrene was inoculated subcutaneously into a group of mice and the development of the tumor was observed. The growth of this tumor is rather slow, 60 weeks being the end point of the experiment.

Everybody has stressed the critical importance of the time factor, and important differences were claimed whether the *C. parvum* is injected two days before or two days after the tumor inoculation. It has emerged from many presentations—including those of Dr. Bomford and Dr. Wrba—that with respect to metastases, there is also a critical moment in timing. Dr. Bomford clearly showed that if *C. parvum* was administered several days after tumor inoculation, the number of nodules in the lung reached almost the same level as nontreated animals. Thus, in treatment with *C. parvum*, the time factor seems to be important, at least in the experimental models.

How would it be possible to control the time factor for administration of *C. parvum* in a tumor which can be judged only by the mortality rate or by palpation, which means when the tumor is already grossly established? Could Dr. Wrba's negative results be relevant to this specific problem, in the sense that it is not possible to define with precision what time would be the most appropriate for the administration of *C. parvum?*

WRBA: We used this methylcholanthrene system, but there are many other ways in which to induce a cancer. We used this particular system because it works well and reliably, giving us 100% tumors between 9 and 15 weeks after tumor grafting. This experiment can be controlled carefully.

On the other hand, I feel that this conception of immunostimulation increasing stimulation and decreasing tumor growth, or decreasing the risk of metastasis, seems too simple. There are other factors involved. In this system, we are looking for protective means against carcinogenesis, and there are different ones. Nobody knows the critical moment or the critical effect on the immunosurveillance in this system of carcinogenesis. It is known that protection can be achieved in different systems by the application of *C. parvum.* However, we know nothing about the timing of the schedule.

I would not agree that the results from the last experiment I described in my presentation were negative. We cannot be sure; after another couple of months perhaps I will be able to say that the results are positive.

HALPERN: Was the *C. parvum* injected every week into animals, or only once?

WRBA: It was injected simultaneously, and was done several times over about six weeks.

HALPERN; It would be interesting if these experiments could be followed, because it is a good model due to the fact that the tumor is autologous and slightly antigenic.

It would be interesting, especially for extrapolation to humans, if the *C. parvum* could be given for a long period of time. A dosage such as giving the injections once a week or every 10 days during the observation time is likely to be adequate for such an experiment. It could happen that one of the injections might coincide with the critical moment, and improve the results. This situation might yield information of crucial importance.

WRBA: I agree, but I should not like to make any extrapolation to humans now. The next experiment should be done with monkeys.

WHISNANT: Repeating an earlier comment to Dr. Wrba, I found his experiments very encouraging, for there is some anxiety that using a T-cell suppressor may decrease the immunosurveillance—whatever that may be—and give rise to increased carcinogenity and an increased incidence of spontaneously-arising tumors.

In answer to my earlier inquiry, Dr. Wrba has assured me that in all cases the mice had no more tumors than the untreated controls. *C. parvum* never led to an increased incidence of methylcholanthrene tumors. That is an important "reversal" of his experiments. Apparently, *C. parvum* does not lead to increased incidence of methylcholanthrene-induced tumors. I think that is a positive result.

WRBA: There is no danger in the use of *C. parvum* in this sense.

HALPERN: I think Dr. Bomford's study on the effect of *C. parvum* on lung metastases is of great relevance, and the problem of the radiosensitivity of the effects of *C. parvum* should be stressed in this connection. This may have also some relevance to human application. I was very interested in his results, and am looking forward to reading his paper when it appears in the *National Journal of Cancer*. He used a most interesting model, and his results show dramatically the effect of *C. parvum* on cancer dissemination. He carried out his study in a quantitative manner, which is most satisfactory.

WANEBO: With respect to the timing of injection of the *C. parvum*, Prof. Dimitrov said that if it was injected prior to enucleation of the tumor, there was no prevention of lung-metastases development. However, if injection into the tumor was by means of intralesional injection, then there was regression of pulmonary metastases; if he injected after the tumor had been removed, there was prevention of metastases.

It seems rather a paradox that *C. parvum* can be injected in the presence of active antigen, such as the growing tumor, and not have prevention of metastases. Yet, on the other hand, there is regression when injection is made into the tumor nodule itself.

DIMITROV: We have never done experiments with removal of the tumor. We only injected *C. parvum* into the tumor and, when the tumor regressed, there were no metastatic lesions in the lungs. Our experiments were very simple, and we carried out no manipulations with the tumors.

WANEBO: I was referring to the statements made about injecting *C. parvum* prior to enucleation of the tumor. Was this quoting someone else's experiment?

DIMITROV: No, all we did was to inject *C. parvum* subcutaneously every third day for five consecutive injections. The tumor was implanted at the same site, after five consecutive s.c. injections. The tumor developed, indicating that *C. parvum* was present too.

WANEBO: If the *C. parvum* was given prior to the tumor being removed, metastases formed? Is that correct?

DIMITROV: Yes, that is right.

WANEBO: On the other hand, if *C. parvum* was injected into the tumor, there was no metastatic formation?

DIMITROV: Yes, that is right.

WANEBO: It is something of a paradox that it is possible to have *C. parvum* in the presence of the tumor—the antigen—even though they are not close together, which I assume is the situation, and there is metastatic formation. Yet, if the tumor is removed—the third part of the experiment—and the *C. parvum* is then given, metastatic formation is prevented.

DIMITROV: No, we never removed the tumor; we made no surgical manipulation at all. We had two groups of animals only: first, a group given *C. parvum* before implantation, and, second, a group given *C. parvum* intralesionally after the tumor reached a size of about 1 cm, but not less than 0.6 cm.

WANEBO: If the tumor was implanted into the same site where the *C. parvum* has been injected, there was no effect on metastases?

DIMITROV: No effect at all; there was no regression.

WANEBO: The *C. parvum* has to be in the presence of tumor antigen; it has to be injected into the tumor to prevent the metastases?

DIMITROV: That is right.

HALPERN: Dr. Milas reported some interesting results concerning the effect of *C. parvum* on metastases. I consider his results to be of great importance as a model for studying the effects of *C. parvum* on tumor dissemination.

I understood from Dr. Milas's presentation that he believes that immunologic factors are involved in the regression of metastases in his system. Dr. Bomford emphasized that the clearing of tumors in the lungs may be the main effect of activated macrophages, and he partially eliminated the possibility of immunological action. However, from Dr. Milas's presentation I gained the impression that he is more in favor of immunologic factors being involved? Is that correct?

MILAS: All of us would certainly agree that it is still too early to talk about a definite mechanism(s) by which *C. parvum* exerts antitumor activity. My impression is that the activity is indeed mediated through the immune system. There are many reports suggesting this, and I shall mention only two observations from my own studies: (a) tumors that regress in mice treated with *C. parvum* or *C. granulosum* are heavily infiltrated with lymphocytes, histiocytes, and macrophages, and (b) mice immunologically suppressed by whole-body irradiation do not respond to treatment with *C. granulosum*. Macrophages and even lymphocytes from mice treated with *C. parvum* have been shown to be capable of destroying tumor cells in an immunologically nonspecific manner, but there is also evidence that treatment with this bacterium augments a specific antitumor response. Therefore, it seems reasonable that both of these modes of action may take place within the same tumor host.

HALPERN: As your model is suitable for quantitative measurements, was there evidence for enhancement in any of the studies?

MILAS: In our studies using a methylcholanthrene-induced fibrosarcoma and two spontaneous mammary carcinomas in mice, we have observed no case of immunological enhancement so far.

WHISNANT: With regard to the radiation studies, have any of the experienced clinical investigators—such as Prof. Israel, or someone else—observed clinical changes in trials which might be explained by the radiation resistance?

CHOUROULINKOV: I should like to give some information about the experiments with the Lewis lung adenocarcinoma in C_{57} Bl mice now in progress in my laboratory. We inoculated the tumors subcutaneously and the *C. parvum* intraperitoneally. There was some complete regression of the tumor and complete protection. The number of metastases was lower in treated animals in comparison with controls.

With regard to the mode of action on the metastases, it seems to me that there may be only cytostatic activity. My reasons for this conclusion are that histological analysis of the lung showed no lymphocytes, no histiocytes, and no reaction when *C. parvum* was inoculated intraperitoneally.

HALPERN: Prof. Chihara showed an interesting phenomenon obtained with lentinan—a peculiar substance, apparently a specific T-cell stimulator—which shows an important effect on a certain type of sarcoma. Sarcoma-180 was used mainly, if not exclusively, in his experiments. Am I correct or did you extend your investigations to other types of tumors? Would you comment on the antitumor effects of lentinan?

CHIHARA: Certainly. We mainly used sarcoma-180. However, we have examined the effects of lentinan on other types of tumors. To some extent, lentinan has antitumor activity against SR-C$_3$H sarcoma, CCM adenocarcinoma, and MM-102 carcinoma in mice. Tokuzen and Nakahara [(1973). *Cancer Res.* **33**:645] observed the complete regression of an autochthonous tumors by lentinan when the autochthonous grafts of spontaneous mammary tumor were implanted together with sarcoma-180 cells. Recently, Tsukagoshi *et al.* [Tsukagoshi *et al.* (1973). *Abstr. 8th Internat. Congr. of Chemotherapy* **B**:156; Tsukagoshi *et al.* (1974). *Proc. Japan Cancer Assoc.* **33**:393; Ohmi *et al.* (1974). *Proc. Japan Cancer Assoc.* **33**:641] reported that the antitumor polysaccharide, PS-K, from a basidiomycetes was effective against ascites hepatoma AH-13 in rat and syngenic leukemia P-388 in mice, as well as sarcoma-180, and that PS-K protected the immunosuppressive effect of cyclophosphamide. Ohmi *et al.* [Ohmi, (1974). *Proc. Japan Cancer Assoc.* **33**:641] reported that PS-K had considerably therapeutic effects on uterine carcinoma in human patients when used in combination with radiotherapy.

Part VI
Corynebacterium parvum
in Human Tumors

29

A Chemotherapeutic Perspective on Clinical Trials with *Corynebacterium parvum*

STEPHEN K. CARTER and MILAN SLAVIK

Introduction

Cancer is one of the oldest diseases afflicting mankind, and the efforts at treatment have been recorded as long ago as the use of arsenic pastes in ancient Egypt. Today, cancer is second only to cardiovascular disease as the major cause of death in the United States. Each year, an estimated 650,000 new cases are diagnosed, and over 1 million known patients continue treatment. The major difficulties in mounting a rapid scientific assault on cancer are that it encompasses more than 100 clinically distinct diseases and is inextricably linked to fundamental life processes which still are not completely understood.

Several modes of therapy, including surgery, radiotherapy, and chemotherapy, are effective against cancer and have been developed to a point of practical use as either single or combined modalities. In many instances, cure can be achieved through removal or destruction of localized cancer, before it has spread to distant areas, by surgery and/or radiotherapy. Surgery is sometimes more successful when both the tumor and involved regional lymph nodes are excised. Radiotherapy is used to destroy localized tumors which are not accessible to surgery.

STEPHEN K. CARTER and MILAN SLAVIK, National Cancer Institute, National Institutes of Health, Bethesda, Maryland 20014.

Unfortunately, although they may eradicate the primary disease, the local modalities often fail as a result of the spread of the disease to other parts of the body. One of the great therapeutic needs is a modality capable of controlling such disseminated disease. For many years, chemotherapy has shown the only potential in this mode of treatment, but immunotherapy has recently come to the fore with its potential for controlling tumor cells anywhere in the body.

Cures, or at least possible cures, by antitumor drugs alone have been achieved in such diseases as choriocarcinoma, Burkitt's lymphoma, acute lymphocytic leukemia, testicular cancer, and Hodgkin's disease. Chemotherapy combined with surgery and/or radiotherapy promises cures in many patients with childhood solid tumors, such as Wilms' tumor, embryonal rhabdomyosarcoma, and Ewing's sarcoma. In other tumors, chemotherapeutic agents produce a significant degree of tumor-cell kill that is reflected in a high rate of objective tumor regression and enhanced survival, although cure cannot be shown at the present time. These tumors include adenocarcinomas of the breast and ovary, non-Hodgkin's lymphoma, multiple myeloma, chronic leukemias, and acute granulocytic leukemia. In many other diseases, chemotherapy can achieve objective regression and palliative benefits in one-fifth to one-third of the treated patients.

While immunotherapy has not shown the established therapeutic activity of chemotherapy, its potential effectiveness appears high, and widespread clinical trials are only now beginning.

Over the years, the Division of Cancer Treatment has functioned as a drug development program and has evolved a three-phase methodology for the clinical evaluation of new agents.

Phase I trials are limited to clinical pharmacology. The aim is to establish the maximum tolerated dose (MTD) at the schedule used and to determine the parameters of toxicity. If a MTD can be determined, and toxic effects are predictable, treatable, and/or reversible, Phase II trials can begin.

Phase II trials survey clinical activity of drugs against a panel of 10 signal tumors, including "fast-growing" and "slow-growing" types: (1) adenocarcinoma of the breast, (2) adenocarcinoma of the colon, (3) bronchogenic carcinoma, (4) adenocarcinoma of the pancreas, (5) ovarian cancer, (6) malignant melanoma, (7) acute myelocytic leukemia, (8) acute lymphocytic leukemia, (9) lymphomatous disease, (10) malignant glioma. Adenocarcinoma of the breast and colon and bronchogenic carcinoma represent the slow-growing tumors, which are most resistant to chemotherapy; acute leukemia and lymphoma represent the fast-growing, more chemotherapeutically sensitive, tumors. Objective response must be clearly evaluable in at least 15–30 patients with each signal tumor, generally by measurable indicator lesions.

Phase II trials examine other important parameters of drug action. If the agent is a new chemical structure, greater interest is shown. Currently, high priority is given to cell-cycle-insensitive agents that can kill nonproliferating cells. Considerable emphasis is placed on drugs that can attack tumor cells in pharmacologic sanctuaries, such as the central nervous system. Indications of suitability for combination chemotherapy (e.g., lack of bone-marrow toxicity) also increase interest in moving an agent forward in clinical trial.

If acceptable activity is shown, based on the characteristics of the drug and response in any of the signal tumors, Phase III trials are initiated to establish definitively the role of the agent in the clinical oncologist's armamentarium.

Heat-killed cells of *Corynebacterium parvum* are a powerful stimulant of the reticuloendothelial system (Prévot *et al.*, 1973) and, as such, have been postulated as being valuable in the treatment of cancer. The experimental antitumor activity of *C. parvum* has been shown in various systems (Halpern *et al.*, 1966; Lamensans *et al.*, 1968; Woodruff and Inchley, 1971), although in most of these it has been necessary to inject *C. parvum* before the tumor cells in order to show effective protection (Fisher *et al.*, 1970). Some activity has been observed against established tumors (Milas and Mujagić, 1972; Smith and Woodruff, 1968).

Although preliminary studies with *C. parvum* date from 1967 (Israel and Halpern, 1972), widespread clinical trials are just beginning. At this time, it might be valuable to consider *C. parvum* as a new anticancer drug and determine how an immunostimulant might fit into the three classical phases of clinical evaluation.

Phase I Studies

Phase I studies are usually limited to clinical pharmacology in patients with advanced solid tumors resistant to all currently available therapy. These patients should have relatively "normal" organ function and must not have received such extensive prior therapy that toxicologic evaluation would be difficult. The estimated survival of patients must be at least 2 months to allow complete evaluation of toxicity. Measurable or evaluable disease is not required, and a favorable clinical response, although gratifying and significant when it occurs, is not essential at this stage.

An outline of some basic Phase I study principles is given in Fig. 1. Drug doses are expressed in mg/m^2, because body-surface area has better correlation to certain metabolic and excretory functions than body weight (Pinkel, 1958). Moreover, body-surface area can be used as a common denominator for drug dosage in adults and children, and for drug dosage in different animal species (Pinkel, 1958; Shirkey, 1965; Schein *et al.*, 1970; Freireich *et al.*, 1966).

As in any clinical study, the design of a Phase I trial must consider a number of critical variables, such as: (1) initial dose, (2) dose schedules, (3) dose-escalation procedure, (4) number of patients treated on any dose schedule, (5) data collection, (6) pharmacology, (7) criteria for moving to Phase II studies. This presentation, rather than specifically answering questions on each variable, is

1. Initial dose chosen from large-animal toxicology studies.

2. Doses not escalated in the same patient.

3. Dose escalation, initially rapid, with increments of escalation smaller as the toxic range is approached.

4. Treat 3 patients at each nontoxic level and treat 6 patients at each level showing any toxicity.

5. Antitumor response, or lack thereof, is not part of the decision-making process to move drug into Phase II studies.

Fig. 1. Phase I study principles.

intended to stimulate discussion by examining the advantages and disadvantages of different approaches used in Phase I drug studies and by asking how they might apply to an immunotherapeutic agent like *C. parvum*.

Initial Dose

The initial dose for Phase I study may be chosen on the basis of (1) rodent data, (2) large animal data, or (3) clinical data obtained with an analogue or from foreign clinical trials.

Several studies, particularly in Europe, the Soviet Union, and Japan, have used rodent data to predict an initial dose. For example, a protocol of the Pharmacology Committee of the Soviet Ministry of Health states that 1/30 of the maximum, tolerated, cumulative dose for rats, given in mg/kg over 15 days, is used for alkylating agents, while lower starting doses are recommended for drugs from other chemical classes.

Most of the European countries accept the approach of using 3 animal species, including 1 nonrodent species, in preclinical toxicity studies. Since the most sensitive species is used for predicting the initial dose, a rodent species might be the predictive one.

Freireich *et al.* (1966) reviewed a large volume of experimental data and demonstrated a close relationship between the LD_{10} in rodents and the TD in man when the values are given on a mg/m^2 basis. However, their conclusions strongly emphasized the dangers of attempting direct extrapolation of animal toxicity data to MTD in man. They did not suggest that it would be wise to convert mouse or rat LD_{10} to mg/m^2 and start clinical trials in man at one-third this level. However, calculation of the MTD on this basis has been recommended and used in Europe (Kenis, 1969).

Large-animal toxicity data have been widely used for predicting the initial dose in man. These species include the cat, which is used in the USSR and is regarded as particularly predictive for hematologic toxicity, and the guinea pig, employed in European countries. However, the best experience using large-animal predictive models has been achieved with the dog and monkey in the United States. The dose levels in these species that might be used in choosing an initial Phase I dose are: (1) highest nontoxic dose (HNTD); (2) toxic dose, low (TDL); (3) toxic dose, high (TDH); and (4) lethal dose (LD).

One-third of the TDL in the most sensitive species, expressed in mg/m^2 of body surface, has been the basis of the initial dose for years at the NCI. However, critical questions remain: Is this really the best starting level? Is it safe enough? Can it be improved? At the present time, the Cancer Therapy Evaluation Program is addressing these questions by statistical analysis of the applicability of animal toxicity data to prediction of drug toxicity in man.

Clearly, a starting dose with subcutaneous (s.c.) *C. parvum* does not need to be chosen from animal studies, since human data already exist. However, administration of intravenous (i.v.) *C. parvum* may pose a different problem. In almost all studies to date, *C. parvum* has been given as s.c. in a dose of 4 mg of dried, heat-killed bacteria suspended in saline containing formaldehyde. Weekly doses have been given for periods of several months and, in one group of patients, for years. More than 500 patients have been treated using this schedule (Israel and Halpern, 1972; Halpern and Israel, 1971; Israel, 1974; Israel and Edelstein, 1974), but apparently the choice of dose and schedule was totally empiric.

Burroughs Wellcome Company (1973) recommends that i.v. administration should not exceed 0.5–1.0 mg/kg by infusion over several hours. In reports of their studies, monkeys given either 2.0 or 20 mg/kg i.v. tolerated the single injection without serious toxic effects, while rabbits injected i.v. with 1.4 mg had a low grade, but definite febrile, response. If one considers any degree of toxicity defining the TDL (as is done at NCI), the monkey TDL may be as low as 24 mg/m^2, with a shallow dose–response effect, because 340 mg/m^2 gives no more serious effects. Since the recommended i.v. starting dose is 18–37 mg/m^2, it appears that the TDL in monkeys is being used as the human starting dose. This is probably safe, given the apparent shallowness of the dose–response curve for toxicity.

Dose Schedules

The choice of an initial schedule for Phase I study is aided by information from various sources, including schedule-dependency data in rodent tumor systems, data on cell-cycle sensitivity and mechanism of action, pharmacology investigations, and schedules used in studies of large-animal toxicology. The commonly used schedules in NCI-sponsored Phase I studies are: (1) single dose, (2) daily × 5 or 10, (3) twice weekly, (4) weekly, (5) continuous infusion.

These schedules generally result from schedule-dependency studies in mice, which raises a question of whether the extrapolation to man is relevant without correlation with metabolism and drug disposition. *C. parvum* has been given, almost exclusively, on a weekly schedule, and this choice was totally empirical

(Israel and Edelstein, 1974). Is this schedule optimal? Should we undertake new Phase I studies with other schedules, and how should they be chosen?

Dose-Escalation Procedures

Dose escalation in Phase I studies may either be done in one patient or be restricted to separate patients. The first procedure is more economical in patient resources, but risks cumulative toxicity, while the second has quite the opposite effect. Also, the techniques of escalation might be different as shown on Fig. 2. The modified Fibonacci search scheme for dose escalation has been used extensively in the Division of Cancer Treatment. It tends to fail with drugs that have a shallow response curve and fails totally if the initial dose is too low. It would probably be inappropriate for an immunostimulant such as *C. parvum.*

Number of Patients Treated

The number of patients who can be treated at any given dose level in a Phase I study ranges from 1–10, or more. However, economic feasibility and statistical significance are two extreme determinants. The Division of Cancer Treatment requires at least 3 patients at each dose level.

Data Collection

In the collection of data, a question might be raised whether or not standard criteria of toxicity and a unified system of data reporting should be used. The investigator's personal freedom to report the study in his own way versus procedures offering better statistical analysis, possibly by computer, should be the main determinants to be balanced.

100% Increments	Fixed 100 mg increments	Modified Fibonacci increments	50% Increments
100	100	100	100
200	200	200	200
400	300	350	300
800	400	525	450
1600	500	700	675
3200	600	925	1000
6400	700	1225	1500
12800	800	1625	2250
25600	900	2050	3375
51200	1000	2750	5000

Fig. 2. Four approaches to dose escalation in Phase I study, starting with an initial dose of 100 mg.

```
1. Determine the maximum dose tolerated.

2. Elucidate parameters of toxicity.

3. Establish biological activity.

4. Elucidate potential therapeutic activity.
```

Fig. 3. End points in Phase I study.

Pharmacology

The question of including pharmacokinetic studies is critical in the design of Phase I studies. If they are to be included, at which dose level should they be implemented in the study? Should comparative pharmacology be done in order to elucidate the toxicity and/or lack of activity in Phase I studies?

Pharmacologic studies in Phase I trials can be initiated at the first dose level, at the level showing initial toxicity, or at the MTD. The advantages of starting these studies at the initial level include early indications of unique pharmacologic situations, early hints of improper choice of schedule, and early comparative pharmacology with other animal species. A disadvantage of starting at the initial dose is the potential waste of resources at doses insufficient for biologic activity. The pharmacology of immunostimulants appears to be poorly understood, and thought must be given to the requirements for pharmacological information in this area.

Criteria for Passage to Phase II Studies

What is the definition of failure in a Phase I study? Does it mean only that the drug produced unpredictable and irreversible toxicity in man, which was not predicted in animal toxicity studies? Or, should lack of activity also be considered?

A Phase I study of an anticancer drug has at least four potential end points (Fig. 3). The classical end points are MTD determination and elucidation of the parameters of toxicity. Establishment of biological activity and therapeutic activity are more specifically the role of a Phase II evaluation.

There are several critical questions that should enter into Phase I study with *C. parvum* (Fig. 4). Is it necessary to push the doses, both s.c. and i.v., to the maximum level tolerated? The rationale of a "MTD" has been the cell-kill hypothesis as elucidated by Skipper, but it may not apply to immunostimulants that are postulated to kill tumor cells by zero-order kinetics, rather than by the first-order kinetics of cytotoxic compounds. It may be enough to simply establish an immunologically active dose, although it would be ideal to establish

1. Should the maximum dose tolerated be established?

2. Would it be satisfactory to establish an "immunologically active dose" or a maximum immunopotentiating dose?

3. Is there a dose–response effect (regarding immunologic activity; regarding anti-tumor activity?

Fig. 4. Critical questions in Phase I study of *Corynebacterium parvum.*

a maximum immunopotentiating dose. The latter would probably require determination of a MTD.

The elucidation of a maximum immunopotentiating dose would permit calculation of a dose–response curve for immunologic activity. The dose–response curve would be important for correlation with antitumor activity, if it exists, and it would be of great interest for all immunostimulating agents to see if the dose–response effect for immunologic activity correlates with the dose–response effect for antitumor activity. It would seem that such knowledge ought to be required so that an "optimal" dose can be used in undertaking any large-scale adjuvant trials.

Phase II Studies

Phase II trials have traditionally been the screen for antitumor activity. Inherent in any screen is a clear end point of response and a critical level of activity demonstrated by this response, which allows passage of the compound to the next step. The sensitivity of the activity level is determined by many factors, including the activity of established agents, the capacity to study drugs at the next level, and the overall psychological expectation from the program involved and the related scientific community. This latter aspect is often the determining factor in how critical individuals will be of a screen, regardless of its intrinsic scientific validity.

The DCT Drug Development Program has decided to use as its screen the panel of 10 signal tumors cited previously. It is felt that this disease-oriented Phase II approach is superior to the often used, general Phase II trial, in which a wide range of tumor types are treated, but only a few of these in patient numbers large enough for meaningful results.

Phase II studies with *C. parvum* could be approached on a variety of lines (Fig. 5). One approach would be to use *C. parvum* as a single agent in advanced disease. The end points could be antitumor response, change in immunologic reactivity, and impact on survival. It may be unfair to expect an immuno-stimulant to shrink a bulky metastatic tumor by greater than 50%, but it would be reassuring to obtain some evidence of its cell-kill potential before committing hundreds of patients to controlled adjuvant trials.

A second approach is to use *C. parvum* in combination with chemotherapy in advanced disease, as has been done by Israel and his colleagues and by Mayo Clinic investigators with BCG. This is an acceptable approach, but it requires well-designed, controlled trials because the end point is the superiority of chemotherapy plus immunotherapy over chemotherapy alone. An end point of survival alone in such a study is the most difficult parameter to evaluate for a number of reasons. First, survival assumes a fixed or homogeneous zero point that is rarely, if ever, achieved in advanced-disease studies. A patient being treated for the second relapse, after initial surgery followed by chemotherapy, may have a very different survival potential in comparison to a newly diagnosed patient with advanced disease being treated for the first time. Unless the treatment groups are well stratified before randomization, survival differences among the treatment groups in this approach are open to skeptical interpretation.

The best end point in such a study would be a clear-cut, higher response rate for chemo–immunotherapy and/or a prolonged duration of remission. Another problem with a survival end point is that therapy given after relapse from the study treatment can also impact on survival and, unless it is fixed in some way, can make interpretation difficult.

The third approach to Phase II studies with *C. parvum* is to employ it in early disease as an adjuvant after surgery or radiotherapy. However, this is a time-consuming and expensive approach. The end point in such a study, besides immunologic reactivity, is a disease-free interval and/or survival. This kind of evaluation requires long-term follow-up and is expensive of patient resources, since the trials must be well controlled, unless one is looking for gigantic therapeutic effects. This type of trial should be reserved for Phase III studies, where a material that has shown reliable evidence of "activity" is tested at an optimum-dose schedule intended to make a meaningful impact on the course of early disease.

Several critical questions immediately arise in considering an optimal Phase II approach for an agent such as *C. parvum* (Fig. 6). The most important one is whether "immunologic activity" without antitumor response can be considered a meaningful positive effect. If not, trials with *C. parvum* alone in advanced disease may not be reasonable. Sooner or later, for all immunostimulants, it will

---

1. Used as a single agent in advanced disease.

2. Used in combination with chemotherapy in advanced disease: (a) controlled trial; (b) uncontrolled trial.

3. Used in early disease as an adjuvant after surgery or radiotherapy.

Fig. 5. Phase II approaches with *Corynebacterium parvum*.

1. Can antitumor response in advanced disease be reasonably used as an end point?

2. Is "immunologic activity" without antitumor response a meaningful positive?

3. Is activity in a tumor site specific, or can activity in one tumor type predict the activity in others, i.e., in how many tumor types should *C. parvum* be tested?

Fig. 6. Critical questions in Phase II study of *Corynebacterium parvum*.

be essential to determine whether the tests for immunologic activity have a meaningful correlation with clinical activity.

Another question is whether the antitumor activity of an agent such as *C. parvum* is site specific, or directed at all tumor sites. This question will bear upon the number of tumor sites that should be evaluated in Phase II trials. As indicated earlier, a variety of signal tumors are used to assess anticancer potential of cytotoxic agents. If *C. parvum* is to be tested with chemotherapy, the issue becomes much more complicated and, clearly, tests would be needed in a range of tumors before one could assume an adequate evaluation.

Phase III Studies

Phase III studies have traditionally been controlled studies which attempt to define the role of a new drug or regimen in therapeutic practice. These studies may entail a comparative study with a standard agent or an attempt to use the new drug in combination with other agents. The principles of random allocation and pretherapeutic stratification play important roles in the design of Phase III studies, as they do in Phase II studies.

Discussion

Recently, the chemotherapy program of the NCI has been expanded and integrated into the NCI Division of Cancer Treatment under the new emphasis of the National Cancer Plan. The immediate objectives of the DCT program are to increase the number of patients responding to cancer therapy and prolong the length of the disease-free period of remission. The ultimate goal is the cure or control of cancer.

The increased scope of the DCT program includes not only the drug development program and clinical testing aspects of the former chemotherapy program, but also the improvement of therapy by combined-modality approaches. These efforts will proceed largely on disease-oriented lines, with the major emphasis on effective treatment for the solid tumors that are the major cause of cancer deaths in the United States.

The major thrust in combined-modality treatment will seek an integration of chemotherapy and/or immunotherapy with surgery and/or radiotherapy. The philosophical base of the combined-modality approach is the recognition that surgery and radiotherapy have reached a plateau in their ability to cure solid tumors. These localized modalities kill tumor cells only where they are applied, and it is not technically feasible to increase the scope of their application on tumors in which they are effective. They fail to cure many patients, even when they remove all the tumor visible to the naked eye or diagnostic x-ray film. The reason for this failure is felt to be the presence of disseminated disease foci at the time of surgical excision of the primary tumor, which many times includes the surrounding tissue and part of the regional lymph nodes.

Chemotherapy, used optimally, has the potential to eradicate these metastatic foci. Immunotherapy may have the same potential. The drug regimens showing the highest degree of activity in advanced disease will be the prime candidates for use in the combined-modality approach. The degree of cell kill necessary to shrink a bulky, solid tumor mass by greater than 50% is quite large. If this degree of cell kill could be directed against the relatively small tumor burden remaining after surgical excision, perhaps eradication of the last neoplastic cell can be achieved.

The proposed therapeutic strategy for increasing cure rates in solid tumors through chemotherapy involves the integration of drugs into combined-modality approaches for primary treatment. In this scheme, new drugs or drug combinations would be tested in advanced disease, and those showing positive results would be studied in the primary therapy of disseminated disease. An optimum regimen developed in this manner would then be integrated into a combined-modality treatment in local and regional diseases. A similar strategy needs to be established for immunostimulating agents.

The Phase III trials of *C. parvum,* assuming activity is observed in Phase II studies, will have to be integrated into this strategy. The future of cancer therapy must lie in combined approaches if significant new successes are to be achieved. The immunostimulants, such as *C. parvum,* offer a new approach to the control of neoplastic cells that are beyond the scope of the local modalities of surgery and radiotherapy. A purely empirical approach to clinical testing of these agents is not sufficient. It is essential that the sponsors of clinical trials and those who perform the trials plan together an overall approach to clinical evaluation.

References

Burroughs Wellcome Company (1973). Information for investigators: *Corynebacterium parvum* (Wellcome, CN. 6134), Research Triangle Park, North Carolina.

Fisher, J. C., Grace, W. R., and Mannick, J. A. (1970). The effect of nonspecific immunostimulation with *Corynebacterium parvum* on patterns of tumor growth. *Cancer* **26:** 1379–1382.

Freireich, E. J., Gehan, E. A., Rall, D. P., Schmidt, L. H., and Skipper, H. E. (1966). Quantitative comparison of toxicity of anticancer agents in mouse, rat, hamster, dog, monkey, and man. *Cancer Chemother. Rep.* **50:**219–244.

Halpern, B. N. and Israel, L. (1971). Etude de l'action d'une immunostimuline associée aux Corynébactéries anaérobies dans les neoplasies expérimentales et humaines. *C. R. Acad. Sci.* **273**:2186–2190.

Halpern, B. N., Biozzi, G., Stiffel, C., and Mouton, D. (1966). Inhibition of tumor growth by administration of killed *Corynebacterium parvum. Nature (Lond.)* **212**:853–854.

Israel, L. (1974). Clinical results with corynebacteria. *Symposium on Cancer and Immunity* (G. Mathé, ed.) (Centre National de la Recherche Scientifique), Paris.

Israel, L. and Edelstein, R. (1974). Nonspecific immunostimulation with *C. parvum* in human cancer. *Symposium on Immune Mechanisms in Neoplasia.* M. D. Anderson Hospital and Tumor Institute, Houston.

Israel, L. and Halpern, B. N. (1972). Le *Corynebacterium parvum* dans les cancer avancés. Première evaluation de l'activité thérapeutique de cette immunostiumline. *Nouv. Presse Med.* **1**:19–23.

Kenis, Y. (1969). Dose schedules and modes of administration of chemotherapeutic agents in man. *Recent Results Cancer Res.* **21**:54–61.

Lamensans, A., Stiffel, C., Mollier, M. F., Laurent, M., Mouton, D., and Biozzi, G. (1968). Effet protecteur de *Corynebacterium parvum* contre la leucemie greffée AKR. *Rev. Fr. Etud. Clin. Biol.* **13**:772–776.

Milas, L. and Mujagić, H. (1972). Protection by *Corynebacterium parvum* against tumor cells injected intravenously. *Eur. J. Clin. Biol. Res.* **17**:498–500.

Pinkel, D. (1958). The use of body-surface area as a criterion of drug dosage in cancer chemotherapy. *Cancer Res.* **18**:853–856.

Prévot, A. R., Halpern, B. N., Biozzi, G., Stiffel, C., Mouton, D., Morard, J. C., Bouthillier, Y., and Decreusefond, (1973). Stimulation du système réticuloendothélial par les corps microbiens tués de *Corynebacterium parvum. C. R. Acad. Sci. (Paris)* **257**:13–17.

Schein, P. S., Davis, R. D., Carter, S., Newman, J., Schein, D. R., and Rall, D. A. (1970). The evaluation of anticancer drugs in dogs and monkeys for the prediction of qualitative toxicities in man. *Clin. Pharmacol. Ther.* **11**:3–40.

Shirkey, H. C. (1965). Drug dosage for infants and children. *J. Am. Med. Assoc.* **193**:443–446.

Smith, L. H. and Woodruff, M. E. A. (1968). Comparative effects of two strains of *Corynebacterium parvum* on phagocytic activity and tumor growth. *Nature (Lond.)* **219**:197–198.

Woodruff, M. E. A. and Inchley, M. P. (1971). Synergistic inhibition of mammary carcinoma transplants in A-strain mice by antitumor globulin and *C. parvum. Br. J. Cancer* **25**:584–593.

30

Action of *Corynebacterium parvum* on the Phagocytic Activity of the Reticuloendothelial System in Cancer Patients (Preliminary Results)

E. ATTIÉ

Abstract

A new method of exploring the phagocytic function of the RES was applied in clinical trials. Microaggregated human-serum albumin labeled with ^{125}I is now produced industrially and distributed by the Centre National de Transfusion Sanguine, Paris, and is at the disposal of researchers wanting to study the phagocytic function of the RES. First results show that the method can be applied to clinical investigation and is faithful. In the first patients with evolving cancers tested, we found an increase in the activity of the phagocytic function of the RES. This test is very useful in measuring the effect of immunotherapy by

E. ATTIÉ, Institut Gustav-Roussy, Villejuif, France.

BCG, *Corynebacterium parvum,* or poly IC, or of immunodepressive drugs such as cortisone.

Introduction

The utilization of *Corynebacterium parvum* or BCG, or the two together in active, nonspecific immunotherapy in patients with cancer made it necessary to devise a quantitative technique to measure the effect of this immunotherapy. It is such a technique and some preliminary results in man that are the subject of this study.

One of the factors in the progression of cancer is host resistance. This factor has remained very vague until now, when new quantitative methods of exploration promise its precise measurement. Our hypothesis is that, to a first approximation and apart from hormone-dependent cancers, host resistance is the result of the activity of the lymphoreticuloendothelial system.

To explore this system, we now have available new precise quantitative techniques, one of which is the study of the phagocytic function of the RES by following the clearance of ^{125}I-labeled microaggregated human-serum albumin in the blood.

The method was developed and tested on animals by Halpern *et al.* (1958), and we wanted to apply it to man.

Materials and Methods

A quantity of 2 mg of microaggregated human-serum albumin is injected per 100 mg of body weight of animal (guinea pig). Samples of blood are taken from the retro-orbitary sinus after 2, 5, 8, 12, 16, 20, and 30 min. The radioactivity is counted, and the logarithm of the number of counts is plotted. If the preparation of albumin microaggregate is homogeneous, a straight line is obtained showing that the phenomenon is exponential. The slope of the line is obtained by the formula

$$\frac{\log B - \log A}{T_2 - T_1} = K$$

where B is the radioactivity at time T_2 and A the radioactivity at time T_1, expressed in counts per minute. This gives a quantitative appreciation of the phenomenon.

A second way of expressing the results is to plot them on semilogarithmic paper, with the time as the abscissa and the radioactivity as the ordinate. The period of time, P, during which radioactivity decreases to half its value, gives the same quantitative appreciation of the phagocytic activity of the Kupffer cells. The relation between K and P is given by the formula

$$\frac{0.693}{K} = P$$

To apply this method to routine clinical trials, an industrial production of the microaggregated human-serum albumin was needed. We tried to utilize available products—CAI furnished by Saclay and made by Sorin in Italy, a Dutch product made by Philips Duphar, and Albumotop H from Squibb. We carried out many experiments, and we discussed the problem with the producers, trying to obtain a homogeneous product. They attempted to satisfy us, but were not successful, and we finally concluded that the solution of the problem of fabrication of a homogeneous product was very difficult.

Figure 1 shows examples of curves obtained on animals with the available commercial products. They are not straight lines; rather, there are two components, showing that the product contains at least two populations of particles, and no conclusion can be reached.

We then began to work with Mr. Drouet of the Centre National de la Transfusion Sanguine. After many trials, adopting the technique described by Brinner (1968), we obtained a product which is perfect for the purpose (Fig. 2).

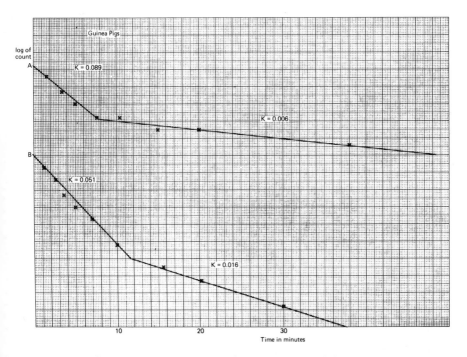

Fig. 1. Log of the radioactive count of microaggregated human-serum albumin tested in animals.

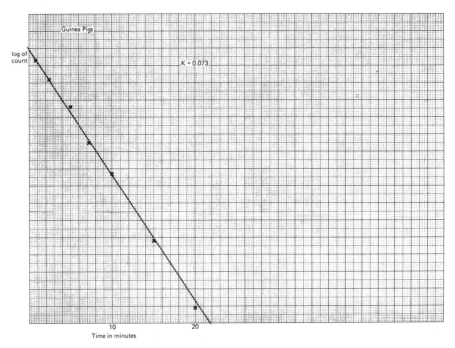

Fig. 2. Log of the radioactive count of a homogeneous albumin microaggregate.

Application to Man

For two days, one day before exploration and on the morning of the exploration, the thyroid of the patient was blocked by 50 drops of lugol. Microaggregated human-serum albumin (5 mg/kg of body weight), labeled with ^{125}I, was injected intravenously, and 6 ml of blood was taken at 2, 6, 10, 15, 20, and 30 min. The blood was permitted to sediment or was centrifuged. At each time period, 1 ml of plasma was taken in each of two tubes, and the radioactivity was counted. Mean values of the two counts were used in plotting the curve. An example tested in man is shown in Fig. 3.

A first approximation of the normal value of the period, P, was done on patients cured by radiotherapy after suffering from Hodgkin's disease for many years and now in good health, all clinical and laboratory examinations being normal for many years. The numbers on the right show the values of P in minutes:

Patient No. 19 (male, Hodgkin's disease, cured) 10
Patient No. 20 (male, age 52, control) 11
Patient No. 21 (male, age 60, Hodgkin's disease, cured) 10.2
Patient No. 15 (male, age 54, Hodgkin's disease, cured) 9.2
Patient No. 28 (male, age 35, Hodgkin's disease, cured) 10.2

Thus, for the time being, we consider the normal value of P to be between 9–11. The work of Halpern *et al.* (1958) led us to expect a value around 9.9, supporting our results.

Some control measurements were conducted to assess the fidelity of the test. Two measurements were made at two-week intervals in three subjects. The numbers on the right show the values of P in minutes:

Patient No. 19 10
2 weeks later 10
Patient No. 21 .... 10.2
2 weeks later 10.6
Patient No. 28 .... 10.2
2 weeks later 9.8

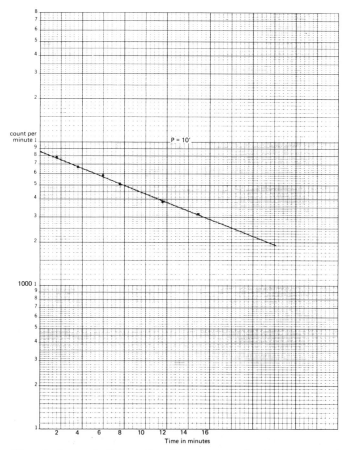

Fig. 3. Log of the radioactive count of microaggregated human-serum albumin, labeled with ^{125}I, tested in man.

The conclusion is that the test is reproducible.

Our first observation in applying the test to patients with evolving cancer—and contrary to our expectation—was a decrease of the period P, meaning an increased activity of the RES. These findings, which are in accord with the pathological findings of Black and Speer (1958), are shown in Table I.

The mechanisms of this increase in the phagocytic function of the RES are obscure, and further investigations have to be carried out to determine if this increase in the phagocyte function is related to the state of the host or if it is a result of circulating cancer cells in the blood, or of material from these cells. For the moment, we must conclude, on the basis of lymphocyte transformation with phytohemagglutinin in cancer patients—which seems to lead to an immunodepression, especially of T lymphocytes, that there seems to exist a dissociation between the T lymphocytes and the phagocytic function of the RES in patients with evolving cancers.

To determine the effect of immunotherapy on the phagocytic function of the RES, the technique of Mathé et al. (1968) was used. The technique consists of two applications of BCG during the week and weekly intramuscular injections of "reticulostimuline," a preparation of C. parvum made by Institut Pasteur. The following examples give the results obtained for P (expressed in minutes):

Patient No. 9 (male, age 30, Hodgkin's disease, evolving) 3
    after one week of immunotherapy 6.8
    after two weeks of immunotherapy 7
Patient No. 26 (male, age 60, Hodgkin's disease, cured) 11.4
    after one week of immunotherapy 9.4

Based on only these two preliminary cases, it appears that when the period (as in case No. 26) is normal, immunotherapy has the effect of stimulating the phagocytic function of the RES. However, when the period is greatly accelerated, immunotherapy seems to bring it closer to the normal value.

Another substance used in immunotherapy, poly IC, was explored. The numbers on the right show the values of P in minutes:

Patient No. 22 (female, acute lymphoblastic leukemia) 7.5
    11 days after poly IC 7.5

In this example, poly IC does not seem to affect the RES.

The following example shows the effect of cortisone associated with purinethol. The value of P is in minutes and appears on the right:

Patient No. 27 (male, lymphoblastosarcoma transformed
    in acute lymphoblastic leukemia) 6.4
    2 weeks after cortisone and purinethol 11.8

We must mention that a few patients explored by this method experienced chills and elevated temperatures, but returned to normal after an intravenous injection of soludecadron.

Table 1. Application of the Human-Serum Albumin Test to Patients

Patient	Sex	Age	Disease	P, min[a]
1	M		Chronic lymphocytic leukemia	3.6
4	F	21	Hodgkin's disease, evolving	2.8
5	F	24	Acute lymphoblastic leukemia in apparent remission	4.4
6	M	39	Seminoma of the testis	4.2
7	M	43	Generalized melanoma	8
8	F	32	Mycosis fongoïde	3.1
9	M	30	Hodgkin's disease, evolving	3
10	M	68	Cancer of the thyroid, differentiated with metastases disseminated	1.8
11	F	40	Anaplastic cancer disseminated in the abdomen	3.2
12	M	34	Hodgkin's disease, evolving	2.3
13	F	58	Hodgkin's disease, evolving	6.5
14	F	34	Lymphoblastosarcoma	5
22	F		Acute lymphoblastic leukemia	7.5
27	M		Lymphoblastosarcoma transformed in acute lymphoblastic leukemia	6.4

[a]In studying these results, we found an acceleration which is important in many cases and pronounced in all cases, except that of melanoma in patient No. 7. We must add to this case the two following cases of acute myeloblastic leukemia:

Patient No. 23   F   56   9.3
Patient No. 24   M   37   8.25

Apart from these exceptions, it seems that the RES was stimulated in patients with evolving cancers.

Conclusion

The method of explorating the phagocytic function of the RES has been applied in clinical trials. The microaggregated human-serum albumin, labeled with ^{125}I, is now produced industrially and distributed commercially by Centre National de la Transfusion Sanguine* and is at the disposal of researchers wanting to study the phagocytic function of the RES. First results show that the method can be applied to clinical investigation and is faithful. In the first patients with evolving cancers tested, we found an increase in the activity of the phagocytic function of the RES.

This test is very useful in measuring the effect of BCG, *C. parvum,* or poly IC immunotherapy, or of immunodepressive drugs such as cortisone.

*6 rue Alexandre Cabanel, Paris 15, France.

Acknowledgments

We want to thank Miss Stiffel of the team of Professor Halpern, Dr. Schneider of the team of Professor Mathé, and Mr. Drouet of the Centre National de la Transfusion Sanguine for their help, and Professors M. Tubiana, B. Halpern, and G. Mathé for their support.

References

Aschoff, L. (1924). Reticuloendothelial system. In: *Lectures on Pathology,* Hoeber, New York.

Benacerraf, B., Biozzi, G., Halpern, B., and Stiffel, C. (1957). Physiology of phagocytosis of particles by RES. In: *Symposium on Physiopathology of the RES,* p. 52 (B. Halpern, ed.), Blackwell Scientific Publications, Oxford.

Biozzi, G., Benacerraf, B., and Halpern, B. (1953). Quantitative study of granulopectic activity of the reticuloendothelial system. *Br. J. Exp. Pathol.* **34**:44.

Black, M. M. and Speer, F. D. (1958). Sinus histiocytosis of lymph nodes in cancer. *Surg. Gynecol. Obstet.* **106**:163–175.

Brinner, W. H. (1968). Preparation of ^{125}I-labeled microaggregated human serum albumin for use in studies of reticuloendothelial function in man. *J. Nucl. Med.* **9**:482–485.

Donovan, A. (1967). Reticuloendothelial function in patients with cancer. *Am. J. Surg.* **114**:230–238.

Halpern, B. and Mouton, D. (1958). Phagocytic function of the RES and experimental tumors. In: *Reticuloendothelial Structure and Function,* p. 259 (J. H. Heller, ed.), Ronald Press Co., New York.

Halpern, B., Biozzi, G., Pequignot, G., Stiffel, C., Delaloye, B., and Mouton, D. (1958). La cinétique de l'épuration sanguine des suspensions colloidales comme mesure de la circulation hépatique. *Rev. Fr. Etud. Clin. Biol.* **3**:549–557.

Halpern, B., Benacerraf, B., Biozzi, G., and Stiffel, C. (1964). Facteurs régissant la fonction phagocytaire du RES. *Rev. Hematol.* **9**:621–642.

Halpern, B., Biozzi, G., and Stiffel, C. (1970). Le système réticuloendothélial et l'invasion tumorale. In: *Mechanisms of Invasion in Cancer. UICC Monograph Series,* Vol. 6, (Pierre Denoix, ed.).

Magarey, C. J., Baum, M., Mackay, W. D., Quantock, D. C., and Vernon-Roberts, B. (1968). Cancer and its treatments and the reticuloendothelial system in man. *Br. J. Surg.* **55**:872.

Mathé, G., Amiel, J. L., Schwarzenberg, L., Schneider, M., Cattan, A., Schlumberger, J. R., Hayat, M., and de Vassal, F. (1968). Démonstration de l'efficacité de l'immunothérapie active dans la leucémie aiguë lymphoblastique humaine. *Rev. Fr. Etud. Clin. Biol.* **13**:454–459.

Old, L. J., Benacerraf, B., Clarke, D. A., Carswell, E. A., and Stockert, E. (1961). The role of the reticuloendothelial system in the host reaction to neoplasia. *Cancer Res.* **21**: 1281–1301.

Stern, K. (1960). The reticuloendothelial system and neoplasia. In: *Reticuloendothelial Structure and Function,* p. 233 (J. H. Heller, ed.), Ronald Press Co., New York.

Stiffel, C., Halpern, B., and Mouton, D. (1960). Recherches sur le mécanisme de l'immunité non spécifique produite par les mycobactéries. *Rev. Fr. Etud. Clin. Biol.* **5**: 876–880.

31

Corynebacterium parvum: Preliminary Report of a Phase I Clinical and Immunological Study in Cancer Patients

RICHARD C. REED, JORDAN U. GUTTERMAN,
GIORA M. MAVLIGIT, ANDREW A. BURGESS,
and EVAN M. HERSH

Introduction

Immunopotentiating agents are being used with increasing frequency in the therapy of human malignancy. The most thoroughly investigated of these materials in clinical trials is *Bacillus Calmette Guérin* (BCG). Therapy with BCG (with or without active specific immunization) has been reported to prolong remission and/or survival of patients with childhood lymphoblastic leukemia (Mathé *et al.*, 1969), adult myeloblastic leukemia (Powles *et al.*, 1973; Vogel and

RICHARD C. REED, JORDAN U. GUTTERMAN, GIORA M. MAVLIGIT, ANDREW A. BURGESS, and EVAN M. HERSH, Department of Developmental Therapeutics, The University of Texas System, Cancer Center, M. D. Anderson Hospital and Tumor Institute, 6723 Bertner Avenue, Houston, Texas 77025.

Supported by Contract N01-CB-33888, Grant No. CA 14984-01 and by Burroughs Wellcome Company, Triangle Park, North Carolina, and Career Development Award 71007-01 from the USPHS (J.U.G.).

Chan, 1974; Gutterman *et al.*, 1974b), chronic myelogenous leukemia (Sokal *et al.*, 1973), malignant lymphoma (Sokal *et al.*, 1974), as well as malignant melanoma (Bluming *et al.*, 1972; Gutterman *et al.*, 1973; Gutterman *et al.*, 1974b). It may also increase the remission rate in malignancy (Gutterman *et al.*, 1974a; Donaldson, 1972).

Although our clinical experience with BCG administered by scarification has demonstrated the potential effectiveness of nonspecific active immunotherapy in human malignancy (Gutterman *et al.*, 1973, 1974a,b), there are several difficulties inherent in the use of living materials. For example, the dose of living BCG is difficult to standardize because of differences in numbers of viable and nonviable organisms in various preparations and from various lots. In addition, dead BCG organisms and/or free antigen, which predominate in the currently available preparations, have demonstrated suppressive effects on cell-mediated immunity (Mackaness *et al.*, 1973) and, therefore, may not be beneficial to the cancer patient. The infectious nature of BCG also results in the complication of systemic BCG disease, at least after intratumoral injection (Sparks *et al.*, 1973). It may also be useful to develop other immuno-adjuvants because (1) different adjuvants have different mechanisms of action; (2) different adjuvants may be given by different routes, thereby having different regional effects; (3) different malignancies may respond to different adjuvants because mechanisms of immunological control may vary; (4) different adjuvants may have different toxicities, and because (5) some of these factors may permit the development of effective combined adjuvant therapy.

C. parvum is an active immunopotentiating agent in various animal tumor models (Halpern *et al.*, 1966; Woodruff and Boak, 1966; Currie and Bagshawe, 1970). *Corynebacterium granulosum* (a closely related species) administered intravenously was more effective than *C. granulosum* administered subcutaneously in the therapy of artificially induced pulmonary metastases (Milas *et al.*, 1974a). In addition, intravenous, but not subcutaneous *C. parvum* is associated with regression of established subcutaneous disease in a rat fibrosarcoma model (Milas *et al.*, 1974b). In humans, *C. parvum* given subcutaneously with chemotherapy is effective in prolonging the survival of patients with metastatic solid tumors as compared to patients who received chemotherapy alone (Israel and Halpern, 1972).

Based on these data and the need for other nonspecific immuno-adjuvants, we conducted a Phase I clinical and immunological study of *C. parvum* in patients with advanced malignancy. The study defined the toxicity of this agent and demonstrated that *C. parvum* can be given safely, on repeated occasions, by both the intravenous and subcutaneous routes. Augmentation of *in vitro* lymphocyte blastogenic responses to T-cell mitogens, no change in established delayed-hypersensitivity, and a transient decrease in circulating lymphocytes and monocytes were observed after intravenous administration.

Materials and Methods

Sixty-six patients were entered in this Phase I study between November 23, 1973 and April 30, 1974. All patients had widely disseminated malignancy and were considered to have a limited life expectancy (1–6 months). All patients had previously failed to respond to, or had relapsed on, a Phase II or III chemotherapy or chemo-immunotherapy protocol. Informed consent was obtained from each patient.

Thirty-one patients were treated with subcutaneous (s.c.) *C. parvum.* There were 12 males and 19 females with a median age of 51 years (range 18–79). Thirty-five patients were treated with intravenous (i.v.) *C. parvum.* There were 18 males and 17 females with a median age of 50 years (range 17–72).

The types of malignancies of the treated patients are listed on Table I. Of the 66 patients, 35 (53%) had malignant melanoma, 13 had acute leukemia, and 18 had malignant lymphoma, breast cancer, squamous-cell cancer, colon cancer, or thyroid cancer.

Drug, Dosage, and Schedule

A formalin-killed preparation of *C. parvum* was supplied by the Burroughs-Wellcome Company of Research Triangle Park, North Carolina. Lots used in these studies were #335K and #7691. Each multidose vial contained 7 mg/ml of formalin-killed *C. parvum* in suspension and was stored at 4°C until used. For s.c. injections, *C. parvum* was given into the deltoid or gluteal areas. Doses greater than 1 ml were divided into multiple injection sites. The i.v. doses of *C. parvum* were mixed with 200 ml of D_5W and were infused over a period ranging from 1–4 h.

Table I. Diagnoses of Patients in Phase I Study of *Corynebacterium parvum* Therapy

Type of malignancy	Route of administration[a]	
	Subcutaneous	Intravenous
Malignant melanoma	15	20
Acute leukemia	7	6
Sarcoma	2	7
Malignant lymphoma	2	—
Miscellaneous solid tumors	5	2

[a]Number of patients in group.

Table II. Phase I Study of *Corynebacterium parvum*: Doses Administered

Dose level, mg/m^2	Subcutaneous[a]	Intravenous[a]
1	—	6
2	6	10
3	6	6
4.5	6	—
5	—	6
6.75	8	—
7.5	—	7
10	5	—

[a]Number of patients in group.

The dose escalations used in this study are shown on Table II. Since 4 mg given s.c. once a week appeared to offer therapeutic benefit without major toxicity in man (Israel and Halpern, 1972), we elected to start at a s.c. dose of 2 mg/m^2. Six patients were entered at dose levels of 2, 3, and 4.5 mg/m^2, respectively. Eight patients were treated with 6.75 mg/m^2 and, 5 patients were treated with a dose of 10 mg/m^2. Half the patients were treated approximately weekly, and the other half were treated once a month. Since most of the Phase I chemotherapy drugs which these patients also received were given for 5 consecutive days (days 1–5 of the study), patients who received *C. parvum* approximately weekly were actually treated on days 7, 12, and 17 of each 21–28-day cycle. Dosages were kept constant for each patient.

Since it seemed likely that greater toxicity would be associated with i.v. administration and since there were no published data regarding this route, the initial i.v. dose of *C. parvum* was 1 mg/m^2. Six patients were treated with 1 mg/m^2, ten with 2 mg/m^2, six with 3 mg/m^2 and 5 mg/m^2, respectively, and seven with 7.5 mg/m^2.

Clinical Evaluation and Follow-up

Patients were evaluated using the following methods: physical examination; complete blood count, including differential white blood count and platelet count; liver and renal function tests; chest x-ray; fibrinogen–fibrin split products; plasma hemoglobin; and serum haptoglobin. These studies were done to detect possible organ damage, hemolysis, or coagulopathy induced by immunological reactions to *C. parvum,* such as the Schwartzman phenomenon.

The physical examination, blood counts, and blood chemistries were repeated approximately every two months for patients receiving subcutaneous doses of *C. parvum.* During the initial phases of the study, the above evaluation was done prior to the i.v. administration of *C. parvum* and was repeated either immediately after, or 24 h after infusion. Changes in levels of formed-blood elements were evaluated statistically by the Wilcoxon signed-rank test. After it was determined that there was no immediate effect on any of these parameters, except for the circulating formed elements of the blood (see results), the extensive evaluation was repeated monthly.

Immunological Evaluation

Forty-eight hours prior to *C. parvum* administration, skin tests were applied by intradermal injection of six established delayed-hypersensitivity antigens, as previously described. The antigens were dermatophytin, dermatophytin-0, *Candida,* streptokinase-streptodornase, mumps, and a purified protein derivative of tuberculin (PPD) (Gutterman *et al.,* 1973). The average diameter of induration of two right-angle measurements at 24 and 48 h was recorded in millimeters. A positive skin test was interpreted as any measurable induration, which from a practical point was 2 mm or greater. The skin tests were repeated monthly for the first three months and every three months thereafter.

Lymphocyte blastogenic responses to a variety of mitogens and antigens were carried out as described previously (Hersh *et al.,* 1970). Freshly drawn, defibrinated venous blood was dextran-sedimented to obtain leukocyte-rich serum. One million lymphocytes in 1 ml of autologous serum and 2 ml of medium were stimulated with various doses of phytohemagglutinin (PHA), concanavalin A (Con-A), pokeweed mitogen (PWM), and streptolysin "0" (SLO).

Table III. Phase I Study of *Corynebacterium parvum:* Number of Doses per Patient

Number doses given	Number of patients	
	Subcutaneous	Intravenous
1	31	35
2	27	28
3	23	22
4	22	14
5	20	6
6	15	2
7	12	2
8	11	
9	8	
10	4	
11	2	
12	2	

**Table IV. Symptoms Associated with Intravenous
Administration of *Corynebacterium parvum***

Symptoms	% Patients	% Infusions
Chills	87	70
Fever $> 101°F$	75	60
Nausea and vomiting	55	40
Headache	24	12
Malaise	24	12
Hypotension[a]	6	2
Hypertension[b]	6	2

[a]Hypotension was mild, no case under 90/60.
[b]Hypertension was mild, no case over 150/100.

The cultures were incubated at 37°C in 5% CO_2 in air for 5 days, and 2 μCi of ^{3}H-thymidine (SA 1.9 Ci/nmole) were added during the last 3 h. Incorporated thymidine was measured by liquid-scintillation counting. Net counts per minute (cpm) of stimulated cultures were determined by subtraction of the amount of thymidine incorporated by 10^6 unstimulated lymphocytes. The stimulation index was determined by dividing the gross counts of the stimulated culture by those of the unstimulated control. The significance of differences between lymphocytes blastogenic response before and after *C. parvum* was tested by the Wilcoxon signed-rank test.

Results

The number of doses given by each route of administration is indicated in Table III. The maximum number of s.c. injections was 12, and the maximum number of i.v. doses given was 7. Administration of additional doses is continuing on schedule.

The side effects encountered with the i.v. route of administration are shown in Table IV. While in the treatment program, 87% of the patients had chills within 4 h after infusion. Chills started approximately 2 h after the initiation of the infusion, regardless of the speed of the infusion. Although the majority of the chills were mild, 30% of the chills were vigorous, lasting as long as 20–30 min. Occasionally, a patient reported mild recurrent chills after a time interval of a few minutes to a few hours following the cessation of the first chill. Only 70% of the infusions were associated with chills. There was a tendency for the chills to decrease in severity, or to disappear, with repeated infusions. This tendency was also noted for the other side effects listed in Table IV. Patients receiving the higher doses (5–7.5 mg/m^2) did not experience an increased severity or higher incidence of side effects. The decreased severity of side effects with repeated doses and the lack of increased severity with increasing doses may be partly explained by the fact that the intravenous infusion time was progressively decreased as the study continued. Thus, the patients who were given 1 mg/m^2, received the *C. parvum* over a 4-h period. As this dose was repeated in these patients and as new patients were entered at higher doses, the infusion time was progressively decreased to one hour. Currently, we feel that a 1-h infusion is safe and may be associated with less toxicity than the 3- to 4-h infusion.

Initially, attempts were made to control the chills with diphenhydramine. However, this achieved only minimal effectiveness. Morphine sulfate given subcutaneously was more effective in rapidly aborting the rigors, but patients receiving morphine seemed to experience more intense and prolonged nausea and vomiting.

Fever usually started 4–12 h after infusion and ranged up to 105°F. The fevers usually subsided within 3–6 h. However, after receiving the initial dose of *C. parvum*, two patients had fever lasting for 24–36 h. With subsequent doses, both patients experienced fever of 3–6 h duration.

Mild hypotension (not less than 90/60) occurred in two patients. The first patient was a 61-year-old female with disseminated melanoma who received 2 mg/m^2 of *C. parvum*. She had this side effect only with the first infusion, and not with the two subsequent infusions. The second patient was a 29-year-old female with disseminated melanoma who received 3 mg/m^2 of *C. parvum*. She had this side effect with the first two infusions, and not with subsequent infusions. Two patients had transient episodes of mild hypertension (not exceeding 150/100). Although all of the cardiovascular changes seen so far have been mild, their occurrence points out that careful evaluation of cardiovascular status of patients prior to the intravenous administration of *C. parvum* must be carried

Table V. Local Symptoms and Signs Associated with Subcutaneous Administration of *Corynebacterium parvum*

Reaction	% Patients
Soreness	100
Induration	60
Erythema	40
Lymphadenopathy	0

out, and a medical decision regarding the use of this agent must be made in each case. The remainder of the side effects noted were mild, of limited duration, and required no symptomatic therapy.

Patients receiving s.c. *C. parvum* experienced the local reactions shown in Table V. All patients experienced soreness at the site of injection, starting immediately after the injection and lasting for several hours to a few days. The soreness, as well as erythema and induration, was mild and easily tolerated without symptomatic therapy. Two patients experienced local soreness which persisted the entire time between doses of *C. parvum*. The first patient received 4.5 mg/m^2, with a total dose of 8 mg in 1.14 ml initially given all at one s.c. site. By dividing the dose to two sites, the local soreness was lessened, but still persisted between doses. The second patient received 10 mg/m^2, for a total of 19 mg, given at two subcutaneous sites. It has been necessary to lengthen the time interval between s.c. doses in this patient. Further evaluation to ascertain whether this represents delayed hypersensitivity to the *C. parvum* or a local toxic phenomenon will be carried out by intradermal testing with *C. parvum*.

Although fever, malaise, and headache occurred in most patients receiving s.c. *C. parvum*, these symptoms were mild and rarely required symptomatic therapy. In one patient, it was necessary to prolong the interval between doses because of the occurrence of nausea, vomiting, headache, and fever of several days duration. One patient receiving s.c. *C. parvum* refused to continue therapy because of severe discomfort at the local injection site.

Preliminary evaluation of the immunological data on the i.v. *C. parvum*

Table VI. Comparison of Delayed Hypersensitivity to Recall Antigens of Patients on *Corynebacterium parvum* and a Historical Control Group[a]

Response to therapy	No change or decrease[b]		Increase[c]	
	Chemotherapy + *C. parvum*	Chemotherapy alone	Chemotherapy + *C. parvum*	Chemotherapy alone
Remission	0/2	5/21	2/2	21/26
Stable	4/10	10/28	6/10	18/28
Progression	12/13	37/37	1/13	0/37
Total number	16/25	52/91	9/25	39/91
percent	(64)	(57)	(36)	(43)

[a]Data from Hersh *et al.* (1972).
[b]Refers to skin-test reactivity; number of positive tests decreased or median diameter of battery decreased > 50%.
[c]Number of positive tests increased or median diameter increased > 100%.

Table VII. Delayed-Hypersensitivity Responses to Recall Antigens before and after *Corynebacterium parvum* Therapy

No change		Increase		Decrease	
Number positive tests	Number of patients	Number positive tests	Number of patients	Number positive tests	Number of patients
0–0[a]	5[b]	0–1	2	1–0	2
2–2	2	0–2	3	2–0	2
4–4	1	1–2	1	2–1	1
		1–3	1	3–0	1
		2–3	1	3–1	1
				3–2	1
				5–3	1
Total	8		8		9

[a]Number of positive skin tests before and after *C. parvum*. Second number is last post-therapy test. The battery of 5 skin tests included dermatophytin, dermatophytin-0, *Candida*, Varidase, and mumps.
[b]Number of patients with indicated pre–post *C. parvum* changes or lack of changes in skin-test reactivity.

patients showed that delayed-hypersensitivity responses to the battery of established recall antigens correlated predominantly with the response of the patient to chemo-immunotherapy (Table VI). Nine of 25 patients tested while on i.v. *C. parvum* showed an improvement in skin-test response. This was defined as an increased number of, or >100% increase in the diameter of the tests. Two patients showed an improvement in their disease while being treated, and both also had increased skin-test responses. Ten patients had stable diseases, and 6 of these had increased skin-test responses. Of the 13 patients with progressive diseases, only one showed an increase response to the battery of recall antigens. Table VI compares these results with a similar study done previously (Hersh *et al.*, 1972) in patients receiving chemotherapy alone. A very similar pattern of skin-test reactivity and prognosis was seen in these patients. This impression was confirmed by the data shown in Tables VII and VIII. Thus, the numbers of patients whose delayed-hypersensitivity reactions increased, decreased, or remained unchanged were approximately equal. Also, the total numbers of positive skin tests and the mean and median diameters of all skin tests did not change in the 4-month follow-up period in the 25 patients treated with i.v. *C. parvum*. No clear-cut relationship of dose to response was noted.

The lymphocytes of 11 patients treated with i.v. *C. parvum* were studied for lymphocyte blastogenic responses to various ranges of PHA, PWM, and Con-A,

Table VIII. Delayed-Hypersensitivity Responses before and after *Corynebacterium parvum* Therapy

Test periods[a]	1	2	3	4
Number of tests[b]	115	115	100	55
Number positive	30	30	21	14
% Positive	26	26	21	25
Diameters[c]				
Median	0	0	0	0
Range	0–23	0–23	0–17.5	0–26
Mean	2.11	2.44	1.96	3.24
S.D.	4.55	4.88	4.78	6.96

[a]Test periods: 1, immediately pretherapy; 2, 3, and 4, post-therapy at 1- to 4-week intervals.
[b]This represents a complete tabulation of all individual tests done in these patients.
[c]No significant differences between different test periods.

Table IX. Association of Lymphocyte Blastogenic Responses with Therapy with Intravenous *Corynebacterium parvum*

Mitogen	Concentration[a]	Parameter	Net CPM[b]		S.I.[c]	
			pre	post[d]	pre	post
PHA[a]	1.0	mean	70.9	90.2	161.0	88.9
		S.D.	51.4	35.8	166.3	62.3
		median	60.9	90.4	69.4	60.0
PHA	0.5	mean	53.7	102.2	107.9	117.0
		S.D.	38.0	72.4	121.1	121.7
		median	49.4	75.3	61.7	84.9
PHA	0.1	mean	9.2	35.6	20.6	30.9
		S.D.	11.8	51.7	30.4	46.7
		median	2.3	6.2	8.6	10.5

[a]Relative concentration of phytohemagglutinin-M (PHA) 1.0 = 0.05 ml per 3-ml culture. Standard dilution of PHA (5 ml/vial).
[b]Counts per minute per 10^6 lymphocytes $\times$ 10^{-3}.
[c]Stimulation index, CPM in PHA culture divided by CPM in control.
[d]Significance data: PHA, CPM at 0.1 concentration significantly higher post-*C. parvum* by Wilcoxon's signed-rank test, $P = 0.05$; 0.5 and 1.0 not significant.

and to individual doses of SLO and KLH. The data are tabulated in Tables IX–XI for the 3 nonspecific mitogens. The data shown are the immediate pre-*C. parvum* evaluation and the last post-*C. parvum* evaluation done, usually at 1–2 months. Responses to the lowest *in vitro* concentration of PHA and to all three doses of Con-A increased after *C. parvum* therapy (Tables IX and X), while responses to PWM (Table XI) and SLO did not change significantly. These data suggest that *C. parvum* may augment T-cell responsiveness, at least to mitogens *in vitro*.

The patients treated i.v. with *C. parvum* all had blood counts immediately before and either immediately (0–4 h) or 24 h after the injection. Blood counts were subsequently obtained at approximately weekly intervals. The data on the immediate and 24-h counts are shown in Tables XII–XIV. Follow-up data are not shown, since changes at 1 week or later were attributed to drug effect from the associated chemotherapy. No effects at 0–4 or 24 h were seen on the hemoglobin or platelet counts. The lymphocyte counts fell significantly at 24 h, but not at 0–4 h, while the monocyte count fell at 0–4 h, but not at 24 h. There was no significant change in the granulocyte count. Interpretation of these data is complicated by the fact that the patients in this study were generally somewhat leukopenic as a result of prior therapy and advanced disease. No clear-cut relationship of dose to response was noted.

Table X. Association of Lymphocyte Blastogenic Responses with Therapy with Intravenous *Corynebacterium parvum*

Mitogen	Concentration[a]	Parameter	Net CPM[b]		S.I.[c]	
			pre	post[d]	pre	post
Con-A[a]	1.0	mean	17.9	33.3	32.3	28.5
		S.D.	17.4	30.4	36.0	20.3
		median	12.2	30.8	20.4	32.3
Con-A	0.5	mean	15.6	36.3	27.5	34.2
		S.D.	10.3	32.7	19.5	37.3
		median	17.2	28.0	25.0	28.4
Con-A	0.1	mean	5.5	11.3	9.8	14.6
		S.D.	6.0	14.8	11.1	29.1
		median	2.4	3.1	7.4	4.2

[a]Relative concentration of concanavalin A (Con-A) 1.0 = 80 μg/3 ml culture.
[b]Counts per minute per 10^6 lymphocytes $\times 10^{-3}$.
[c]Stimulation index.
[d]Significance data: Con-A, CPM at 1.0, 0.5, and 0.1 concentrations, significantly higher post-*C. parvum* by Wilcoxon's signed-rank test, $P = 0.05$.

Table XI. Association of Lymphocyte Blastogenic Responses with Therapy with Intravenous *Corynebacterium parvum*

Mitogen	Concentration[a]	Parameters	Net CPM[b] pre	Net CPM[b] post	S.I.[c] pre	S.I.[c] post
PWM[a]	1.0	mean	25.0	31.7	65.4	21.9
		S.D.	16.6	28.4	48.7	15.0
		median	21.2	29.2	38.9	26.6
PWM	0.5	mean	28.8	29.8	61.8	80.1
		S.D.	23.9	27.2	68.8	28.5
		median	28.6	24.5	30.5	20.1
PWM	0.1	mean	29.4	50.3	60.7	67.6
		S.D.	25.2	38.8	52.9	68.9
		median	18.1	37.0	46.3	39.9

[a]Relative concentration of pokeweed mitogen (PWM), 1.0 = 0.05 ml per 3 ml (standard vial diluted with 5 mg).
[b]Counts per minute per 10^6 lymphocytes $\times 10^{-3}$.
[c]Stimulation index.
[d]No significant differences pre- vs post-treatment.

Table XII. Changes in Absolute Lymphocyte Counts Associated with *Corynebacterium parvum* Therapy

Parameter	Pre-therapy	Immediate post-therapy	24 h post-therapy
Number of studies	66	38	28
Median	600[a]	450[b]	400[c]
Range	10–2300	0–2100	10–1200
Mean	670	530	400
S.D.	330	360	320
Number decline			
100–249		3	7
250–499		5	7
500–999		5	6
≥ 1000		1	–
Number increase			
100–249		12	3
250–499		2	1
≥ 500		1	–
No change or < 100		9	4

[a]Absolute lymphocyte count in cells per mm^3.
[b]Pre- vs. immediate post-therapy evaluations were not significantly different.
[c]Pre- vs. 24-h post-therapy evaluations were significantly different by Wilcoxon's signed-rank test, $P = 0.01$.

Table XIII. Changes in Absolute Monocyte Counts Associated with *Corynebacterium parvum* Therapy

Parameter	Pre-therapy	Immediate post–therapy	24 h post-therapy
Number of studies	66	38	28
Median	0^a	0^b	0^c
Range	0–500	0–300	0–1000
Mean	193	115	267
S.D.	131	96	288
Number decline			
10–99		5	2
100–199		4	2
200–299		2	–
⩾ 300		2	1
Number increase			
10–99		1	2
100–199		2	3
200–299		–	–
⩾ 300		–	1
No change or < 10		22	16

[a]Absolute monocyte count in cells per mm^3.
[b]Pre- vs. immediate post-treatment evaluations were significantly different by Wilcoxon's signed-rank test, $P = 0.05$.
[c]Pre- vs. 24-h post-treatment evaluations were not significantly different.

Table XIV. Changes in Absolute Granulocyte Counts Associated with *Corynebacterium parvum* Therapy

Parameter	Pre-therapy	Immediate post-therapy	24 h post–therapy
Number of studies	66	38	28
Median	2300^a	2250^b	1450^c
Range	0–11.2	0–11.7	0–8.9
Mean	2570	2750	2200
S.D.	2240	2510	2380
Number decline			
100–249		5	2
250–499		4	1
500–999		5	1
⩾ 1000		3	3
Number increase			
100–249		6	2
250–499		5	1
500–999		3	3
⩾ 1000		4	7
No change or < 100		3	8

[a]Absolute granulocyte count in cells per mm^3.
[b]Pre- vs. immediate post-treatment evaluations were not significantly different.
[c]Pre- vs. 24-h post-treatment evaluations were not significantly different.

Discussion

This preliminary analysis of an ongoing Phase I study suggests that *C. parvum* is safe when given by either the intravenous or the subcutaneous route.

C. parvum administered i.v. was clearly associated with more systemic toxicity than s.c. *C. parvum.* However, in general, the chills and fever experienced with intravenous *C. parvum* decreased with repeated doses. The reasons for this are not clear. It is conceivable that this decrease is due to an increase in anti-*C. parvum* antibody, with rapid clearing of opsonized material from the circulation. Antibody-titer studies are now underway to clarify this. The major side effects of chills and fever also did not increase with increasing doses of *C. parvum,* at least with the dose range reported in this paper. Although cardiovascular side effects were mild and uncommon, caution should be used in patients with a previous history of cardiovascular or pulmonary disease, and a medical decision regarding the risks of mild hyper- or hypotension must be made in each case.

The biological significance of the decreases in circulatory lymphocytes and monocytes following a dose of intravenous *C. parvum* is not understood. A similar decrease in circulating lymphocyte counts has been observed in the mouse (Woodruff and Dunbar, 1973). Trapping of lymphocytes and/or monocytes in the spleen or other areas may account for some of these changes (Zatz *et al.,* 1973). Whether these phenomena would occur after repeated intravenous infusion in man is not known. The change in monocytes was immediate, while in the lymphocytes it was delayed. The former might indicate a rapid response of the RES to antigen, while the latter might reflect the results of stress. The changes in lymphocyte and monocyte count were moderate, even though this population was both lymphopenic and monocytopenic, presumably as a result of advanced disease and prior therapy.

In a small subset of the patients treated with i.v. *C. parvum,* the *in vitro* lymphocyte blastogenic response to the T-cell mitogen PHA and to Con-A increased, while PWM and SLO responses did not change. Many possibilities exist to explain this, including mobilization of T cells, selective depletion of B cells, maturation of T cells, etc. Also, the effects of the chemotherapy that the patients received must also be considered. This is in contrast to observations made by Scott (1972), in which *C. parvum* given to mice was associated with a profound decrease in T-cell function. The doses used in the animals, however, were larger than those used in our studies. Despite suppression of T-cell function, these doses have been associated with profound antitumor effects in the animals. It is conceivable that higher doses of *C. parvum* may suppress, while smaller doses may augment, T-cell function. Since T cells, B cells, and macrophages have all been implicated in the destruction of human and animal tumors— depending on the model studied and the assays used (Freedman *et al.,* 1970; Lamon *et al.,* 1972, O'Toole *et al.,* 1973; Basic *et al.,* 1974), careful evaluation and correlation of the immunologic and clinical effects of *C. parvum*, administered in different doses, by different routes, and in different schedules will be very helpful in the development of optimal therapeutic programs. One of the weaknesses of the current study is that no measurements of macrophage function or macrophage activation were carried out. Studies of particle clearance from the peripheral blood, the local cutaneous-inflammatory response, and pulmonary-macrophage exudation can all be conducted in man and should add considerably to our knowledge of adjuvant action.

In patients receiving *C. parvum*, the delayed-hypersensitivity reactivity to recall antigens did not change during therapy and was not significantly different from a previously studied group of patients receiving chemotherapy alone. This also suggests that the antitumor activity observed in animal systems may, in part, be due to a nonlymphocyte mechanism such as macrophage activation. Further evaluation of skin-test response at higher doses and with a longer follow-up period may reveal changes in skin-test responses.

Our previous experience with BCG combined with chemotherapy in advanced melanoma suggests that one of its major actions is to increase the response rate in the areas regional to the BCG administration (Gutterman *et al.*, in press). The concept of regional immunotherapy, a prerequisite for maximal suppression of tumor growth in many (Milas *et al.*, 1974a,b; Zbar *et al.*, 1971), but not all (Yron *et al.*, 1973), animal tumor models, may be an important consideration for future design of immunotherapy trials. Thus, the use of intravenous *C. parvum* for patients with lung cancer or pulmonary metastases could have great potential. Phase II studies with detailed immunological evaluation are now indicated to test these hypotheses and to determine the spectrum of activity of *C. parvum* in the treatment of patients with both solid tumors and leukemia.

Despite the apparent safety of *C. parvum*, the side effects—as described in this paper—are significant. Therefore, the development of subcellular fractions of *C. parvum* which retain the antitumor activity, but have reduced side effects, are needed.

Other areas which require investigation are a careful study of the kinetics (on a day to day basis) of the immunological effects of *C. parvum* on host-defense mechanisms and characterization of the immune response to *C. parvum* itself and how this interrelates to its immunopotentiating action.

Addendum: Since this analysis, 6 patients have received 10 mg/m^2 *C. parvum* i.v. Acute toxicity does seem to be more severe at this dose and includes recurrent chills and high fever lasting up to 36 h, severe myalgias, muscle weakness, and cyanosis during and immediately after the infusion. Also one patient receiving 7.5 mg/m^2 *C. parvum* underwent a generalized Schwartzman reaction with acute azotemia and severe thrombocytopenia, which did not clear until 10 days after its occurrence.

Summary

A Phase I clinical and immunological study of *Corynebacterium parvum* immunization was carried out in 66 patients with advanced metastatic malignancy. The study is still in progress, and this paper discusses preliminary observations. Thirty-five patients received intravenous (i.v.) *C. parvum* in doses ranging from 1 to 7.5 mg/m^2, given either once or twice per month. Thirty-one patients received subcutaneous (s.c.) *C. parvum* in doses ranging from 2 to 10 mg/m^2, given weekly or monthly. Chills and fever higher than 101°F developed in 87% and 75% respectively of the patients treated with i.v. *C. parvum*. Transient, mild hypotension was noted in 6% of the patients (90/60), but no life-threatening morbidity was observed. Soreness at the site of injection and mild fever less than 101°F were experienced by 100% and 90% of patients who received s.c. *C. parvum*. Other side effects included nausea and vomiting in 55% and headache in 24% of the i.v. group, and local induration and/or nodule formation in 60% of the s.c. group. Toxic side effects did not increase in frequency, intensity, or duration with increasing doses within the dose range studied. There was no impairment of liver, renal, or coagulation function attributable to *C. parvum* in any of the 66 patients. In general, both i.v. and s.c. *C. parvum* were well tolerated. No serious or life-threatening complications or side effects were observed. On the other hand, occasional patients did have severe symptomatic toxicity lasting over 24 h, making the therapy difficult to tolerate. *In vitro* lymphocyte blastogenic responses to T-cell mitogens appeared to be augmented by *C. parvum* administered i.v. There was no definite change in delayed-hypersensitivity responses to a battery of recall antigens. Peripheral blood monocyte and lymphocyte counts showed a moderate decrease 4–24 h following an i.v. dose of *C. parvum*. *C. parvum* given i.v. or s.c. appears to be a safe material for use in human cancer therapy. Careful monitoring of vital functions during, and for 24 h after, i.v. administration of *C. parvum* is mandatory.

Acknowledgments

We acknowledge the excellent technical assistance of Mrs. Annette Matthews, Ms. Cathy Dandridge, Ms. Karen Terry, Ms. Shirley Malarchuk, and Ms. Clarice Murray. In addition, we acknowledge the support and helpful discussions of Dr. J. Whisnant and Burroughs Wellcome Company, Triangle Park, North Carolina.

References

Basic, I., Milas, L., Grdina, D. J., and Withers, H. R. (1974). Destruction of hamster ovarian cell cultures by peritoneal macrophages from mice treated with *Corynebacterium granulosum. J. Natl. Cancer Inst.* 52:1839–1842.

Bluming, A. A., Vogel, C. L., Ziegler, J. L., *et al.* (1972). Immunological effects of BCG in malignant melanoma: two modes of administration compared. *Ann. Intern. Med.* 76: 405–411.

Currie, G. A. and Bagshawe, K. D. (1970). Active immunotherapy with *Corynebacterium parvum* and chemotherapy in murine fibrosarcoma. *Br. Med. J.* 1:541–544.

Donaldson, R. C. (1972). Methotrexate plus *Bacillus Calmette-Guerin* (BCG) and isoniazid in the treatment of cancer of the head and neck. *Am. J. Surg.* 124:527–534.

Freedman, L. R., Cerottini, J. C., and Brunner, K. T. (1970). *In vivo* studies of the role of cytotoxic T cells in tumor allograft immunity. *J. Immunol.* 109:1371–1378.

Gutterman, J. U., Mavligit, G., McBride, C., Frei, E. III, and Hersh, E. M. (1973). Active immunotherapy with BCG for recurrent malignant melanoma. *Lancet* 1:1208–1212.

Gutterman, J. U., Mavligit, G. M., Gottlieb, J. A., Burgess, M. A., McBride, C. M., Einhorn, L. A., Freireich, E. J., and Hersh, E. M. (1974a). Chemoimmunotherapy of disseminated malignant melanoma with dimethyl triazeno imidazole carboximide (DTIC) and *Bacillus Calmette-Guerin* (BCG). *New Engl. J. Med.* 291:592–597.

Gutterman, J. U., Rodriguez, V., Mavligit, G. M., Burgess, M. A., Gehan, E., Hersh, E. M., McCredie, K. B., Reed, R. C., Smith, T., Bodey, G. P., and Freireich, E. J. (1974b). Chemoimmunotherapy of acute leukemia, prolongation of remission in acute myeloblastic leukemia with BCG. *Lancet* 2:1405–1409.

Halpern, B. N., Biozzi, G., Stiffel, C., and Mouton, D. (1966). Inhibition of tumor growth by administration of killed *Corynebacterium parvum*. *Nature (Lond.)* 212:853–854.

Hersh, E. M., Harris, J. E., and Rogers, E. A. (1970). Influence of cell density on response of leukocytes and column purified lymphocytes to mitogenic agents. *Reticuloendothel. Soc.* 7:567.

Hersh, E. M., Curtis, J. E., Butler, W. T., Rossen, R. D., and Cheema, A. R. (1972). Host defense failure. In: *The Etiology and Pathogenesis of Malignant Disease in Environment and Career*, pp. 407–427, The Williams and Wildins Co., Baltimore, Md.

Israel, L. and Halpern, B. (1972). *Corynebacterium parvum* in advanced human cancers. First evaluation of therapeutic activity of this stimulin. *Nouv. Presse Med.* 1:19–23.

Lamon, E. W., Skurzak, H. M., Klein, E., and Wigzell, H. (1972). *In vitro* cytotoxicity by a nonthymus-processed lymphocyte population with specificity for a virally determined tumor cell surface antigen. *J. Exp. Med.* 136:1072–1079.

Mackaness, G. B., Auclair, D. J., and Lagrange, P. H. (1973). Immunopotentiation with BCG. I. The immune response to different strains and preparations. *J. Natl. Cancer Inst.* 51:1655–1667.

Mathé, G., Amiel, J. L., Schwarzenberg, L., *et al.* (1969). Active immunotherapy for acute lymphoblastic leukemia. *Lancet* 2:697–699.

Milas, L., Hunter, N., and Withers, H. R. (1974a). *Corynebacterium granulosum* induced protection against artificial pulmonary metastases of a syngenic fibrosarcoma in mice. *Cancer Res.* 34:613–620.

Milas, L., Gutterman, J. U., Basic, I., Hunter, N., Mavligit, G., Hersh, E. M. and Withers, H. R. (1974b). Immunoprophylaxis and immunotherapy for a murine fibrosarcoma with *C. granulosum* and *C. parvum*. *Int. J. Cancer* 14:493–503.

O'Toole, C., Perlmann, P., Wigzell, G., Unsgaard, G., and Zetterlund, C. G. (1973). Lymphocyte cytotoxicity in bladder cancer. No requirement for thymus-derived effector cells? *Lancet* 1:1085–1089.

Powles, R. L., Crowther, D., Bateman, C. J. T., *et al.* (1973). Immunotherapy for acute myelogenous leukemia. *Br. J. Cancer* 28:365–376.

Scott, M. T. (1972). Biological effects of the adjuvant *Corynebacterium parvum*. I. Inhibition of PHA, mixed lymphocyte and GVH reactivity. *Cell. Immunol.* 5:459–468.

Sokal, J. E., Aungst, C. W., and Grace, J. T., Jr. (1973). Immunotherapy in well controlled chronic myelocytic leukemia. *NY State J. Med.* 73:1180–1185.

Sokal, J. E., Aungst, C. W., and Snyderman, M. (1974). Prolongation of remission in stage I and II lymphoma by BCG vaccination. *Proc. Am. Assoc. Cancer Res.* 15:13.

Sparks, F. C., Silverstein, M. J., Hunt, J. S., Haskell, C. M., Pilch, Y. H., and Morton, D. L. (1973). Complications of BCG immunotherapy in patients with cancer. *New Engl. J. Med.* **289**:827–830.

Vogel, W. R. and Chan, Y-K. (1974). Effect of *Bacillus-Calmette Guerin* (BCG) in prolongation of remissions in acute myeloblastic leukemia (AML). *Lancet* **2**:128–131.

Woodruff, M. F. A. and Boak, J. L. (1966). Inhibitory effect of injections of *Corynebacterium parvum* on the growth of tumor transplants in isogenic hosts. *Br. J. Cancer* **20**:345–355.

Woodruff, M. F. A. and Dunbar, N. (1973). The effect of *Corynebacterium parvum* and other reticuloendothelial stimulants on transplanted tumors in mice. In: *Immunopotentiation* (Ciba Foundation Symposium 18), Associated Scientific Publishers.

Yron, I., Weiss, D. W., Robinson, E., *et al.* (1973). Immunotherapeutic experiments in mice with the methanol extraction residue (MER) fraction of BCG: solid tumors. *Natl. Cancer Inst. Monogr.* **39**:33–35.

Zatz, M., White, A., and Goldstein, A. (1973). Alterations in lymphocyte populations in tumorigenesis. I. Lymphocyte trapping. *J. Immunol.* **111**:706–711.

Zbar, B., Bernstein, I. D., and Rapp, H. J. (1971). Suppression of tumor growth at the site of infection with living *Bacillus Calmette-Guerin*. *J. Natl. Cancer Inst.* **46**:831–839.

DISCUSSION

WANEBO: It is difficult to know how to begin to discuss this series of papers. Dr. Carter has illustrated an interesting and important set of guidelines which all of us could follow when we begin our studies on patients using *Corynebacterium parvum* and other immunostimulants.

I might suggest that it would be useful to start now to use a two-pronged approach combining the beginning of Phase II with Phase I. Although this is a little different from the classic approach, it seems necessary with certain tumors.

We are investigating the effects of *C. parvum* on three tumors: lung, colon, and gastric cancers. The protocols are still in the formulation stage, but we have started to use them on a few patients.

The group with colon cancers is comprised of patients with nonresectable, recurrent or residual disease, or metastatic disease. Our previous experience with about 300 patients with advanced colon cancers treated with chemotherapy gave us useful historical information on which to base this protocol: Patients' advanced rectal colon cancer can be categorized into 4 distinctive groups or patterns: local recurrence, liver metastases, intra-abdominal metastases, or generalized disease; of course, intermediate patterns can also occur.

Our plan is to compare radiation with chemotherapy, here termed My FuCA, which is mytomycin C_1, 5 FU, and cytosine arabinoside. *C. parvum* will be given in a randomized fashion to patients in these two major treatment groups. We have initiated a Phase II study because of the short-term nature of this disease, most of these patients living less than a year. We used the dosage, at least initially outlined, by Dr. Israel, which we hope to modify with our own Phase I study, and the results from studies such as those of Dr. Reed.

We are also studying *C. parvum* in a Phase II program on operable lung cancer. Our conceptual approach was to take patients with stage 1 lung cancer. This is an operable cancer, patients having a solitary nodule either less than 3 cm or larger than 3 cm, but without mediastinal nodal metastases. These patients receive a radical lobectomy, or a pneumonectomy, at which time the node status is ascertained.

We have just started to use *C. parvum* with or without a cytotoxin in this group. Normally, a patient with a solitary nodule has a five-year survival prognosis of about 40%. The prognosis is greater than 40% for the smaller nodules, and less for the larger ones.

The second, a more significant group, has a greater number of patients. Over the course of a year, we saw 20 cases belonging to the first group and over 200 belonging to the second and third groups.

In the second group we are comparing cytoxin versus an intensive chemotherapy, and each group is further stratified or randomized for *C. parvum*. This group has about a 10% five-year survival rate.

The last group consists of patients with locally advanced disease, which is not resectable. Again, chemotherapy in high or low doses, with or without *C. parvum,* is being used.

For the purpose of illustration one patient's history is presented, though little can be inferred from this. The patient had a resectable adenocarcinoma of the lung. There were positive nodes. Initially, when he was operated on last December, he was completely anergic to DNCB, although his tuberculin was positive. At the beginning of the trial with *C. parvum* in February, he was completely negative to DNCB. At the five-week level, he developed a strong positivity to DNCB, even at a small dose; this was after five treatments with 4 mg of *C. parvum* in divided doses administered subcutaneously at four separate extremities. After about eight injections of *C. parvum,* this patient's blastogenic response to PHA, and appropriate mitogen, increased to a normal pattern. The amounts of his T and B cells were not changed, however, during the whole course of treatment.

We are just beginning to look at a Phase I study with *C. parvum,* and we hope to have detailed information on that in the near future.

With reference to Dr. Attié's paper, one of the issues which arises in the use of an invasive measurement for reticuloendothelial function is the potential toxicity. I wonder about the practical use of this when it is necessary to follow a patient with repeated doses. Can this microaggregated albumin be used in subsequent doses, and what overall toxicity might be expected? If such toxicity is too extensive, or too formidable, is it possible to use an *in vitro* test with the same agent?

Dr. Reed's paper is a magnificent start in the study of immune responses, as well as the toxicity of *C. parvum*. I think it will be a classic study.

As to the fever seen in these patients, I wonder whether there is a possibility of, for example, endotoxin being completely excluded from the preparation? Second, are there differences in the toxicities of the formalin-treated *C. parvum* and the heat-treated variety? This should be investigated.

It is interesting that blastogenic response, in general, shows an increase, rather than a decrease, which certainly suggests that there is T-cell stimulation. I had the impression from some of the experiments performed on animals that there was T-cell loss, as suggested by the loss of cortical lymphocytes in some of the histologic studies. However, it seems that, whatever PHA is stimulating, T-cell stimulation is increased.

BAND: Our experience with *C. parvum* is too recent to enable us to report on more than the toxicity data on a few patients. So far, we have treated seven patients at doses of 4 mg and 8 mg of *C. parvum*, given weekly by intramuscular injections. Tolerance to the drug has generally been good. Pain at the site of injection occurs commonly, though it tends to decrease with each subsequent injection and to disappear after the third or fourth injection. We are now mixing, at Dr. Israel's suggestion, *C. parvum* with 1 ml of hyaluronidase and xylocaine. Fever and a flu-like syndrome, lasting for 24–48 h, have been observed in two patients.

I would like to mention, in relation to Dr. Carter's questions, that the effects of nonspecific systemic immunotherapy, at this time, are too subtle to be quantitated in terms of tumor regression. Therefore, criteria of response to immunotherapy will have to be developed on a basis different from the standard criteria of response to chemotherapeutic drugs.

KOCHMAN: Our study consisted of investigating the effects of *C. parvum*, given subcutaneously, on the responsiveness of cancer patients' lymphocytes to mitogens, such as PHA, Con-A, or pokeweed. No significant difference was observed between untreated and treated patients. Most of our patients had lung carcinoma and some had been treated with cobalt irradiations.

We measured the mitogen effect by evaluation of DNA-labeled thymidine and uridine (RNA) incorporation. However, when vaccination against *Salmonella* was carried out with *Eberthella typhosa* with paratyphoid A and paratyphoid B *Salmonella*, there was a double titer of antibodies after the addition of *C. parvum* as compared to untreated patients.

From the results obtained, we conclude that administration of *C. parvum* consistently increased the antibody production, but did not affect the reactivity of lymphocytes to mitogens *in vitro*.

I should emphasize that the results mentioned were obtained on a rather small population.

WHISNANT: Those of us who have *recently* become involved in the burgeoning effort of cancer immunotherapy must stop, express our appreciation, and our respect for the pioneering and advanced work presented here. The early observations relating to anaerobic bacteriology, animal immunostimulation mechanisms of tumor rejection, and the clinical response all constitute the bequest of a firm foundation on which we can work. Rather than comment on the prototypic studies or even the studies presented here, I should like to briefly discuss some ideas for additional experiments. The inheritance which is ours should stimulate us to make clinical applications, but also to discover underlying principles and the basic biology of the immunostimulated host.

Four areas in which clinical protocols for cancer immunotherapy may make significant contributions are: (1) tumor immunity; (2) pharmacology and immunopharmacology; (3) host bacterial flora and their immunologic significance; and (4) the genetics of host immunity and tumor resistance.

The interest in *tumor immunity* has been apparent. We certainly hope that significant prolongation of life can be achieved with *C. parvum* vaccine. In addition, however, clinical protocols should be designed to find out (a) the role of lymphocyte killing and/or macrophage activation; (b) whether local, as opposed to systemic, or nodal, as opposed to splenic, immunostimulation is sufficient for therapy; (c) whether CEA or other fetal-like tumor-specific antigen—antibody levels and interactions are affected; (d) whether changes in homocytotropic antibody levels brought about by *C. parvum* play a role in tumor rejection. Moreover, the rather unique situation of tumor regression by an agent which causes T-cell suppression forces us to reevaluate our present understanding of tumor immunity. The recent observation by Dr. Martin Scott that splenectomy abolishes the *C. parvum* T-cell suppression is particularly relevant to this point [Scott, M. (1974). *Cell. Immunol.* 13:251].

The *pharmacologic,* including endocrine and metabolic, changes being studied in cancer patients are legion. Based on the observations of histamine sensitization and phenobarbital intolerance in mice treated with *C. parvum,* our patients theoretically may manifest (a) alteration in β-adrenergic reactivity, similar to anaphylactic hypersensitivity or allergies; (b) changes in levels of enzymes in monocytes or other cells; (c) increased or decreased half-lives of barbiturates, antihistamines, or chemotherapeutic agents; and, most assuredly, (d) cyclic AMP activation or inactivation. It is possible that some of these changes will give us basic information about the duration of the action of *C. parvum,* or about how this vaccine affects the immune response.

One of the most difficult problems in our clinical protocols will be the assessment of immune reactivity. This has been amply demonstrated by Dr. Reed's results. It would seem that the variability in pretreatment parameters is very large and that it will therefore be difficult to assess the response. An alternative to this apparent defect may rest in the elucidation of some of the base-line variabilities. If host immunologic status is due in part to the ongoing natural load of *bacterial colonization,* then *C. parvum* vaccination may be looked on as some increment in host immunostimulation. The variation in anaerobic corynebacterial colonization has been emphasized in recent studies by Hattori and Mori [Gann, (1973). **64**:7] and by Whiteside and Voss [*J. Invest. Dermatol.* **60**:94]. As the classification and immunochemistry of these organisms become better defined, it should be possible to study, and perhaps manipulate, the flora of the tumor-bearing animal or patient and to relate these changes to host immunostimulation. Certainly, we should be aware that results in conventional SPF or germ-free animals, as well as in patients on antibiotics or with septicemia, may not be entirely comparable. One other implication of bacteriologically oriented studies may be the definition of cross-reactive "tumor antigens" in the organisms themselves. In this case, it would not be surprising to achieve much better results with some tumors than with others.

The fourth item, host genetics, may not be applicable to clinical studies at present, for genes in man are not well defined. Genetic susceptibility, even to a virus infection, has only recently been reported and localized on its chromosome. Nevertheless, host immune response—under genetic control—will likely introduce variability into our studies. I solicit your suggestions for possible ways to learn more about this during our studies.

ADLAM: I have two questions. First, people are concerned that repeated intravenous injections of a material such as *C. parvum* could produce anaphylactic shock in recipient patients. Does Dr. Reed have any evidence of this occurring in his patients?

Second, in the studies on the blood cell numbers, were red cells counted? I am thinking about Dr. McBride's work with mice in which he demonstrated auto-immune hemolytic anemia following *C. parvum* treatment.

REED: In answer to the second question, we did blood counts, hemoglobins, hematocrits, and red cells; there was no significant change. One patient we infused showed a drop in his hemoglobin value in relation to the infusion of the *C. parvum*. However, he had also received chemotherapy; so the hemoglobin drop may have been due to that. As a result, we started studying the serum haptoglobins and plasma hemoglobins. We found no evidence of the destruction of red cells.

We have had no indication that anaphylaxis may be related to subsequent doses of *C. parvum*. I tried to point out that the symptoms decrease as the number of infusions increases—symptoms such as chills, fever, and so on.

HALPERN: For five years, we have been following the history of a few patients who received intradermal injections of *C. parvum*. We have never seen any allergic type of reaction in these patients during all this time. I was surprised not to find such reactions, because I expected them. However, it appears from animal experiments that *Corynebacterium* has a very low potency to sensitize in the manner of the typical allergic reaction known as type 1.

32

Results Obtained with Active Immunotherapy Using Corynebacteria *(Corynebacterium parvum* or *Corynebacterium granulosum)* in the Treatment of Acute Lymphoid Leukemia

L. SCHWARZENBERG and G. MATHÉ

Stimulation of immune defenses in animals can be induced before or after the establishment of a tumor; immunostimulation before the establishment of a tumor can be called immunoprophylaxis, and stimulation of immune reactions provoked after the tumor is established can be called immunotherapy.

Immunostimulation can be specific or nonspecific; it is called specific when intact or modified tumor cells or tumor-associated antigens are administered; it is nonspecific when immunity adjuvants are used. Using subcutaneously grafted

L. SCHWARZENBERG, Institut de Cancérologie et d'Immunogénétique, Hôpital Paul-Brousse, Villejuif, France, and G. MATHÉ, Service d'Hématologie de l'Institut Gustav-Roussy, Villejuif, France.

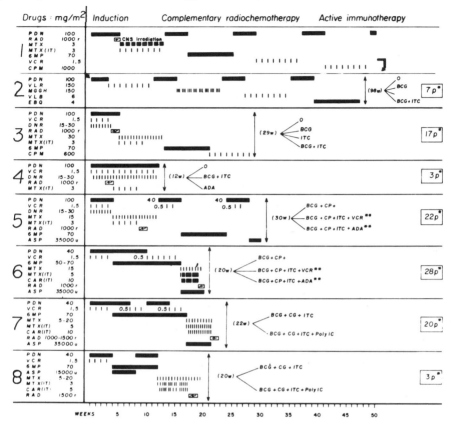

Fig. 1. Different protocols used in treating leukemic patients. PDN = prednisone; RAD = irradiation; MTX = methotrexate; IT = intrathecal; 6MP = 6-mercaptopurine; VCR = vincristine; CPM = cyclophosphamide; VLR = vinleurosine; MGGH = methylglyoxal-*bis*(guanylhydrazone); VLB = vinblastine; EQB = ethylene iminobenzoquinone; DNR = daunorubicine; ASP = L-asparaginase; CAR = arabinoside cytosine; ITC = irradiated tumor cells; ADA = adamantadine; CP = *Corynebacterium parvum;* CG = *Corynebacterium granulosum.*

L1210 leukemia as the first model to evaluate the possible effectiveness of active immunotherapy, we have shown that immune stimulation can be followed by a regression of the grafted tumor. A study of the efficiency of this treatment indicated that (1) systemic immunity adjuvants (BCG) given alone are rarely—and, if so, only slightly—effective, while irradiated-tumor cells are more frequently active; systemic immunity adjuvants can potentiate the effect of the cells (even when they are given at different sites and possibly at different times) (Mathé *et al.,* 1969); (2) The effectiveness of active immunotherapy is limited, and the most important limiting factor is the number of tumor cells. Systemic immunity adjuvants or irradiated tumor cells, or both, are only effective if the number of grafted leukemic cells does not exceed 10^5 (Mathé, 1968).

The experiments cited above suggested that the optimum condition for efficiency of active immunotherapy in acute leukemia is when the patient has the smallest possible number of leukemic cells. To achieve this condition, we reduced the cell number by chemotherapy, inducing an apparently complete remission. We then tried to further reduce tumor-cell loss with sequential complementary systemic chemotherapy. In addition, we administered intrathecal chemotherapy and central nervous system irradiation because of the high incidence of meningeal relapses in acute lymphoid leukemia patients and the well-known isolation of the central nervous system from systemic immune reactions.

A first trial was conducted in patients previously subjected to chemoradiotherapy, successively using all drugs available at the time. A randomized study of these patients (and a control group having received no previous treatment) proved the favorable effect of active immunotherapy. Following this, different protocols were used (Fig. 1) for the patients to benefit from the recent progress made in chemotherapy and immunotherapy. Thus, in protocols 5 and 6, *Corynebacterium parvum* was systematically administered to

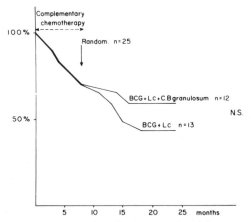

Fig. 2. **Results obtained in protocol 9.** Patients were randomized into two groups; both were treated with BCG + irradiated leukemic cells; one of the two groups was also treated with *Corynebacterium granulosum*. The results, though apparently better for the last group, are not statistically significant. (Lc = leukemic cells.)

all patients during the immunotherapy phase of the treatment; in protocols 7 and 8, *Corynebacterium granulosum* replaced *C. parvum;* in protocol 9, the patients were randomized into two groups, each given BCG and irradiated leukemic cells, but one of them was also given *C. granulosum* (Fig. 2). The results, though not statistically significant, seem to be in favor of the group which received *C. granulosum.*

C. granulosum was injected intramuscularly in doses of 750 μg in children and 1500 μg in adults, once a week, on the same day as the administration of BCG and irradiated leukemic cells.

The administration of *C. granulosum* was often accompanied by a sharp pain at the site of injection and was sometimes followed by fever, which in some cases led to the interruption of its administration. During the protocol adopted, another randomization was carried out in order to judge the value of this immunity adjuvant when added to BCG and irradiated allogenic leukemic cells.

References

Mathé, G. (1968). Immunothérapie active de la leucémie L1210 appliquée après la greffe tumorale. *Rev. Fr. Etud. Clin. Biol.* **13**:881.

Mathé, G., Pouillart, P., and Lapeyraque, F. (1969). Active immunotherapy of L1210 leukemia applied after the graft of tumor cells. *Br. J. Cancer* **23**:814.

33

Therapeutic Trial with Reticulostimulin in Patients with Ear, Nose, or Throat Cancers

E. MAHÉ, J.-S. BOURDIN, J. GEST, R. SARACINO,
M. BRUNET, G. HALPERN, B. DEBAUD,
and F. ROTH

Abstract

The authors are studying the effects of subcutaneous injections of *Corynebacterium parvum* in male patients with acute ear, nose, or throat tumors and poor prognosis. These patients had no treatment other than ^{60}Co radiation; patients who had undergone surgery or chemotherapy were excluded. Increases in the survival rate were observed, but as this trial is still going on, the authors cannot draw any final conclusions.

Introduction

We present the first clinical results of a therapeutic trial with reticulostimulin. This trial on patients with cancer of the ear, nose, or throat (ENT) is still in progress. In this paper, we shall discuss the compound which we have been using, the criteria of choice for our patients, our protocol for this trial, the tests which

E. MAHÉ, J.-S. BOURDIN, J. GEST, R. SARACINO, M. BRUNET, G. HALPERN, B. DEBAUD, and F. ROTH (deceased), Centre René Huguenin, St. Cloud, France.

were considered to assess our results, and the first partial clinical results of about three years of study.

The Compound

The compound is a suspension of bacteria: first anaerobic *Corynebacterium parvum* and then anaerobic *Corynebacterium granulosum* were killed by heating and formaldehyde was added. Our trial studied the effects of this compound, which we call "reticulostimulin," on the local evolutive persistence, relapse, or appearance of new metastatic localizations in patients with ENT cancers.

Choice of Patients

The Disease

We chose ENT localizations without any particular immunological problem because the evolution is usually short, allowing a quick judgment. We excluded from this trial cancers of the endolarynx and other localizations, e.g., the lips and the mouth floor, which could be treated by surgery with some hope of a cure. We also excluded localizations which were amenable to chemotherapy.

The cases we studied are listed below, classified according to the nomenclature of the U.I.C.C.:

> Malignant tumors of the tongue, No. 141 (A.B.C.K.), except cases suitable for surgery
> Malignant tumors of the gums, No. 143 (A.K.B.)
> Malignant tumors of mouth floor, No. 144 (A.K.), except cases suitable for surgery
> Malignant tumors of the buccal cavity, No. 145 (A.B.C.K.)
> Malignant tumors of oropharynx, No. 146 (A.B.C.D.E.K.)
> Malignant tumors of hypopharynx, No. 148 (B.C.D.K.) and extended piriform fossa
> Malignant tumors of pharynx, No. 149
> Malignant tumors of pharyngolaryngeals, No. 165
> Malignant tumors of subhyoidal epiglottis, No. 166 (anterior face)

All the patients had been treated at the Centre René Huguenin with external or interstitial radiotherapy for one or more lesions, all of which were confirmed histologically. Most often, they were epidermoid carcinomas.

Carcinological Treatment before the Trial: Irradiation (Dr. Debaud)

Irradiation doses, delivered with cobalt-60 and photons according to several modalities depending on localization, were on the average 6000–7500 rad.

To allow the inflammatory phenomena which very often accompany irradiation to disappear and to permit an unobstructed assessment of results, the trial with reticulostimulin was not begun until 6 weeks after the end of the radiation treatment. The first biological and immunological checkup was done at this time, before the start of the therapeutic trial.

Patients

Only male patients, less than 75 years old, with correct kidney functions, were studied. We did not include patients who lived far away or whose social condition made it impossible to follow them regularly (patients outside the Paris area). We did not study patients for whom chemotherapy was considered mandatory.

Biological and Immunological Checkup (Dr. Saracino)

This checkup included a standard list which could be repeated easily at fixed intervals:

> CBC with absolute percentage of lymphocytes and monocytes
> Sedimentation rate
> Lymphocyte-transformation test
> Protein electrophoresis with: Cetavlon, Burnstein, Kunkel zinc test
> Intradermal reaction with tuberculin, and prick test with tuberculin
> Tests exploring cellular immunity (D.N.C.B. intradermal reaction with *Candida albicans,* mumps antigen, Melitin, etc.)

The interval between checkups was established according to the clinical and radiological surveillance. After the initial checkup, done at the end of the irradiation, the same checkup was repeated after 6 weekly injections, that is, in the seventh week, and then every three months.

The Therapeutic Trial

The compound seems to be without toxicity. Our way of injection for this trial was subcutaneous.

Posology

We used 1 mg for each injection for an adult weighing between 50 and 100 kg, i.e., two subcutaneous injections of 0.5 ml at the superior-blade level homo-laterally.

Periodicity of injections was one injection weekly during the first six weeks, then one injection every 15 days.

Duration of the Trial

Since there is a theoretical possibility of inactivation due to stimulation of antireticulostimulin antibodies, the injections were given every 15 days during the entire duration of the trial. No other treatment was required. The trial was performed in a double blind manner: the physician examining the patient did not know whether or not the patient was being treated with reticulostimulin. Lots (saline placebo or active compound) were drawn as soon as the patients' initial treatment was completed. Patients were than labeled "ready for trial" and were randomized into two groups, one being treated with reticulostimulin and the other receiving saline as placebo. The drawing of lots was balanced for each group of four patients.

Criteria

The criteria for efficiency were: (a) lessening of local relapses, (b) persistence of local evolution, and (c) observation of new localizations or metastases. These criteria are very closely linked to survival, and we could therefore summarize them through a study of survival rates. Nevertheless, we recorded these events very carefully.

A study of the survival rates for these localizations at the Centre René Huguenin was made for 1959–1966, and gave the following results:

Survival after 1 year 75%
Survival after 2 years 35%
Survival after 3 years 21%
Survival after 4 years 15%
Survival after 5 years 14%

These rates were estimated by actuarial methods. It is therefore a pragmatic formulation which can be kept according to the nature of the compound, with explication criteria, with the data of the numerical exploration done before treatment and rejected afterward, and these data can be interpreted only after the full results of the trial.

Method

For each new patient, there was the usual file with complete information on the lesions, their qualification, pathology, and other general characteristics (age, environment, etc.). Each patient was seen again in general consultation with the full staff at the end of the radiation treatment, when the decision to try reticulostimulin was made.

An immunological checkup was done 8 days before the end of the radiation treatment, and again before the start of the trial. Patients were assigned to groups according to a random list. The surveillance and follow-up were identical for all patients. Patients were seen again during the sixth week, and then every three months until the end of the trial. This surveillance was clinical, radiological, immunological, and pathological.

Follow-up file No. 9 was used at each consultation. Relapses, new localizations, metastases, and other treatments required (derivative surgery, digestive, or respiratory) were recorded.

Number of Patients

Since we were dealing with a pragmatic formulation, we took the survival rate after two years, i.e., 35%, as reference. We expected to note an improvement of 20% with risks of alpha 100%, beta 5%, and gamma 5%, and this has led us to keep 35 patients in each group, 70 patients altogether. We saw an average of 80–100 patients with these diseases every year. The duration of the trial was three years.

General Organization and Surveillance of Evolution (Dr. Mahé)

Tolerance of the Treatment

Systemic Reactions

We had no systemic reactions (no fever and no general pain). Some patients had a local pain at the site of injection.

Local Reactions

We had only three cases of local reactions. In one case, we noticed some nodes at the site of injection, but they later disappeared spontaneously. In two other cases, we noted a herpes zoster during the first injections, but we could not find any direct relationship between this disease and the injection of reticulostimulin.

Elementary asepsis precautions (disinfection with alcohol) allowed us to avoid any local superinfection.

Status of the Trial

This trial started on February 8, 1971. To date, 68 patients have been chosen to enter the trial (70 were considered). Of these 68 patients, some received (and continue to receive) injections of reticulostimulin, while others (according to randomization) received injections of placebo (1 ml of saline).

In this trial, 68 patients were studied regularly for three years. According to the requirements for statistical significance, two more patients will have to be taken into the trial, and a detailed analysis of this trial will not be possible until after the data for the last patient become available after two years in the trial. Of the 68 patients, 34 of whom were treated with reticulostimulin, 38 have died: 19 in the group treated with reticulostimulin and 19 in the group without reticulostimulin. Also, three of the patients still alive have had relapses, two of them in the group treated with reticulostimulin.

Status According to Localization

Among the 68 patients in the trial, we have the following localizations:

Malignant Tumors of the Tongue

Of the 12 cases in this group, 6 were cancers located at the base of the tongue, and 6 at the sides or in the mobile part of the tongue. In the first of these groups, 3 cases received reticulostimulin and 2 are still alive, while in the placebo group, 2 out of 3 are dead. In the second group, 3 received reticulostimulin. Of these, only 1 is alive, while in the control group, 2 out of 3 are alive.

Malignant Tumors of the Floor of the Mouth

Three cases were investigated. Two cases received reticulostimulin; only 1 is alive. There were 2 fatalities in the control group.

Tumors of the Oropharynx and the Oral Cavity

This group comprised 34 cases. It is the most important and can be subdivided as follows: tonsils, 16 cases; soft palate, 1 case; tonsil sulcus, 5 cases; glossoepiglottic sulcus, 8 cases; oral cavity, 4 cases. Among the 16 tonsil cases, 9 received reticulostimulin with 6 fatalities, as compared to 3 fatalities out of 7 in the control group. Of the 5 patients with tonsil sulcus, 2 received reticulostimulin, and 1 died. Of the 3 patients in the control group, 2 died. In the group of 8 patients with carcinoma of the glossoepiglottic sulcus, 2 received reticulostimulin, and 1 died. In the control group, 4 patients out of 6 died. Finally, among the group of tumors of the oral cavity, which includes 2 uvula and 2 intermaxillary comissures, the 2 uvula cases received the placebo and are alive. Of 2 patients with the intermaxillary comissures, one received the placebo and the other reticulostimulin. Both are alive.

Malignant Tumors of the Hypopharynx

Of the 19 cases, 17 had very large malignant tumors of the piriform sinus, beyond any surgical possibility. Eight of them were treated with reticulostimulin; of these, 5 died. Nine patients received the placebo, and of these, 7 died. Two cases in this group had a localization in the posterior wall of the hypopharynx. Both of them received reticulostimulin and are alive.

Discussion

Of course, since this trial is still going on, we cannot draw any conclusions from these first results as to the effectiveness of the reticulostimulin. We can only cite three observations: (1) The tolerance to the compound is excellent and we evidenced no adverse systemic or local reactions. (2) There was no significant difference between the survival rates of the two groups studied, but we should temper this assertion by pointing out that the series are not strictly homologous and superimposable. (3) Many parameters of the bio-immunological data are being studied, but with the trial still going on, no usable conclusions can as yet be drawn. However, it seems to us in the field of immunobiology that the statistical analysis of the results by Dr. Brunet will provide some very interesting information to help delineate the course of further research.

References

Amiel, J. L., Litwin, J., and Bérardet, M. (1969). Essais d'immunothérapie active non spécifique par *Corynebacterium parvum* formolé. *Rev. Fr. Etud. Clin. Biol.* **14**:909–912.

Fisher, J. C., Grace, W. R., and Mannick, J. A. (1970). The effect of nonspecific immune stimulation with *Corynebacterium parvum* on patterns of tumor growth. *Cancer* **26**: 1379–1382.

Halpern, B. N., Biozzi, G., Stiffel, C., and Mouton, D. (1966). Inhibition of tumor growth by administration of killed *Corynebacterium parvum*. *Nature (Lond.)* **212**:853–854.

Israel, L. and Edelstein, R. (1975). Nonspecific immunostimulation with *Corynebacterium parvum* in human cancer. In: *Immunological Aspects of Neoplasia*, M. D. Anderson Hospital and Tumor Institute at Houston. Baltimore, Williams and Wilkins (in press).

Israel, L. and Halpern, B. (1972). Le *Corynebacterium parvum* dans les cancers avancés. Première evaluation de l'activité thérapeutique de cette immunostimuline. *Nouv. Presse Med.* **1**:19–23.

Lamensans, A., Stiffel, C., Mollier, M. F., Laurent, M., Moulton, D., and Biozzi, G. (1968). Effet protecteur de *Corynebacterium parvum* contre la leucémie greffée AKR. Relations avec l'activité catalasique hépatique et la fonction phagocytaire du système réticuloendothélial. *Rev. Fr. Etud. Clin. Biol.* **13**:773–779.

Mathé, G., Amiel, J. L., Schwarzenberg, L., Schneider, M., Cattan, A., Schlumberger, J. R., Hayat, M., and De Vassal, F. (1969). Active immunotherapy for acute lymphoblastic leukemia. *Lancet* **1**:697–699.

Milas, L., Hunter, N., Mason, K., and Withers, H. R. (1974). Immunological resistance to pulmonary metastases in C_3 Hf/Bu mice bearing syngenic fibrosarcoma of different sizes. *Cancer Res.* **34**:61–71.

Neveu, T., Branellee, A., and Biozzi, G. (1964). Propriétés adjuvantes de *Corynebacterium parvum* sur la production d'anticorps et sur l'induction d l'hypersensibilité retardée envers les protéines conjuguées. *Ann. Inst. Pasteur, Paris* **106**:771–777.

O'Neill, G. J., Henderson, D. C., and White, R. G. (1973). The role of anaerobic coryneforms on specific and nonspecific immunological reactions. I. Effect on particle clearance and humoral and cell-mediated immunological responses. *Immunology* **24**:977–995.

Woodruff, M. F. A. and Inchley, M. P. (1971). Synergistic inhibition of mammary carcinoma transplants in A-strain mice by antitumor globulin and *C. parvum*. *Br. J. Cancer* **25**:584–593.

34

The Effect of Intravenous
and Intramuscular Injection
of *Corynebacterium parvum*

M. F. A. WOODRUFF, G. J. A. CLUNIE,
W. H. McBRIDE, R. J. M. McCORMACK,
P. R. WALBAUM, and K. JAMES

Introduction

A series of investigations into the effect of killed *Corynebacterium parvum* preparations on the growth of isogenic tumor transplants in mice has demonstrated inhibition of tumor growth following even a single injection of an appropriate strain of this systemic adjuvant (Woodruff and Boak, 1966; Woodruff and Inchley, 1971; Woodruff *et al.*, 1972; Woodruff and Dunbar, 1973). The mechanism underlying this phenomenon has not been defined by these experiments. The demonstration that inhibition of tumor growth by *C. parvum* injection in T-cell-deprived mice occurs to an extent comparable to that in *C. parvum*-treated, normal mice (Woodruff *et al.*, 1973) lends support to the hypothesis that its effects on tumor growth depend primarily on macrophage stimulation. However, the administration of *C. parvum* to both tumor-bearing

M. F. A. WOODRUFF, G. J. A. CLUNIE, W. H. McBRIDE, R. J. M. McCORMACK, P. R. WALBAUM, and K. JAMES, The Departments of Surgery and Bacteriology, The University of Edinburgh Medical School, Edinburgh, United Kingdom.

and normal mice may have an enhancing effect on the response of both thymus-dependent and independent antigens (James *et al.*, 1974).

It is clear that the effect of *C. parvum* on tumor growth is most marked following intravenous or intraperitoneal injection, the subcutaneous route being much less effective (Woodruff and Inchley, 1971; Woodruff *et al.*, 1974). Other measures of response to *C. parvum*—such as increased phagocytic activity, as judged by the clearance of intravenously injected colloidal carbon from the blood stream, rise in anti-*C. parvum* antibody titers, and splenomegaly—also indicate the superiority of intravenous or intraperitoneal injection when compared with subcutaneous administration (Woodruff *et al.*, 1974).

On the basis of this experimental work, a cautious clinical trial of *C. parvum* was started in Edinburgh early in 1973. The route of administration was primarily intravenous, and the aims of the trial were to determine any immediate toxicity and to assess any beneficial or deleterious effects on tumor growth. Thirty patients were treated in the period from January 1973 to April 1974, 20 suffering from bronchogenic carcinoma, 6 from malignant melanoma, and 4 from mammary carcinoma.

Materials and Methods

Two basic therapeutic protocols were followed. The first group of 22 patients received a single intravenous injection of a formalin-killed suspension of *C. parvum* designated CN6134, batch WEZ174, which has been used throughout the series and in much of the experimental work previously reported. Initial patients, in whom there was clinical evidence of significant residual tumor, received a dose of *C. parvum* (1 mg/kg body weight) administered in 500 ml 1N saline over the course of 3–4 h. The infusion was stopped if any side effects were observed, and the total dose of *C. parvum* actually given ranged from 15 to 47.6 mg. This dose (somewhat less than 1 mg/kg) is in sharp contrast with the approximately 70 mg/kg dose given to the experimental animals. Because of toxic effects (which will be discussed in detail later), the protocol was modified, so that more recent patients have received a standard dose of 20 mg *C. parvum* in 100 ml saline over one hour. This lower dose was given both to later patients with major residual tumor and to the first 10 patients in a controlled trial of *C. parvum* following resection for bronchogenic carcinoma. In this trial—where the patients were considered by the operating surgeon to be free from macroscopic evidence of tumor, but were known to have a poor prognosis from previous studies, a random allocation was made, following resection to a treatment or nontreatment group.

In the second protocol, which was used more recently in 8 patients with clinically obvious residual tumors, 20 mg of *C. parvum* was administered intravenously as before, but was followed by 2 mg injected intramuscularly at weekly intervals for 3 months. This course was followed in surviving patients by fortnightly injection for a further 3 months, with monthly injections thereafter.

Results and Discussion

All patients receiving intravenous injections of *C. parvum* developed pyrexial reactions, either during or within 2–3 h of the infusion. These reactions varied from a mild pyrexia with associated general malaise in elderly patients with extensive tumors, to severe systemic disturbances with rigors, nausea, vomiting, and severe headache. Some of the major reactions lasted intermittently for 4–5 days; they were most striking in the younger and fitter patients and with the higher doses used initially. In contrast, reaction to the much smaller intramuscular dose was minimal, with slight discomfort and swelling at the site of injection, lasting 24–36 h in some patients, and no systemic upset.

One 21-year-old patient with disseminated malignant melanoma developed transient, but severe, jaundice with biochemical evidence of hepato-cellular damage 5 days after the intravenous infusion of 20 mg of *C. parvum*. Apart from occasional and slight rises in serum-alanine aminotransferase levels, there was no other evidence of hepato-toxicity in this series.

The response of the patients was followed by a series of investigations on peripheral blood samples taken before treatment, on the day of treatment, and on days 4, 11, 21, 39, and at varying intervals thereafter. Routine hematological investigations showed no changes in hemoglobin and packed-cell volume. Thus, there was no clinical evidence of anemia comparable with the striking falls in packed-cell volume demonstrated experimentally in mice receiving injections of the various *C. parvum* strains effective in inhibiting tumor growth in these animals (McBride *et al.*, 1974). Some of the patients showed a fall in peripheral monocyte count to levels of less than 30% of starting values by day 4–5, with a rebound to higher than starting levels by day 11. However, this finding was by no means consistent, and was not dose related. The reason for these apparent changes is not clear, but it is tempting to postulate that the monocytes are localizing in the tumors.

Serum immunoglobulin (IgG, IgA, IgM, IgE) and α_2-macroglobulin levels were estimated at the same time intervals. No consistent changes were demonstrated in this small series, but one patient with extensive contralateral secondaries following lung resection for bronchogenic carcinoma and a history of asthma showed a sharp rise in IgE levels (63–5448 International Units) by day 5, and a less striking rise (980–1448 mg/100 ml) in IgG levels by day 11. The reason for this response is not clear, and may be peculiar to the individual. However, it is of interest that this man is alive and well, with little evidence of further extension of his secondary tumor, one year after a single intravenous injection of 46.8 mg of *C. parvum*. The response of peripheral blood lymphocytes to the mitogens phytohemagglutinin, Con-A, and pokeweed were studied sequentially in some of the patients. Again, no clear or consistent pattern was demonstrated.

Assays of anti-*C. parvum* antibodies were carried out, using a modification of the latex-agglutination test of Florman and Scoma (1960), which is described in detail elsewhere (Woodruff *et al.*, 1974). Assays in normal persons showed significant background titers of antibody in all persons tested. These basic titers did not differ significantly from the pretreatment levels in the tumor population studied (Table I). This high basic titer is perhaps not surprising in the light of the ubiquitous nature of the corynebacteria and the cross-reactivity demonstrated by different strains (Johnson and Cummins, 1972). When tested for antibodies, all 24 patients receiving intravenous injections of *C. parvum* demonstrated a significant rise in titer ($\log_2 ab > 8$) by day 11 following infusion, persisting to at least day 39. The antibody titer was not related to the dose of *C. parvum*, which varied between 15–47.6 mg. It is not yet clear whether regular intramuscular injections after the initial intravenous dose has any effect on the maintenance of agglutinating-antibody levels, or even whether such antibodies have any beneficial effect in inhibiting tumor growth. However, recent experimental results indicate that both the antitumor effect of *C. parvum* and its effect on macrophage activity, as judged by a modification of the carbon clearance test of Biozzi *et al.* (1954), can occur in the presence of high levels of antibody directed against the organism (Woodruff *et al.*, 1974). Thus, it seems logical to administer *C. parvum* at regular intervals in patients with frank residual tumors, although

Table I. Anti-*Corynebacterium parvum* Assays by the
Latex-Agglutination Test[a]

Number tested		$\log_2 ab \pm$ S.D.[b]
23	Normal males	5.9 ± 1.7
22	Normal females	5.7 ± 2.6
	C. parvum treated	
24	Day 0	5.6 ± 1.9
11	Day 4	6.2 ± 1.5
11	Day 11	9.4 ± 1.5
6	Day 39	10.5 ± 1.9

[a]Woodruff *et al.* (1974).
[b]Results are expressed as the $\log_2$ reciprocal of the antiserum end point dilution.

the optimal dose levels and time intervals between injections remain to be defined.

We can make no striking claims with regard to regression or control of tumor growth in this small and heterogeneous group of patients. In one male with secondary brochogenic carcinoma (already discussed), there may have been some beneficial effect in the year since treatment; in one female with extensive malignant local ulceration of the chest wall following mastectomy for mammary carcinoma, there was an apparent arrest of growth for 7 months. It is apparent that a larger series of patients treated over a longer period of time with careful follow-up will be necessary before any precise statement regarding beneficial or harmful effects can be made. The results of this preliminary study suggest that such an extension of the trial is now justified.

Summary

Following a series of investigations which demonstrated the inhibitory effect of the injection of suspensions of killed *Corynebacterium parvum* on the growth of experimental tumors in mice, a cautious clinical trial of this material was started in Edinburgh in January 1973. The aims of the trial were to determine toxicity in man and to assess the effects on tumor growth. Thirty patients have been treated, 20 suffering from bronchogenic carcinoma, 6 from malignant melanoma, and 4 from mammary carcinoma.

Two therapeutic protocols have been followed. The first group of 22 patients received a single intravenous injection of a formalin-killed *C. parvum*. Because of toxic reactions which led to the stopping of the infusion, the dose administered varied from 15 mg to 47.6 mg.

More recent patients have received a standard dose of 20 mg given intravenously over the course of one hour. This group includes both patients with significant residual tumor, and the first 10 patients in a randomized trial of *C. parvum* following resection of bronchogenic carcinoma.

All patients receiving intravenous injections of *C. parvum* developed pyrexial reactions, either during or within 2–3 h of the start of infusion.

Response of the patients has been followed by investigations on peripheral blood samples, investigated by routine hematological observations, serum protein levels, and responses to mitogens. Assays of anti-*C. parvum* antibodies have shown a significant background titer of antibody in all patients and in normal controls, with marked rise in titer following *C. parvum* infusions.

No striking claims can be made in terms of regression or control of tumor growth in this small and heterogeneous population. It is apparent that a larger series of patients treated over a longer period of time with careful follow-up will be necessary before any precise statement regarding beneficial or harmful effects can be made.

Acknowledgments

We are indebted to the Cancer Research Campaign for generous financial assistance, to the Wellcome Foundation for supplies of *Corynebacterium parvum*, to our clinical colleagues in the Royal Infirmary and the City Hospital, Edinburgh, for referral of patients, and to our colleagues in the Departments of Surgery and Bacteriology of the University of Edinburgh for their participation in these studies.

References

Biozzi, G., Benacerraf, B., Stiffel, C., and Halpern, B. N. (1954). Étude quantitative de l'activité granulopexique du système reticuloendothelial chez la souris. *C. R. Soc. Biol. (Paris)* **148**:431.

Florman, A. L. and Scoma, J. L. (1960). A latex agglutination test for anaerobic diphtheroids. *Proc. Soc. Exp. Biol. Med.* **104**:683.

James, K., Ghaffar, A., and Milne, I. (1974). The effect of transplanted methylcholanthrene-induced fibrosarcomata and *Corynebacterium parvum* on the immune response of CBA and A/HeJ mice to thymus-dependent and independent antigens. *Br. J. Cancer* **29**:11.

Johnson, J. L. and Cummins, C. S. (1972). Cell-wall composition and deoxyribonucleic acid similarities among the anaerobic coryneforms, classical propionibacteria and strains of Arachniapropionica. *J. Bacteriol.* **190**:1047.

McBride, W. H., Jones, J. T., and Wier, D. M. (1974). Increased phagocytic cell activity and anaemia in *C. parvum* treated mice. *Br. J. Exp. Pathol.* **55**:38.

Woodruff, M. F. A. and Boak, J. L. (1966). Inhibitory effect of injection of *Corynebacterium parvum* on the growth of tumor transplants in isogenic hosts. *Br. J. Cancer* **20**:345.

Woodruff, M. F. A. and Dunbar, N. (1973). The effect of *Corynebacterium parvum* and other reticuloendothelial stimulants on transplanted tumors in mice. In: *Immunopotentiation*, p. 287 (Ciba Foundation Symposium), Elsevier–Excerpta Medica–North Holland, Amsterdam.

Woodruff, M. F. A. and Inchley, M. P. (1971). Synergistic inhibition of mammary carcinoma transplants in A-strain mice by antitumor globulin and *C. parvum*. *Br. J. Cancer* **25**:584.

Woodruff, M. F. A., Inchley, M. P., and Dunbar, N. (1972). Further observations on the effect of *C. parvum* and antitumor globulin on syngenically transplanted mouse tumors. *Br. J. Cancer* **26**:67.

Woodruff, M. F. A., Dunbar, N., and Ghaffar, A. (1973). The growth of tumors in T-cell deprived mice and their response to treatment with *Corynebacterium parvum*. *Proc. R. Soc. Lond. B.* **184**:97.

Woodruff, M. F. A., McBride, W. H., and Dunbar, N. (1974). Tumor growth, phagocytic activity and antibody response in *C. parvum* treated mice. *Clin. Exp. Immunol.* **17**:509.

35

Report on 414 Cases of Human Tumors Treated with Corynebacteria

LUCIEN ISRAEL

Abstract

Four-hundred and fourteen cases of human cancers in various clinical situations are reported. Randomized studies in advanced breast cancer and lung cancer, comparing combination chemotherapy with the same chemotherapy and weekly subcutaneous injections of *Corynebacterium parvum,* showed a significant superiority of the latter procedure in survival and resistance to bone-marrow depression and infections. Some uncontrolled studies showed an indication of synergism between *C. parvum* and BCG and a local effect of *C. parvum* injected intratumorally. Recent studies of *C. parvum* injected intravenously each day in a dose of 4 mg and without chemotherapy showed very promising and intriguing results in various disseminated cancers. Four good partial regressions were registered out of 12 patients. Problems relative to immune status and optimal conditions for nonspecific immune stimulation are discussed.

Introduction

Following the experimental reports of Halpern *et al.* (1964, 1966), clinical trials of *Corynebacterium parvum* were initiated in 1967. Some 414 patients

LUCIEN ISRAEL, Centre Hospitalier Universitaire Lariboisiere, Paris, France.

were evaluated for toxicity, and 330 of them were included in controlled or pilot studies.

Patients and Methods

The different clinical categories that were studied are listed in Table I. Except where otherwise stated, corynebacteria were given as a subcutaneous injection in the deltoid region. The dose was 4 mg of killed bacteria suspended in 2 ml of saline with formaldehyde. Corynebacteria were obtained from the Pasteur Institute (courtesy of Prof. Raynaud) from 1967 to April 1973, and then from the Mérieux Foundation (courtesy of Dr. Triau).

Patients were seen weekly. Every two months, they were given skin tests with a battery of recall antigens and with DNCB, to which they were sensitized prior to therapy. They also had bimonthly blood counts, the usual blood chemistries, and urinalyses. Since October 1973, some of them underwent a more extensive immunological monitoring that will be separately reported by Dimitrov and Israel.

Table I. Clinical Material

Type of study	Number of cases
Randomized studies	
Various advanced cancers	70
Bronchogenic epidermoid	68
Bronchogenic oat cells	30
Metastatic breast cancer	46
Sarcomas	13
Resected melanomas	17
Pilot studies	
Ocular melanomas	9
(*C. parvum* + BCG)	
Intranodular *C. parvum*	14
Intravenous *C. parvum* (daily)	12
Intraperitoneal *C. parvum*	4
Uncontrolled studies	
Disseminated melanomas	37
Stage IV lymphomas	10
Miscellaneous	84
Total	414

Table II. Duration of Therapy

Duration, months	Number of cases
1–11	161
12–23	150
24–35	59
36–47	27
More than 48	10

Toxicity and Side Effects

In two cases, local pain and swelling were such that after the first injection, the administration of C. parvum was stopped. Usually the only reaction was a local pain of short duration accompanied, at times, by fever (38–39°C). These side effects tended to decrease with time, and disappeared after 20 weeks.

We did not see any other clinical or biologic reactions. All the biological parameters remained within normal limits, even after three years of therapy (Table II). Intraperitoneal injections were usually tolerated very well. Daily intravenous injections of 4 mg of C. parvum for as long as 90 days have also been well tolerated, except for short-lasting febrile reactions. Intratumoral injections were painful and induced an important local imflammation within a few days, sometimes followed by suppuration.

Results

Early Studies

Tables III and IV summarize the results of our first study (Israel and Halpern, 1972; Israel, 1973). Disseminated solid tumors from various sites were randomized between a group receiving bimonthly courses of a five-drug combination chemotherapy (Israel et al., 1971), which included cyclophosphamide, fluorouracil, methotrexate, vinblastin, and streptonigrin, and a group receiving, in addition, weekly injections of C. parvum (4 mg). C. parvum significantly prolonged the survival of patients treated by chemotherapy, survivors being more than twice as numerous in the treated group at 6 months, 12 months, and 18 months. In the C. parvum group, patients also tolerated much greater amounts of cytostatic drugs without leukopenia and, hence, received more

Table III. Randomized Study of Various Disseminated Carcinomas[a]

Interval from onset of therapy, months	% Survivors, controls	% Survivors, C. parvum	Statistical significance
3	56	89	$P < 0.001$
6	32	59	$P < 0.005$
9	20	49	$P < 0.005$
12	14	36	$P < 0.01$
18	10	23	$P > 0.05$
24	5	9	$P > 0.05$

[a]Same chemotherapy was used in both groups.

chemotherapy. The response rates were similar in the two groups, but the duration of the response was significantly prolonged in the treated group as compared to the controls.

That these results were related to immune phenomena is shown by the fact that PPD-positive patients survived significantly longer than the PPD-negative ones, not only within the control group, but also within the treated group (Table IV). This will be discussed further.

Table IV. Randomized Study of Various Disseminated Carcinomas[a]

Subgroup	Mean survival, months	Significance
PPD-positive, C. parvum	13	$P < 0.05$
PPD-positive, no C. parvum	9.4	$P > 0.05$ $P < 0.0000001$
PPD-negative, C. parvum	7.6	$P < 0.01$
PPD-negative, no C. parvum	3.6	

[a]Mean survival according to pretherapeutic PPD skin tests.

Randomized Studies

We then started studies randomizing patients according to tumor type.

In disseminated bronchogenic squamous-cell carcinoma, the results obtained showed (Table V) that the median survival shifted from 4 months to 9 months ($P < 0.001$), a result which, in our experience, is highly unusual.

Similar results were obtained in oat-cell carcinomas (Table VI), again comparing our five-drug chemotherapy against the same chemotherapy plus weekly injections of *C. parvum*. Owing to the smaller number of patients, the difference just reaches the 0.02 level of significance. But it is again highly suggestive that, at twelve months, 3% of the controls survived versus 30% in the treated group. The duration of response was also more influenced than the response rates.

Our series of sarcomas, although limited, indicates a superior survival in the group treated with *C. parvum* (Table VII).

Our randomized study of metastatic breast cancer (Table VIII) reached the 0.001 level of significance, with more than a twofold difference at 12 months and more than a fourfold difference at 18 months. We excluded patients with skin metastases, pleural metastases, and cerebral metastases. It is noteworthy that we have had complete regression of massive liver metastases, lasting for more than two years.

Our study of resected primary melanomas included a small number of patients. These were stratified according to the presence or absence of regional lymph nodes (that were also resected if involved). One group received no therapy while the other was treated weekly with subcutaneous *C. parvum*. A tendency to an increase in the disease-free interval in the immunotherapy group was seen (Table IX).

Table V. Randomized Study of Disseminated Epidermoid Bronchogenic Carcinomas[a]

Group	Median survival, months	Range	Mean survival, months	Statistical significance
75 patients treated with chemotherapy	4	1–28	5.6	
				$P < 0.001$
68 patients treated with chemotherapy and *C. parvum*	9	2–38	9.8	

[a]Same chemotherapy was used in both groups.

Table VI. Randomized Study of Oat-Cell Carcinomas[a]

Time from onset of therapy, months	% in study, controls (30 cases)	% in study, C. parvum (30 cases)	Difference
3	70	100	
6	26	73	
9	13	40	
12	3	30	$P < 0.05$
15	3	24	
18	0	24	

[a]Response rates: 60% for treated patients, 43% for controls. Same chemotherapy was used in both groups; 4 mg of *Corynebacterium* was given s.c. weekly (life-table analysis).

Table VII. Randomized Study of Sarcomas[a]

Time from onset of therapy, months	% in study, controls (12 cases)	% in study, C. parvum (13 cases)
6	65.2	84
12	43.5	84
18	43.5	58.2
24	0	38.8
30	—	38.8
36	—	0

[a]Same chemotherapy was used in both groups; *C. parvum* was given weekly in a dose of 4 mg.

Table VIII. Randomized Study of Metastatic Breast Cancers[a]

Time from onset of therapy, months	% in study, controls (43 cases)	% in study, C. parvum (46 cases)	Statistical significance
6	62	90	
12	34	75	
18	13	62	$P < 0.001$
24	7	26	

[a]Response rates: 70% in treated patients, 60% in controls. Included are lung, liver, and bone metastases; isolated skin or pleural metastases, as well as cerebral metastases, were excluded from the study. The same chemotherapy was given to both groups; 4 mg of *Corynebacterium* was given s.c. weekly.

Uncontrolled Studies

Two uncontrolled studies are underway that seem worth reporting: (a) Thirty-seven disseminated melanomas, mostly with visceral metastases have been treated with a combination of methyl-CCNU (200 mg/m^2 every 4 weeks), cyclophosphamide (1 mg/m^2 every 4 weeks), bleomycine (15 mg weekly), and *C. parvum* (4 mg weekly). They have been compared to 13 historical controls without *C. parvum,* and there is a difference that could justify a controlled trial

Table IX. Randomized Study of Resected Melanomas[a]

Time from onset of therapy, months	% in study controls (19 cases)	% in study, C. parvum (17 cases)
6	78	94
12	63	87
18	63	78
24	41	58

[a]Stratified for primary alone, or primary plus regional lymph-node involvements. No chemotherapy was given; 4 mg of *Corynebacterium* was injected s.c. weekly (life-table analysis); disease-free interval.

Table X. Disseminated Melanomas (Methyl-CCNU, CTX, and
BLM in Both Groups)[a]

Time from onset of therapy, months	% in study controls (13 cases)	% in study, C. parvum (37 cases)
3	76	100
6	61	81
9	38	55
12	38	49
15	7	32
18	0	28

[a]Response rates: 18% in controls, 30% in treated patients. A dose of 4 mg of *Corynebacterium* was given s.c. weekly. Controls are historical cases.

in such patients (Table X). (b) In addition, we have 10 patients with non-Hodgkin stage IV lymphomas who are all alive and free of disease between 11[+] and 34[+] months. Cyclophosphamide, Vincristine, bleomycine, and streptonigrin were given for 18 months and *C. parvum* for 24 months (Table XI).

Table XI. Stage IV Non-Hodgkin
Lymphomas[a]

Survival with NED
11[+] 12[+] 15[+] 18[+] 19[+] 20[+] 20[+] 21[+] 32[+] 34[+]
No recurrence

[a]No controls were used; chemotherapy with cyclophosphamide, Vincristine, bleomycine, streptonigrin was discontinued at 18 months. A dose of 4 mg of *Corynebacterium* was given s.c. weekly; this treatment was discontinued at 24 months.

Table XII. Resected Ocular Melanomas[a]

Survival with NED
$6^+8^+10^+19^+20^+23^+36^+38^+50^+$

[a]A dose of 4 mg of *C. parvum* was given s.c. weekly for 18 months. A dose of 1 ml of freeze-dried Pasteur BCG was administered i.d. in 4 limbs weekly for 18 months. No controls were used.

Pilot Studies

Nine consecutive ocular melanomas were treated after resection by weekly injections of *C. parvum* (4 mg, s.c.) and Pasteur freeze-dried BCG (0.1 ml intradermally in 4 limbs weekly). The preliminary results (Table XII) are unusual. Except for one patient who died of metastatic rectal carcinoma (and had no chemotherapy at that time), all other patients are free of disease from 6^+

Table XIII. Corynebacteria Injected Intravenously (4 mg Daily) as the Single Agent in Disseminated Disease

Type	Number of injections	Result
Melanoma	30	P.R. (80 days)[a]
Melanoma	31	Progression
Melanoma	19	Progression
Melanoma	55	No change
Gastric cancer	32	P.R. (2 months)[a]
Bronchogenic adeno cancer	16	P.R. (2 months)[a]
Oat cells	23	Progression
Oat cells	41	Progression
Bronchogenic squamous-cell carcinoma	62	No change
Bronchogenic squamous-cell carcinoma	90	No change
Teratoma[b]	35	No change
Bronchogenic adeno cancer	32	P.R. (1 month)[a]

[a]Four partial regressions (P.R.) out of 12 cases.
[b]Complete response with chemotherapy after the *C. parvum* course.

months to 50^+ months. *C. parvum* and BCG can be given together. We have indications derived from the immunological monitoring of these patients that a high degree of immune stimulation was achieved by combining *C. parvum* with BCG.

So far, we have treated 12 patients with intravenous injections of *C. parvum* alone (Table XIII). It is noteworthy that in four cases, partial regression of more than 50% was achieved. After induction with i.v. *C. parvum,* we are now studying higher doses. It is noteworthy also that one complete response following chemotherapy was obtained.

Following the study of Paslin *et al.* (1974), we employed *C. parvum* intratumorally in 14 cases (Table XIV). Twelve complete local regressions were obtained. As with BCG (Israel *et al.,* 1974), we did not see any systemic effect inasmuch as injected nodules continued to grow. These results are similar to those induced using BCG. It must be stated, however, that patients could only be treated for five consecutive days because of local pain, swelling, and suppuration. Intratumoral *C. parvum* in conjunction with i.v. *C. parvum* is now being tested.

Last, we treated four patients with intraperitoneal injections of *C. parvum* (4 mg daily). All had ascitis that was partially removed before injection. The tolerance to this procedure has been very good. The responses (Table XV) are questionable, but our experience is too limited. It could well be that i.p. *C. parvum* should be given to patients without peritoneal involvement.

Immunological Considerations

The immunological changes induced by *C. parvum* in the course of the disease and in various clinical situations will be reported separately by Dimitrov and Israel. Only two points will be emphasized here.

Table XIV. Corynebacteria Injected Intratumorally (4–8 mg Daily for Five Days)[a]

Site	Number	Response
Secondary melanomas	11	11 complete regression
Oat-cell cancer (skin metastases)	2	1 complete regression 1 progression
Gastric cancer (abdominal-wall involvement)	1	1 partial regression

[a]No distant effect.

Table XV. *Corynebacterium parvum* Injected
Intraperitoneally (4 mg Weekly for Ascitis)

Site of origin	Number of injections	Response
Breast	18	No change
Ovary	14	No change
Ovary	20	No change
Mesothelioma	16	Complete local response (?)

(a) The absolute number of blood lymphocytes, and especially of blood monocytes, is very often significantly increased after a few weeks of *C. parvum* therapy.

(b) The protection against the reversal of previously positive skin tests induced by *C. parvum* is significantly higher in patients responding to chemotherapy. The skin tests of chemotherapy responders not treated with *C. parvum* frequently turn negative, presumably as a result of the immunosuppressive effects of the cytostatic agents.

In contrast, the skin tests of patients not responding to chemotherapy or not receiving chemotherapy may become negative, despite continuous *C. parvum* administration. In these cases, evidence of tumor recurrence is readily observed, indicating that this reversal is tumor-induced.

Discussion

Effectiveness of *C. parvum* in Patients with Cancer Immunochemotherapy

Whereas in adjuvant situations our only study in melanomas has shown no significant differences to date, in disseminated cases treated with chemotherapy and *C. parvum*, the survival and the duration of response and—to a lesser extent—the response rate improved significantly. It now becomes critical to study dose schedules in relation to the kinetics of tumor-cell killing, immunosuppressive effect, and adjuvant-induced immune stimulation. It has been generally stated that immunostimulation should not be used in association with chemotherapy and should be restricted only to cases of minimal residual disease. Our data contradict these views. Our experience has led us to the conclusion that in adjuvant studies one should compare immunotherapy to chemotherapy and to immunochemotherapy. It might well be that *C. parvum* is not potent enough, and that chemotherapy alone is too immunosuppressive, whereas a combination of both modalities could adequately control the residual cells.

Mechanisms of Action

It would appear from this report that the immune stimulation and the numbers of immunocytes available are closely interrelated. It has been shown (Dimitrov, 1975) that *C. parvum* significantly increases the colony-stimulating factor in the bone marrow of mice, a result in keeping with our data. Moreover, immunochemotherapy gives better results in patients who have retained their immune status from the onset. It seems probable that *C. parvum* not only is able to make more white cells available, and thus to increase the tolerance to chemotherapy, but is also able to activate macrophages and lymphocytes and also to enhance the specific immune response against the tumor.

As stated earlier, *C. parvum* protects the host from the immunosuppressive effect of chemotherapy, but it cannot prevent the loss of immune competence due to the tumor itself. It is likely that some tumor-induced, nonspecific, humoral factors are responsible for this phenomenon. This is why, at least in the advanced stages, the tumor burden needs to be reduced by chemotherapy for adjuvants to express their optimal activity. In this respect, synergism is seen between chemotherapy and nonspecific immunostimulation.

Prospects

The prospects for *C. parvum* and immunopotentiation, in general, are far from fully explored. The optimal dose schedule and duration of therapy are not known, nor are the most sensitive types of diseases. It is now time for the clinician to answer these questions and to develop better means for monitoring therapy with immunostimulating agents.

References

Dimitrov, N. V. (1975). In this volume.

Halpern, B. N., Prévot, A. R., Biozzi, G., Stiffel, C., Mouton, D., Morard, J. C., Bouthillier, Y., and Decreusefond, C. (1964). Stimulation de l'activité phagocytaire du système réticuloendothélial provoquée par *Corynebacterium parvum. J. Reticuloendothel. Soc.* **1**:77–96.

Halpern, B. N., Biozzi, G., Stiffel, C., and Mouton, D. (1966). Inhibition of tumor growth by administration of killed *Corynebacterium parvum. Nature (Lond.)* **212**:853–854.

Israel, L. (1973). Preliminary results of non-specific immunotherapy for lung cancer. *Cancer Chemother. Rep.* **4**:283–286.

Israel, L. and Halpern, B. N. (1972). Le *Corynebacterium parvum* dans les cancers avancés. Première évaluation de l'activité thérapeutique de cette immunostimuline. *Nouv. Presse Med.* **1**:19–23.

Israel, L., Depierre, A., and Chahinian, P. (1971). Combination chemotherapy for 418 cases of advanced cancer. *Cancer* **27**:1089–1093.

Israel, L., Depierre, A., and Edelstein, R. (1974). Local and systemic effects of intranodular BCG in 25 cases of recurrent melanoma. *Proc. Am. Soc. Clin. Oncol.* **15**:161, Abstr. 711 (March 27–28).

Paslin, D., Dimitrov, N. V., and Heaton, C. (1974). Regression of a transplantable hamster melanoma by intralesional injections of *Corynebacterium granulosum. J. Natl. Cancer Inst.* **52**:571.

DISCUSSION

REED: What route of administration did Dr. Schwarzenberg use for administering *Corynebacterium parvum?*

SCHWARZENBERG: Intramuscular.

OETTGEN: I should like to know what the chemotherapy regimen was in protocols 9 and 10. Was it the same in both, or were they different? Were they different from the earlier protocols?

SCHWARZENBERG: The chemotherapy applied in protocol 9 was not exactly the same as protocol 10: in the former, methotrexate and L-asparaginase were given in association. We then learned that these two drugs are antagonists, so the results were not very good. The results were better when methotrexate was given without L-asparaginase. As a result, there were some modifications in protocols 9 and 10.

WANEBO: In Dr. Mahé's interesting study I noted that although there may be no difference in the two groups treated—that is, of 38 patients who died, half had received *C. parvum* and half had not—at least there is no evidence of enhancement. Am I right about that?

Second, if the patients were categorized exactly according to the international classification, could this give some insight into the results? For example, patients with a certain stage of disease have a much higher recurrence rate and a poorer prognosis than those with a lesser stage. If these two factors could be balanced so that it could be seen whether *C. parvum* had an effect on diseases at the same stage of development, this would be of interest and importance.

MAHÉ: In the actual status of the trial, we have no proof of enhancement. However, two years must be waited to judge the results of the trial. Our results are very closely linked to survival and will be obvious only if there is an improvement of 20%.

All our patients were strictly categorized according to the International T:N classification (of UICC). The subjects belonged to: T_2N_2 (tumor, 2 cm plus bilateral lymphatic nodes); T_2N_3 (tumor, 2 cm plus bound lymphatic node); T_3N_2 (big tumor, 2 cm plus bilateral lymphatic nodes); T_3N_3 (big tumor, 2 cm plus bound lymphatic node).

To clarify this study, no patient in this trial had ever received chemotherapy. These tumors have a *very poor prognosis* and were chosen for this reason; the survival rate is shorter. It will be possible to shortly have an objective test of the efficiency (or nonefficiency) of *C. parvum* in ENT solid tumors.

Should the result be good (an improvement of 20% in the survival rate), we could then use *C. parvum* in homogeneous groups. For example, we could study its effects for one precise localization in patients with cancers at a lesser stage of development.

OETTGEN: Patients with head and neck cancers frequently have a negative DNCB test. Was this test done and, if so, did *C. parvum* increase reactivity to DNCB?

HALPERN: Has anybody carried out systematic DNCB application to see whether *C. parvum* can reverse a negative reaction?

COHEN: The DNCB tests which were carried out are being studied. Dr. Saracino can give the results. However, from the first data we obtained, the differences did not appear to be statistically relevant. The data are being computerized because, as we all know, first impressions are unreliable.

What was the toxicity that caused Dr. Clunie to stop infusion with the high dose of *C. parvum?* Did he try to prevent or restore these toxicities in any way?

CLUNIE: Basically, the reactions were very similar to those described by Dr. Reed. With the slow administration, a pyrexial reaction developed two or three hours after the onset of the infusion. This was also the time at which reactions developed after the short, sharp infusion we gave to later patients. There was pyrexia, nausea, malaise, headache and vomiting—all the symptoms described earlier by Dr. Reed.

The intravenous administration of hydrocortisone was tried at the time of the reactions and aspirin was also tried before, during, and after the administration of *C. parvum,* but these materials provided no real benefit.

ISRAEL: With respect to the intravenous hydrocortisone, aspirin, and so on, we tried not to give the standard drugs of this type to our patients because we know that even aspirin will impair the PHA-blastogenesis in patients and normal controls. We ask patients to tolerate their fever.

CLUNIE: I am sure this is important. Since we evidenced no benefit from their use, I think we should not be using these drugs.

SCHWARZENBERG: In Dr. Israel's results concerning two groups of patients—those submitted to chemotherapy alone and those submitted to chemotherapy plus *C. parvum*—was the chemotherapy administered at the same time in these two groups, or more or less often in patients submitted to *C. parvum?*

ISRAEL: Our protocols were such that there was a bimonthly administration of chemotherapy and a weekly administration of *C. parvum.* We tried to keep these protocols going. In fact, it was easier to keep to the protocol in *C. parvum*-treated patients than in the control group in which there was a greater development of leucopenia.

WHISNANT: Dr. Israel suggested that some of his patients failed to receive some *C. parvum* doses as scheduled because of leucopenia. Was this lymphocytopenia or granulocytopenia, or both? Is there any marrow data on those patients? Is there any way of knowing whether there is a total suppression, or just a redistribution of cells based on the vaccine?

ISRAEL: In patients receiving chemotherapy alone, there was suppression of granulocytes and lymphocytes. Our protocol stated that we had to stop chemotherapy when there were less than 4000 white cells per ml, so that we would not have to wait too long before treatment could be restarted. Therefore, this was not a particularly severe suppression.

Patients without *C. parvum* went below 4000 white cells per ml twice as often as *C. parvum*-treated patients.

WANEBO: Can Dr. Israel comment on the timing of the *C. parvum* in relation to the chemotherapy, and can he make suggestions from his present experience about whether *C. parvum* should be given between chemotherapy doses, or at the same time, or what? What would he recommend?

ISRAEL: This is an important question for which we have no answer, unfortunately. It would take a lifetime's work to find an answer to it. I hope that cooperative trials will help to find such an answer.

The patients received *C. parvum* weekly and chemotherapy bimonthly. *C. parvum* was given at the same time as the chemotherapy. I do not know whether this is the best schedule; I know that there are theoretical considerations against this, inasmuch as proliferation of immunocytes is being induced by immunopotentiation at the same time as they are being killed by simultaneous chemotherapy. At least, this is the theory on the basis of a few experiments, but we see the contrary occurring in our patients.

SCHWARZENBERG: From a theoretical point of view, we have never treated patients with chemotherapy plus immunotherapy; we have treated residual disease with immunotherapy alone. In the United Kingdom, Powles and Hamilton-Fairley treated patients with AML by immunotherapy plus chemotherapy, once a week with the former and once a month with the latter. Immunotherapy was given on the same day as chemotherapy. Their results are statistically significant, being much better for the group treated by the association chemotherapy plus immunotherapy.

GRIFFITH: There are a number of observations I wish to make from the viewpoint of a person responsible for the issue of Wellcome *C. parvum* vaccine for clinical evaluation.

The main purpose of laboratory studies and early clinical investigations is to provide data relevant to the development of an optimum schedule of treatment for patients. An essential requisite for the program is a certain amount of definable consistency in the nature and biological properties of the material used in all studies. Impressive information generated by a laboratory experiment or a clinical trial may be rendered completely irrelevant or prove misleading if specifications on the quality and biological properties of the material used are poor. Under these circumstances, no assessment can be made as to whether similar results can be obtained with other preparations or subsequent batches of similarly prepared material, and opportunities of equating results of laboratory tests with clinical effects are missed. This is particularly important in the case of *C. parvum* vaccines, since biological properties of different preparations vary greatly, or may rapidly alter with storage.

C. parvum vaccine supplied for investigational purposes should be prepared from a seed pool of a carefully selected strain of the organism. The manufacture of each batch should be rigidly controlled and conform with precise manufacturing protocols. The final container material should be subjected to a number of relevant and exacting quality control tests designed to provide reliable information on certain pharmacological, immunological, biological, oncological, and toxicological properties of the batch. The Wellcome Research Laboratories have prepared a large batch of lyophilized vaccine which is reserved for use as a reference in quality control procedures.

The pitfalls of extrapolation from results obtained in laboratory animal studies to the human situation are well known and apply particularly to *C. parvum* vaccine. For instance, Wellcome *C. parvum* vaccine has been given intravenously to three monkeys at a dosage of 20 mg/kg (diluted to 20 ml) over a 20-min period without producing any discernable effects other than increase in spleen weight in two of the monkeys. Prof. Clunie reported today that in patients, an intravenous infusion of a more dilute vaccine, at a dose of less than 1 mg/kg over a period of 2 h, produced fever and rigors and that eventually the dosage for an adult was reduced to 25 mg. At this stage, we can only contemplate whether a 50-mg dose, suitably diluted in saline and infused over 20–60 min, may not eventually be the optimum dose for man.

Table I. Tests Used for Immunoevaluation

Tests for humoral immunity	
Total complement	*Immunoglobulins*
C_3, C_4, C_5	IgG
B lymphocytes (absolute count)	IgM
PWM	IgA

Tests for cellular immunity	
Skin tests	
PPD	Streptokinase-streptodornase
Candidin	DNCB 50
	5.0
	0.5
	PHA
	PWM
	Total lymphocytes
	T lymphocytes
	Total monocytes
	Monocytes NBT
	Monocytes - lysozyme
	Monocytes - chemotaxis
	Migration-inhibition factor

C. parvum vaccine should be regarded as a possible adjunct to standard treatment of neoplastic conditions. Therein lies one of its virtues, inasmuch as it should not interfere with established forms of therapy but may supplement them. It is difficult to contemplate how it can effectively dispose of a heavy tumor load. There may be means by which it can immunologically manipulate tumor-cell destruction at a rate which at least balances the cell-replication rate, as seems to be the case in Prof. Israel's series. However, the attainment of this equilibrium has not yet been demonstrated in animals. I believe that *C. parvum* vaccine will find its role in the treatment of residual, microscopic, tumor foci after removal of main tumor masses by surgery, chemotherapy, or radio-therapy.

SERROU: In two patients with malignant melanomas (T, N+, MO) that were treated by subcutaneous or intranodular injections of *C. parvum,* we observed a stimulation of tumor growth.

First case (Table I): The patient was a 58-year-old woman who, six months previously, underwent an extensive exeresis of a malignant melanoma on the right leg, associated with an inguinal radical lymph-node dissection. She had a recurrence in October 1973 and was treated by a complementary surgical exeresis. With the appearance of new inguinal nodules in December 1973, we decided to start chemo-immunotherapy. The protocol was: first week, Vincristine on days 1 and 2 at 1 mg/m^2 and 50 mg/m^2 of CCNU on days 3 and 4; the second, third, and fourth weeks, the patient received BCG treatment at a dose of 150 mg by scarifications. After the first application of BCG, she presented a fever varying between 38–39°C that lasted for 3 weeks. The temperature disappeared spontaneously before we could demonstrate peripheral localizations of BCG. During this period, there was no noticeable evolution of the inguinal nodules. Due to the fact that we could no longer use BCG because of the patient's very strong reaction to it, we decided to switch to *C. parvum* at a dose of 4 mg twice a week. It was injected subcutaneously and associated with intranodular injections of 8–12 mg of *C. parvum* once a week in all the inguinal nodules. Between the middle of January and the end of February 1974, we noted an extremely rapid increase in nodular masses (30 times more nodules). This increase (Table I) was accelerated by the rhythm of *C. parvum* injections. The patient died three weeks later in a state of diffuse pulmonary metastases. In the course of treatment, we noted that when *C. parvum* was discontinued and chemotherapy resumed because of the local evolution and the start of metastases, there was a significant decrease of inguinal nodules due to the chemotherapy.

Second case (Table II): The patient was a 64-year-old woman who was first treated using surgery for a malignant melanoma on the thoracic wall in the right mammary region. She was then treated with radiotherapy and, finally, with an association of chemotherapy and BCG for one year, according to the modalities described for the preceding patient. In the beginning of October

Table II. Comparative Study of Lymphocyte Stimulation

Number of patients	Test	Before therapy	After 2 months of therapy
13	PHA (stimulation)	13.3 ± 3.6	41.0 ± 8.9
13	C$_3$ (mg %)	129 ± 14.0	86 ± 10.0

1973, the patient presented an icterus due to granulomatous hepatitis caused by BCG. As it was impossible to resume BCG treatment, we decided in January 1974 to use *C. parvum* at a dose of 4 mg twice a week injected subcutaneously. The patient was thus treated for a period of two months. During this treatment, we noted the progressive appearance of numerous small nodules. This was followed by pulmonary metastases, and the patient died very quickly in this state.

Discussion: In two cases of advanced malignant melanomas (T, N+, MO), we noted the appearance of the clinical signs of tumor growth during treatment with *C. parvum*—using strong doses in one case, local treatment in the other case, and systemic treatment in both cases. It is very difficult to prove whether or not this tumor growth was a matter of facilitation since we only used clinical elements, and the growth might have been a rapid evolution over a period of stabilization. However, in both cases, there was a very close relationship between the start of *C. parvum* treatment and the extremely rapid increase in nodules. In addition, we noted in the first patient, as had already been noted in an identical case after BCG treatment, that the nodules rapidly increasing under the apparent influence of immunity adjuvants were extremely

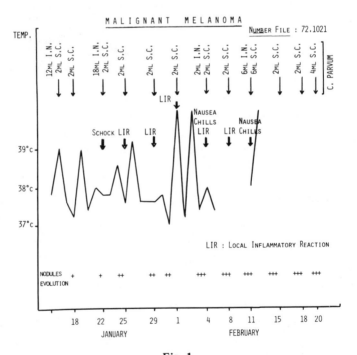

Fig. 1

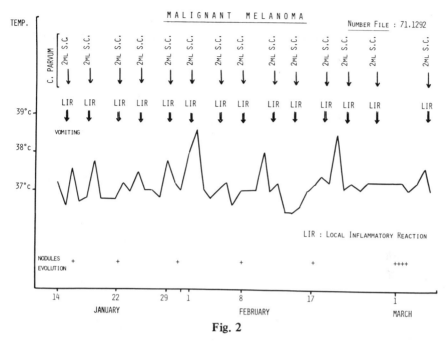

Fig. 2

sensitive to chemotherapy. The proof of tumor facilitation under the influence of *C. parvum* is, therefore, only clinical, and we have no biological element bearing its proof.

It seems clear that if we are to know the eventual complications in the use of adjuvants, these cases, by no means, contraindicate their use in man. In effect, such treatments are chosen for patients often in very advanced stages of disease, or at least presenting neoplasias with very unfavorable prognosis—such as malignant melanomas. It is only in this direction that we can obtain encouraging results in the near future. However, we must proceed with prudence, and such treatment should only be used under strict surveillance in order to evaluate the effects of adjuvants on the immune response, especially on T and B lymphocytes and on blocking factors. It is only under these conditions that we can adapt such treatment as a function of the immune response.

DIMITROV: I am familiar with the two cases presented by Dr. Serrou. We must have immunological monitoring to know what is happening during treatment with any vaccine because of the possibility of the complications described.

I should like to present part of the study done by Dr. Israel and myself on immunological monitoring of patients intravenously injected for five days a week with 4 mg of *C. parvum* for a period of two months. I will not discuss all these tests because there was no real relationship between some of them and the therapy.

Some aspects of cellular immunity and skin tests have already been discussed by Dr. Israel. Our results with lymphocyte stimulation are a little different than those of the Texas group. I do not think that the spontaneous rosette-formation test is reliable.

These are the results from the lymphocyte stimulation with PHA. There are two groups: one representing cases with a low-stimulation index, and the other group representing those with an elevated index, which remained elevated after the therapy was discontinued. This latter group consisted entirely of patients who responded to the immunotherapy.

Table II shows unexpected results. When Dr. Israel and I started this study, we were strongly attacked by the immunologists, particularly for using the third complement. They thought that we should use total complement. We used C_3 because Prof. Halpern and Dr. Biozzi showed that there is increased activity in phagocytosis following injections of *C. parvum*. This indicates that complement may be needed for phagocytosis of some tumor antigens which will result in increased utilization.

This is, in fact, probably what did happen. In all cases, the levels of C_3 were normal before treatment. After treatment, there was a substantial decrease in most of the cases. This indicates that there was probably overutilization of the complement, which may be necessary for the phagocytosis. Of course, this is pure speculation.

These are the only two tests which could be used at this time with certainty as immunological monitoring tests for registration of the immunological response during immunotherapy with *C. parvum*. We may have to wait until some other valuable tests are developed.

Part VII
Concluding Remarks

36

Corynebacterium parvum: Outlook and Future

STEPHEN K. CARTER

Now that I have listened to all of the speakers, I am still not certain that I have answers to all the questions that I raised earlier, but I do have some. I am particularly intrigued by the data on the administration of intravenous *Corynebacterium parvum.* Three separate studies have been presented, each utilizing a different schedule. Professor Woodruff's group may have reached the single dose MTD at 10–15 mg/m^2, as a single dose appears to be about as much as can be tolerated. I wonder whether the M. D. Anderson group, which is now up to 10 mg/m^2 and is trying to repeat their dose once or twice monthly, may not be pretty close to their limit, based on the amount that can be well tolerated as a single dose.

Professor Israel approached the question with a totally different schedule: essentially, chronic daily administration. This appears to be tolerated reasonably well. What gives me cause for guarded optimism is his observation of antitumor responses in advanced solid tumor patients. If I were to see these kinds of data for a new investigational chemotherapeutic agent, I would surely suggest that more detailed Phase II work be initiated in melanoma, gastric, and lung cancers.

The future use of any particular drug or material has to fit into an overall treatment strategy. In this case, the treatment has to be evolved for a specific tumor.

STEPHEN K. CARTER, Division of Cancer Research, National Cancer Institute, Bethesda, Maryland.

DRUG DEVELOPMENT PROGRAM	COMBINED MODALITIES PROGRAM
PRECLINICAL Acquisition ↓ Basic Screen ↓ Verification Screen ↓ Detailed Evaluation ↓ Formulation ↓ Large Animal Toxicology	Develop Experimental Model Systems ↓ Select Models with Biological Properties Which Suggest Lines of Approach to Therapy in Man ↓ Test Procedures for Potential Human Application
CLINICAL Phase I Studies ↓ Phase II Studies ↓ Phase III Studies ISSUES 1. What constitutes adequate clinical trial? 2. How many signal tumors should be used? 3. How many drugs per year can the clinical program handle?	Phase II Studies ↓ Phase III Studies ↓ Phase IV Studies ISSUES 1. How many solid tumor studies can the clinical program handle? 2. Which are the highest priority tumors that the clinical program should handle? 3. What type of studies (Phase II, III, or IV) should be implemented for each disease and what type of chemotherapy should be utilized (new agents, established agents not previously tested, or drug combinations)?

	% Survival
Surgery	32
Surgery + x-ray	47
Surgery + x-ray + chemotherapy	89

Fig. 2. "Cure" rates in Wilm's tumor.
(Data from Gross and Burget.)

Figure 1 is shown again to emphasize our combined-modalities program, in which there are various kinds of clinical trials. One of the critical issues in trying to develop combined-modality studies for any particular disease is what type of studies need to be implemented for each disease and what kind of chemotherapy or immunotherapy should be used within the exigencies of what is optimal for the overall strategy in that particular disease.

Figure 2 reminds us that combined-modality treatment approaches have been used for a long time and have shown success. One of the areas that has been successfully attacked by this means is Wilm's tumor in children. The cure rate historically with surgery alone was only 32%; when x-ray was added, this rose to 47%; and with chemotherapy added—actinomycin D—it rose to 89%. This data was evolved about 15 years ago, indicating that there has been evidence that combined modalities could increase survival above that which can be achieved by an individual modality.

There are some assumptions which we have been using in trying to integrate chemotherapy into a combined modality (Fig. 3). I will broaden my definition of chemotherapy in this instance to any systemic mode of therapy which can either eradicate or arrest tumor cells in any part of the body. Surgery and

Test new drugs and combinations in
advanced disease.

↓

Develop optimal chemotherapy regimen
for primary treatment of disseminated disease.

↓

Integrate optimal chemotherapy regimen
into combined modality approach for
primary treatment of local and regional
disease.

Fig. 3. Proposed strategy for developing
combined-modality therapy for solid
tumors.

radiotherapy are localized modalities, killing tumor cells only where applied. Unfortunately, while these modalities are the major potential curative therapies available, they have failed, or plateaued, in their ability to eradicate tumor cells because cure rates in the major solid tumors have not changed over the last 10 or 15 years.

Our present hypothesis is that these local modalities fail to cure because there are microscopic metastatic foci existing outside of their therapeutic range. If that is so, we need a systemic mode of therapy.

Schabel and Skipper, from the Southern Research Institute, showed the validity of the combined-modalities approach on an experimental tumor, CA755, in mice. This is a solid tumor, showing the classic Gompertzian growth curve of solid tumors. When the tumor is implanted, it begins to grow extremely rapidly, almost logarithmically. At this time it has an extremely rapid doubling time of about 12 h, and its growth fraction is almost 100%—almost all the cells are actively synthesizing their DNA. As the tumor begins to grow and enlarge, the doubling time of the tumor becomes progressively longer, and the growth fraction becomes progressively smaller. The latter is the situation we find in most of the advanced metastatic solid tumors which are being treated with chemotherapy or, by Professor Israel, with intravenous *C. parvum.*

Shrinking such a tumor by more than 50% is a very significant degree of tumor-cell kill, particularly in a situation in which the kinetics are not really favorable. From the few studies in human tumors, we know that the growth fraction is very small and that the doubling time is quite long. Yet, we are able to kill a massive number of cells.

What happens if we take that chemotherapy and employ it in a situation in which only microscopic metastatic foci of tumor exist after the surgeon has removed the bulk of the cancer? If these foci are in a situation in which the growth fraction is large and the doubling time rapid, then perhaps that chemotherapy which could shrink the bulky tumor might well eradicate the microscopic tumor, thus leading to an increase in cure rates.

This is the rationale of many of our adjuvant trials currently ongoing in tumors such as breast cancer, gastrointestinal cancer, melanoma, etc. What is used in these trials can be chemotherapy, immunotherapy, or chemo-immunotherapy, but it must be some modality which has the ability to kill tumor cells wherever they exist.

Figure 3 outlines what I like to call Phase II, III, and IV kinds of studies for combined modality treatment. In advanced disease, we test our new drugs and combinations; we develop the optimal chemotherapy regimen for the primary treatment of disseminated disease, which means that we try to develop the optimal cell-kill potential. Again, this chemotherapy can be broadly defined as chemo-immunotherapy. We then integrate this optimal chemotherapy into a combined-modality approach for the primary treatment of localized and regional disease.

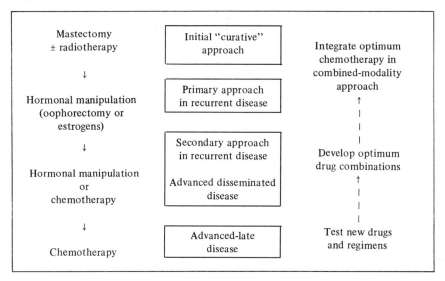

Fig. 4. Proposed integration of chemotherapy into the treatment of breast cancer.

Figure 4 is an example of how this might work in a specific tumor, such as breast cancer. Outlined is the classic treatment flow for breast cancer patients, beginning with surgery, plus or minus radiation therapy, a variety of hormonal manipulations, and, eventually, chemotherapy. In the classic approaches to the treatment of breast cancer, chemotherapy has been reserved for the hormonal failures or for the patient whose disease has progressed so rapidly that it is felt hormonal therapy would not work.

At the most advanced stage, we would test the new drugs and regimens. Then we would move up to the initial advanced disease situation, where we would elucidate the optimal combination. Next we would move to the "localized" stages, where we would be trying out various combined-modality approaches. Figure 5 shows that in breast cancer, we have six active agents, all with 20–30% response rates, and that combinations work in about 60% of the patients with advanced disease. There are a variety of NCI-sponsored studies ongoing that involve surgery plus drugs and oophorectomy plus drugs.

Figure 6 details where experimental models are needed in this combined-modality approach. We need models to identify new and active modalities of treatment, whether drugs or immunopotentiating agents. We need to develop model systems to help us pick out the optimal combinations from the myriad possible combinations which might be evaluated. If we have 10 active drugs for a given tumor, we can have at least 45 two-drug and 120 three-drug combinations. If we consider 4- and 5-drug combinations, the possibilities become nearly infinite. If we then consider that a two-drug combination can be used in a wide

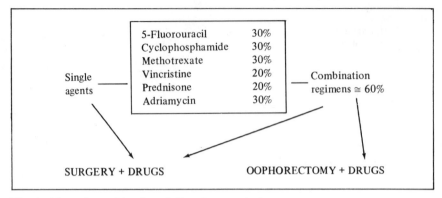

Fig. 5. Plan of combined-modality therapy in breast cancer. Six different single agents produce 20—30% objective response, and combinations of these can approximately yield a 60% response rate.

range of schedules, routes, sequences, and ratios, this produces an astronomical number of possibilities from which the clinician can test only microfractions. We must have experimental models to more rapidly set priorities for clinical testing. Of course, when we want to combine systemic therapy with surgery and radiotherapy, we must have model systems to work in these areas as well as with all of the considerations cited above for combinations.

What is the future? The future for all cancer treatments must be in all of the therapeutic modalities working together to plan an optimal therapeutic strategy for the specific tumor. The surgeon, radiotherapist, immunologist, chemotherapist, and pathologist must all sit down together to blend their expertise, to mold their modality-oriented developmental thrust into a combined-modality approach so that patient resources are used optimally to achieve cure.

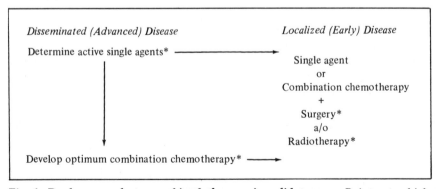

Fig. 6. Dual approach to combined therapy in solid tumors. Points at which model systems could be used are shown by (*).

37

Closing Remarks

BERNARD HALPERN

You should not expect from your chairman a summary of all papers and discussions presented at this meeting because that is not possible. The matters which we discussed here are in full development, and what we get out of a meeting like this is a comprehensive account of today's knowledge. This meeting is only a way station on the road of progress.

I shall therefore restrain myself and give a few personal impressions, not so much about what we have learned, but about what we are looking for.

The first point to be emphasized is that there was a general agreement that *Corynebacterium parvum* has proven to be a particularly promising and valuable immunopotentiating agent. It is practically devoid of pharmacological and organ toxicities in various laboratory animals, including primates, even when administered in doses much higher than the presently used therapeutic doses and also in chronic treatment. The observations made so far in man with *C. parvum* confirm its great safety margin and the absence of organ damages. Since *C. parvum* is a heat-killed vaccine, reviviscence or resurgence of the virulence in the host is excluded.

Second, *C. parvum* belongs to the recently autonomized group of so-called *nonspecific immunopotentiators*. The potentialities of these substances in treatment of infections or viral diseases, theoretically plausible, are still to be explored. Interest has been concentrated on the effects in malignant tumors. In this respect, the experimental data reported from several laboratories are impressive. Treatment with *C. parvum* inhibits and, to a great extent, slows down tumor growth and tumor invasiveness, probably by strengthening the host's immune-defense reactions.

BERNARD HALPERN, Institut d' Immuno-Biologie, Hôpital Broussais, 96 rue Didot, 75674 Paris Cedex 14 (France).

It should be stressed, however, that most of the reported results were obtained when *C. parvum* was administered either shortly before, simultaneously with, or immediately after the tumor inoculum. On that account, the results presented by Dr. Fisher were particularly interesting. In his model, *C. parvum* was applied in already established and developed tumors. We badly need a model for studying the antitumor effects of *C. parvum* under experimental conditions which approach clinical conditions as much as possible.

Another important aspect emerged from the studies of Drs. Bomford, Milas, and Dimitrov, namely, a remarkable inhibitory effect of *C. parvum* on metastatic dissemination. These results, to which may be added our own observations not presented here, are so striking that it would be surprising should they prove not to have clinical implications. Now, what about enhancement? Enhancement has become an unreasonable fear in adjuvant therapy. From what we have heard, with the exception of Dr. Serrou's report concerning two patients with melanomas in which intralesional injection of *C. parvum* was apparently followed by a flare-up effect, no evidence of enhancement was reported, either in experimental animals or in humans. The possibility of enhancement cannot be excluded theoretically and should therefore be watched for with care.

During this meeting, the problem of posology has been discussed at length. At present, clinical posology of *C. parvum* is completely arbitrary and varies from one group to another. Animal toxicology studies ascertained the low toxicity of *C. parvum* (50–100 mg/kg, dry weight, i.p.). On the other hand, studies on animal tumors suggest that relatively high doses are necessary to repress tumor development. A current dose range from 10–25 mg/kg body weight was reported. Lower doses had irregular effects. Although extrapolation to man is highly hazardous, this problem must be taken into consideration as one of priorities. Most of the clinicians have chosen 4 mg in weekly subcutaneous injections as an arbitrary standard. When Professor Lucien Israel and I decided to treat the first cancer patients in 1967, the choice of that dose was motivated by Hippocrates' maxim: *Primum non nocere*. By experimental standards, this dose is much below the active threshold dose. A dose regimen approaching 1 mg/kg body weight would be more realistic on the basis of animal experiments.

Furthermore, posology is directly related to the route of administration. The experimental results suggest that hypodermic injection is of questionable efficiency. The best results were obtained either by the intraperitoneal or the intravenous routes. Intraperitoneal administration is very unusual in man. It is likely that inoculation of a material like *C. parvum* into the peritoneal cavity would produce local inflammations, which may cause problems of their own. We have also heard from several participants about incidents produced by intravenous injection or infusions of *C. parvum:* pyrexia, malaise, headache. Such side effects were predictable, and they will occur with any bacterial vaccine given intravenously. They can be alleviated and easily overcome by adaptation of the infusion technique and by dose adjustment. Doses up to 50 mg have been administered by Edinburgh's team without real organ damage. It remains to be proved that *C. parvum* administered at these doses by the intravenous route produces dramatic clinical effects. Thus far, this evidence is still lacking.

Somebody in the audience mentioned intradermal injections. This suggestion deserves consideration. Immunologists are well aware that this way of immunization is the most effective, not only for antibody synthesis, but also for induction of cell-mediated immunity. Years ago, Mitchison showed that lymphocytes obtained from nodes draining a tumor graft were able to confer passive tumor immunity to a syngenic second recipient. Dr. Fisher [B. Fisher, N. Walmark, and E. R. Fisher (1975). This volume, p. 218] found that local injection of *C. parvum* rendered the lymphocytes from the corresponding nodes cytotoxic toward the tumor cells. We reported similar observations [(1973). *Immunopotentiation* (Ciba Foundation Symposium), London]. A limited personal clinical experience of several years dealing with the treatment of patients by intradermal injection of *C. parvum* into the region drained lymphatically by the tumor convinced me that intradermal administration of *C. parvum* is worth exploring.

One of the problems which has been discussed was how to assess the immunological status of the patient and its responsiveness to immunotherapy. There is a general consensus that anti-tumor defense is conditioned by cell-mediated immunity. Within the last few years, a number of papers have been published about the immunological status of cancer patients, explored by a variety of tests. The aim is to find out whether or not the patient is anergic. The choice of the test agent may vary from one country to another, depending on local endemicities or prophylaxis legislation. A battery of tests, including tuberculin, *Candida,* mumps, and eventually one of the streptococcal antigens, should cover most of the tests in the Western countries. I would hesitate to use dinitrochlorobenzene—a known, potent, contact allergen—routinely, because of the risk of cross-sensitization to other, more common, potential contact allergens.

Besides these common tests, several other more sophisticated procedures have been mentioned. The measurement of the phagocytic activity of the reticuloendothelial system by the clearance of intravenously injected, heat-denatured, and ^{131}I-tagged human-serum albumin has been suggested by Dr. Attié. This technique, developed in my laboratory, has since been used routinely for screening RES stimulants. In our hands, in animal models, the phagocytic activity was found to be stimulated in the first phase of tumor development and depressed in more advanced stages. The method is innocuous, reliable, and accurate. The value of this method for assessing the immunological conditions of patients with cancer remains to be proven. The chemotactic test described by Dr. Wilkinson is certainly of interest as it measures another aspect of cellular immunity. It may help in understanding the mechanism of activation of macrophages by *C. parvum* or other immunological adjuvants.

It is clearly established that *C. parvum* may be considered the most potent bacterial stimulant of the macrophage system presently available [Halpern *et al.* (1964). *J. Reticuloendothelial Soc.* 1:77]. It enhances the antibody synthesis to T-dependent and independent antigens and stimulates cell-mediated immunity. It displays the capacity to increase the resistance to a wide range of experimental tumors. There is now increasing evidence that it is also effective in human neoplastic affections. These experimental and clinical data, remarkable as they are, must be evaluated in the light of the cellular mechanism underlying these activities of *C. parvum*. It is now well documented that *C. parvum* exerts a striking stimulatory activity on lymphoreticular tissues, and, in particular, on macrophages. The "activated" macrophages have been shown to acquire new biological activities: modulation of T-cell function; stimulation of B-cell function; inhibition of tumor-cell division, and lymphocyte trapping.

It remains to be discovered how these various activities are articulated and how they follow one another, culminating in antitumor activity in animals and in man. At this point, I would like to stress the possibilities suggested by the images obtained in cooperation with Dr. Puvion from the Cancer Research Institute of Lille (France) on surface interactions between macrophages activated by *C. parvum* and malignant cells in conventional and scanning electron microscopes. When incubated with YC8 tumor cells, the activated macrophages presented close membrane contacts at either the cell body or by expanded villosities. Most of tumor cells hit by the macrophages showed holes and were probably dead. These phenomena were never observed with nonactivated macrophages under the same conditions. The significance of these phenomena is now being investigated.

Professor Dimitrov and Dr. Toujas have reported that *C. parvum* recruits and stimulates bone-marrow and spleen colony-forming cells. This is an interesting problem in itself. It has been suggested that adjuvants, in general, recruit immunologically reactive cells. The recruitment of blood-forming precursor cells is of particular importance in those cases which are most frequent today—those involving combined chemo- and immunotherapy. As has been reported by Professor Israel and Professor Dimitrov, treatment with *C. parvum* permits much higher doses of cytostatic agents without risk of bone-marrow aplasia.

From what I heard, the experimental data reported at this meeting were well documented and verified. They were highly interesting, not only because of the results obtained, but also because they raised new questions and suggested new problems.

By contrast, the clinical results appeared, on the whole, to be preliminary. One could explain these differences by the fact that *C. parvum* has become available for clinical trials in most countries, France excepted, only recently. Obviously, clinical studies of this type must be carried out with the greatest care, and they are necessarily of long duration.

It was nevertheless gratifying to hear suggestions on ways to conduct such trials. Dr. Reed has presented an excellent pharmacological study protocol, and

Dr. Carter has established signposts to guide the clinical oncologist. In this respect, the comprehensive study of Professor Lucien Israel may also serve as a model. In my opinion, studies with immunopotentiators—and *C. parvum* in particular—in clinical oncology are handicapped by the lack of a commonly accepted rationale and by the lack of international cooperative programs. It is my hope that this gap will be rapidly filled.

In calling this conference the "First International Conference on the Use of *C. parvum* in Experimental and Clinical Oncology," I had in mind that other similar conferences would follow subsequently. Yesterday, someone asked me when I plan to organize the next conference. I was pleased to be asked this question, which I may be allowed to consider a compliment. It is my belief, considering the mass of problems that remain unsolved and the increasing number of papers recently published on this matter, that a new conference should be called in the near future. It could be planned for in about two years.

I would be delighted to welcome you again to this place; but the next conference might also take place to advantage in Great Britain, the United States, Japan, or some other country.

I have been asked to suggest some main problems to be investigated. It is my opinion that four main areas should be prospected:

1. An experimental model allowing us to ascertain antitumor action in neoplasias.
2. The cellular patterns implied in the mechanism of action of *C. parvum*.
3. Attempts to obtain soluble extracts from *C. parvum* and the determination of their activity *in vitro* and *in vivo*.
4. Extensive and well-conducted clinical studies on the effects of *C. parvum* in controlling malignant tumors and their dissemination.

My last word will be to thank you all for having responded readily to my invitation, and for your valuable and skillful contribution to the success of this conference.

Contributors

ADLAM, C., Wellcome Research Laboratories, Langley Court, Beckenham, Kent BR3 3BS (Great Britain)

AMIEL, J.L., Institut de Cancérologie et d'Immunogénétique, Hôpital Paul-Brousse, 14–16 avenue Paul-Vaillant-Couturier, 94800 Villejuif (France)

ANDRE, S., Institut d'Immuno-Biologie, Hôpital Broussais, 96 rue Didot, 75674 Paris Cedex 14 (France)

ATTIÉ, E., Institut Gustave Roussy, 16 bis avenue Paul-Vaillant-Couturier, 94800 Villejuif (France)

AYME, G., Institut Français d'Immunologie, Marcy l'Etoile, 69260 Charbonnières-les-Bains (France)

BAŠIĆ, I., Section of Experimental Radiotherapy, The University of Texas System Cancer Center, 6723 Bertner Ave., Houston, Texas 77025 (USA)

BOMFORD, R., Department of Experimental Immunobiology, Wellcome Research Laboratories, Langley Court, Beckenham, Kent BR3 3BS (Great Britain)

BOURDIN, J.-S., Centre René Huguenin, 5 rue Gaston Latouche, 92211 St. Cloud (France)

BRUNET, M., Centre René Huguenin, 5 rue Gaston Latouche, 92211 St. Cloud (France)

BURGESS, A.A., Department of Developmental Therapeutics, The University of Texas System Cancer Center, 6723 Bertner Ave., Houston, Texas 77025 (USA)

CARTER, S.K., National Cancer Institute, Bldg 37, Room 6A17, National Institutes of Health, Bethesda, Maryland 20014 (USA)

CASTRO, J.E., Department of Surgery, Royal Postgraduate Medical School of London and Hammersmith Hospital, Du Cane Road, London W 12 (Great Britain)

CERUTTI, I., Laboratoire de Virologie, Hôpital St. Vincent de Paul, 74 avenue Denfert-Rochereau, 75014 Paris (France)

CHIHARA, G., National Cancer Center Research Institute, Tsukiju-5-chöme, Chuo-Ku, Tokyo (Japan)

CHOUROULINKOV, I., Institut de Recherches sur le Cancer, Boite Postale 8, 94800 Villejuif (France)

CLUNIE, G.A., Department of Surgery, University Medical School, Teviot Place, Edinburgh EH8 9AG (Great Britain)

COHEN, I.R., Department of Cell Biology, The Weizmann Institute of Science, Rehovot (Israel)

COQUET, B., IFFA-CREDO, Saint Germain sur l'Arbresle, 69210 l'Arbresle (France)

CREPIN, Y., Institut d'Immuno-Biologie, Hôpital Broussais, 96 rue Didot, 75674 Paris Cedex 14 (France)

DAZORD, L., Centre Anti-cancéreux E. Marquis, Pontchaillou, 35000 Rennes (France)

DEBAUD, B., Centre René Huguenin, 5 rue Gaston Latouche, 92211 St. Cloud (France)

DIMITROV, N.V., Hahnemann Medical College, Department of Hematology, 230 N. Broad Street, Philadelphia, Pennsylvania 19102 (USA)

ELIOPOULOS, G., Institut d'Immuno-Biologie, Hôpital Broussais, 96 rue Didot, 75674 Paris Cedex 14 (France)

FAUVE, R., Institut Pasteur, 28 rue du Dr Roux, 75015 Paris (France)

FELDMAN, M., Department of Cell Biology, The Weizmann Institute of Science, Rehovot (Israel)

FISHER, B., Department of Surgery, University of Pittsburgh Medical School, Pittsburgh, Pennsylvania 15261 (USA)

FISHER, E.R., Institute of Pathology, Shadyside Hospital, Pittsburgh, Pennsylvania 15232 (USA)

FLOC'H, F., Laboratoires de Recherches, Société des Usines Chimiques Rhône-Poulenc, Vitry-sur-Seine (France)

FRAY, A., Institut d'Immuno-Biologie, Hôpital Broussais, 96 rue Didot, 75674 Paris Cedex 14 (France)

GEST, J., Centre René Huguenin, 5 rue Gaston Latouche, 92211 St. Cloud (France)

GOLDMAN, C., Institut Mérieux, Marcy l'Etoile, 69260 Charbonnières-les-Bains (France)

GUÉLFI, J., Centre Anti-cancéreux E. Marquis, Pontchaillou, 35000 Rennes (France)

GUTTERMAN, J.U., Department of Developmental Therapeutics, The University of Texas System Cancer Center, 6723 Bertner Ave., Houston, Texas 77025 (USA)

HALL, J.G., Chester Beatty Cancer Research Institute, Clifton Avenue, Belmont, Sutton, Surrey SM2 5PX (Great Britain)

HALLE-PANNENKO, O., Institut de Cancérologie et d'Immunogénétique, Hôpital Paul-Brousse, 14–16 avenue Paul-Vaillant-Couturier, 94800 Villejuif (France)

HALPERN, B., Institut d'Immuno-Biologie, Hôpital Broussais, 96 rue Didot, 75674 Paris Cedex 14 (France)

HALPERN, G.M., 227 Boulevard Saint-Germain, 75007 Paris (France)

HERSH, E.M., Department of Developmental Therapeutics, The University of Texas System Cancer Center, 6723 Bertner Ave., Houston, Texas 77025 (USA)

HUNTER, N., Section of Experimental Radiotherapy, The University of Texas System Cancer Center, 6723 Bertner Ave., Houston, Texas 77025 (USA)

ISHIMURA, K., National Cancer Center Research Institute, Tsukiju-5-ch'ôme, Chuo-Ku, Tokyo (Japan)

ISRAEL, L., Consultation de Médecine, Hôpital Lariboisière, 2 rue A. Paré, 75475 Paris Cedex 10 (France)

JAMES, K., Department of Bacteriology, University Medical School, Teviot Place, Edinburgh EH8 9AG (Great Britain)

JOLLÈS, P., Laboratoire de Biochimie, 96 Boulevard Raspail, 75006 Paris (France)

KNIGHT, P.A., Department of Bacteriology, Wellcome Research Laboratories, Langley Court, Bechenham, Kent BR3 3BS (Great Britain)

KORONTZIS, M., Laboratory of Proteins, University of Paris V, 45 rue des Saints-Pères, Paris (France)

LIKHITE, V., Torndike Memorial Laboratory, Harvard Medical Unit, Boston, Massachusetts 02118 (USA)

LORINET, A.M., Institut d'Immuno-Biologie, Hôpital Broussais, 96 rue Didot, 75674 Paris Cedex 14 (France)

LUCKEN, N., Department of Bacteriology, Wellcome Research Laboratories, Langley Court, Beckenham, Kent BP3 3BS (Great Britain)

MAEDA, Y.Y., National Cancer Center Research Institute, Tsukiju-5-chöme, Chuo-Ku, Tokyo (Japan)

MAHÉ, E., Centre René Huguenin, 5 rue Gaston Latouche, 92211 Saint Cloud (France)

MARAL, R., Laboratoires de Recherches, Société des Usines Chimiques, Rhône-Poulenc, Vitry-sur-Seine (France)

MASON, K., Section of Experimental Radiotherapy, The University of Texas System Cancer Center, 6723 Bertner Ave., Houston, Texas 77025 (USA)

MATHÉ, G., Institut de Cancérologie et d'Immunogénétique, Hôpital Paul-Brousse, 14–16 avenue Paul-Vaillant-Couturier, 94800 Villejuif (France)

MAVLIGIT, G.M., Department of Developmental Therapeutics, The University of Texas System Cancer Center, 6723 Bertner Ave., Houston, Texas 77025

McBRIDE, W., Department of Surgery, University Medical School, Teviot Place, Edinburgh EH8 9AG (Great Britain)

McCORMACK, R.J.M., Department of Surgery, University Medical School, Teviot Place, Edinburgh EH8 9AG (Great Britain)

MIGLIORE-SAMOUR, D., Laboratory of Proteins, University of Paris V, 45 rue des Saints-Pères, Paris (France)

MILAS, L., Section of Experimental Radiotherapy, The University of Texas System Cancer Center, 6723 Bertner Ave., Houston, Texas 77025 (USA)

MOORE, A.R., Division of Tumour Immunology, Chester Beatty Cancer Research Institute, Royal Cancer Hospital, Downs Road, Sutton, Surrey SM2 5PX (Great Britain)

MUSETESCU, M., Institut Français d'Immunologie, Marcy l'Etoile, 69260 Charbonnières-les-Bains (France)

MYNARD, M.C., Institut Français d'Immunologie, Marcy l'Etoile, 69260 Charbonnières-les-Bains (France)

OLIVOTTO, M., Department of Experimental Immunology, Wellcome Research Laboratories, Beckenham, Kent BR3 3BS (Great Britain)

O'RANGERS, J.J., Institut de Recherches sur le Cancer Boite Postale 8, 94800 Villejuif (France)

PRÉVOT, A.R., Institut Pasteur, 25 rue du Dr Roux, 75015 Paris (France)

PUVION, F., Institut de Recherches sur le Cancer, INSERM U124, 59000 Lille (France)

RABOURDIN, A., Institut d'Immuno-Biologie, Hôpital Broussais, 96 rue Didot, 75674 Paris Cedex 14 (France)

REED, R., Department of Developmental Therapeutics, The University of Texas System Cancer Center, 6723 Bertner Ave., Houston, Texas 77025 (USA)

REID, D.E., Wellcome Research Laboratories, Langley Court, Beckenham, Kent, BR3 3BS (Great Britain)

ROTH, F., Centre René Huguenin, 5 rue Gaston Latouche, 92211 St. Cloud (France)

ROUMIANTZEFF, M., Institut Français d'Immunologie, Marcy l'Etoile, 69260 Charbonnières-les-Bains (France)

SADLER, T., Department of Surgery, Royal Postgraduate Medical School of London and Hammersmith Hospital, Du Cane Road, London W 12 (Great Britain)

SARACINO, R., Centre René Huguenin, 5 rue Gaston Latouche, 92211 St. Cloud (France)

SCHWARZENBERG, L., Institut de Cancérologie et d'Immunogénétique, Hôpital Paul-Brousse, 14–16 avenue Paul-Vaillant-Couturier, 94800 Villejuif (France)

SLAVIK, M., National Cancer Institute, National Institutes of Health, Bethesda, Maryland 20014 (USA)

SPARROS, L., Institut d'Immuno-Biologie, Hôpital Broussais, 96 rue Didot, 75674 Paris Cedex 14 (France)

TORKINGTON, P., Wellcome Research Laboratories, Langley Court, Beckenham, Kent, BR3 3BS (Great Britain)

TOUJAS, L., Centre Anti-cancéreux E. Marquis, Pontchaillou, 35000 Rennes (France)

TREVES, A.J., Department of Cell Biology, The Weizmann Institute of Science, Rehovot (Israel)

WALBAUM, P.R., Department of Bacteriology, University Medical School, Teviot Place, Edinburgh EH8 9AG (Great Britain)

WERNER, G., Société Rhône-Poulenc, 5 Quai J. Guesde, 94200 Ivry-sur-Seine (France)

WHITE, R.G., Department of Bacteriology and Immunology, University of Glasgow, Western Infirmary, Glasgow W1 (Great Britain)

WIENER, E., Wellcome Research Laboratories, Langley Court, Beckenham, Kent BR3 3BS (Great Britain)

WILKINSON, P.C., Department of Bacteriology and Immunology, University of Glasgow, Western Infirmary, Glasgow W1 (Great Britain)

WITHERS, H.R., Section of Experimental Radiotherapy, The University of Texas System Cancer Center, 6723 Bertner Ave., Houston, Texas 77025 (USA)

WOLMARK, N., Department of Surgery, University of Pittsburgh Medical School, Pittsburgh, Pennsylvania 15261 (USA)

WOODRUFF, M.F.A., Department of Surgery, University Medical School, Teviot Place, Edinburgh EH8 9AG (Great Britain)

WRAB, H., Institut für Kresbsforschung der Universität Wien, Borschkegasse 8A, 1090 Vienna (Austria)

Discussants

ADAM, A., Institut de Biochimie, Bâtiment 432, 91405 Centre d'Orsay (France)

ARNOULD, M., Institut d'Immuno-Biologie, Hôpital Broussais, 96 rue Didot, 75674 Paris Cedex 14 (France)

BAND, P.R., Department of Medicine, Clinical Science Building, The University of Alberta, Edmonton (Canada)

BIOZZI, G., Institut du Radium, Fondation Curie, Section de Biologie, 26 rue d'Ulm, 75231 Paris Cedex 05 (France)

BOIRON, M., Hôpital Saint-Louis, 2 place du Dr. Fournier, 75010 Paris (France)

BOURDON, G., Institut d'Immuno-Biologie, Hôpital Broussais, 96 rue Didot, 75674 Paris Cedex 14 (France)

CHANY, J., Laboratoire de Virologie, Hôpital St. Vincent de Paul, 74 avenue Denfert-Rochereau, 75014 Paris (France)

CHARBONNIER, C., Institut Mérieux, 17 rue Bourgelat, 69002 Lyon (France)

CHATEAUREYNAUD, P. INSERM U89, Domaine de Carreire, 33000 Bordeaux (France)

CIORBARU, R., Institut de Biochimie, Bâtiment 432, 91405 Centre d'Orsay (France)

DAVIES, A.J.S., Chester Beatty Cancer Research Institute, Clifton Avenue, Belmont, Sutton, Surrey SM2 5PX (Great Britain)

DEL GUERCIO, P., Institut d'Immuno-Biologie, Hôpital Broussais, 96 rue Didot, 75674 Paris Cedex 14 (France)

DESBORDES, J., 34 bis rue de Longchamp, 92200 Neuilly-sur-Seine (France)

GRIFFITH, A.H., Department of Clinical Immunology, Wellcome Research Laboratories, Langley Court, Beckenham, Kent BR3 3BS (Great Britain)

HOLLMANN, K.H., Laboratoire de Microscopie Électronique, Hôpital Broussais, 96 rue Didot, 75674 Paris Cedex 14 (France)

KOCHMAN, S., Faculté de Médecine de Reims, 45 rue Cognacq Jay, 51000 Reims (France)

KREIS, B., Hôpital Cochin, 27 rue du Faubourg Saint-Jacques, 75014 Paris (France)

LEDERER, E., Institut de Biochimie, Bâtiment 432, 91405 Centre d'Orsay (France)

MÉRIEUX, C., Directeur de l'Institut Mérieux, 17 rue Bourgelat, 69002 Lyon (France)

MONSIGNY, M., Centre de Biophysique Moléculaire du CNRS, 45045 Orléans (France)

OETTGEN, H.F., Memorial Hospital, 444 East 68 Street, New York, N.Y. 10021 (USA)

PARAF, A., Institut de Biologie Moléculaire, Université Paris VII, 2 place Jussieu, 75221 Paris Cedex 05 (France)

PETIT, J.F., Institut de Biochimie, Bâtiment 432, 91405 Centre d'Orsay (France)

REYNAUD, R., Institut Pasteur, 25 rue du Dr Roux, 75015 Paris (France)

ROMAÑA BERON DE ASTRADA, C., avenida Dr Andreu 10, Barcelona (Spain)

SACHS, L., Department of Genetics, The Weizmann Institute of Science, Rehovot (Israel)

SERROU, B., Département d'Immunologie, Université de Montpellier, 34000 Montpellier (France)

STIFFEL, C., Institut du Radium, Fondation Curie, Section de Biologie, 26 rue d'Ulm, 75231 Paris Cedex 05 (France)

SYLVESTRE, R., Hôpital Henri Mondor, 51 avenue du Maréchal de Lattre de Tassigny, 94000 Créteil (France)

TRIAU, R., Institut Mérieux, 17 rue Bourgelat, 69002 Lyon (France)

VERLEY, J.M., Laboratoire de Microscopie Électronique, Hôpital Broussais, 96 rue Didot, 75674 Paris Cedex 14 (France)

WANEBO, H.J., Sloan Kettering Institute for Cancer Research, New York, N.Y. (USA)

WHISNANT, J.K., Medical Department of Immunology, Burroughs Wellcome Co., Research Triangle Park, N.C. 27709 (USA)

Index